MOTIVATING SUBSTANCE ABUSERS TO ENTER TREATMENT

MOTIVATING SUBSTANCE ABUSERS TO ENTER TREATMENT

Working with Family Members

Jane Ellen Smith
Robert J. Meyers

SOCIAL SCIENCES

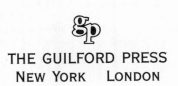

THE GUILFORD PRESS
New York   London

Printed in the United States of America

This book is printed on acid-free paper.

Last digit is print number: 9 8 7 6 5 4 3 2 1

Library of Congress Cataloging-in-Publication Data

Smith, Jane Ellen.
  Motivating substance abusers to enter treatment : working with family
  members / by Jane Ellen Smith & Robert J. Meyers.
    p. cm.
  Includes bibliographical references and index.
  1-59385-052-2 (hbk.)
    1. Substance abuse—Treatment. 2. Substance abuse—Patients—
  Rehabilitation. 3. Motivation (Psychology) I. Meyers, Robert J. II. Title.
  RC564.S566 2004
  362.29—dc22

                                                        2004009472

To my parents, Gloria and John (Bud) Smith,
for the many years in which they have
exemplified respect, love, hard work, and humor;
and to my #1 brother, David J. Smith,
for living his own life in this same rich tradition.

—J. E. S.

To my father, Charles J. Meyers (The Big "C"),
for his love and support.

—R. J. M.

ABOUT THE AUTHORS

Jane Ellen Smith, PhD, is a Professor in the Psychology Department at the University of New Mexico in Albuquerque, where she has also served as Director of Clinical Training. She received her doctorate in Clinical Psychology from the State University of New York at Binghamton. Specializing in both alcoholism and eating disorders, Dr. Smith has written 50 articles or chapters on these topics. She is the coauthor of *Clinical Guide to Alcohol Treatment: The Community Reinforcement Approach* (1995), also with Robert J. Meyers. She has received federal grants from the National Institute on Alcohol Abuse and Alcoholism to test the Community Reinforcement Approach program with homeless individuals.

Robert J. Meyers, PhD, is a Research Associate Professor of Psychology working in the clinical research branch of the University of New Mexico's Center on Alcoholism, Substance Abuse, and Addictions, and is Associate Director of the Life Link Training Institute. Dr. Meyers is the winner of the 2002 Dan Anderson Research Award from the Hazelden Foundation and the 2003 Young Investigator Award from the Research Society on Alcoholism. He has published dozens of scientific articles and several books, including *Get Your Loved One Sober: Alternatives to Nagging, Pleading and Threatening.* Dr. Meyers has been in the addiction field since 1976 and at the University of New Mexico since 1986.

PREFACE

It seems as though *everybody* knows *somebody* who absolutely refuses to get professional help for a serious substance abuse problem. Once the nonabusing family members have tried everything conceivable on their own to convince the addict to seek treatment, they often place desperate phone calls to clinics, hospitals, and substance abuse centers. Sadly, these agencies typically have not had much to offer. Alternatively, other family members enter therapy themselves in an effort to cope with the anxiety and depression that result from living in the midst of a chronic alcohol or drug crisis. When eventually they pointedly ask their therapists for help in getting a resistant individual into treatment, many counselors have found themselves in the uncomfortable position of not knowing how to respond. In the past, the only options for therapists or agencies were either to recommend the highly confrontational Johnson Institute Intervention, or for the client to be sent to an Al-Anon meeting in order to learn how to "detach" from the substance abuser. Perhaps not surprisingly, many clients found these choices unacceptable, and thus were forced to resort again to their old patterns of begging, threatening, or nagging the substance abuser to quit using and to get professional help.

This book was written so that therapists could provide a scientifically supported program that is neither confrontational nor advocates detachment. Instead, CRAFT (Community Reinforcement and Family Training) teaches these family members (Concerned Significant Others) how to change their own behavior toward the substance abuser with the objective of getting the person with the alcohol or drug problem to enter treatment. Importantly, CRAFT never makes Concerned Significant Others (CSOs) feel responsible for the substance abuse problem, but simply offers a method for fostering a solution. CRAFT also addresses two other goals: getting the substance abusers to reduce their substance use in the meantime, and helping CSOs increase their own happiness by targeting problems in various other aspects of their lives.

CRAFT has shown remarkable success across a series of studies with both resistant drinkers and illicit drug users. Upon receiving CRAFT training, the family members (e.g., spouses, parents, siblings, adult children) or friends of substance abusers successfully get their *treatment-refusing* loved ones to begin therapy programs in 64–86% of the cases. These rates are dramatically higher than those of the traditional choices: the Johnson Institute Intervention and Al-Anon. Furthermore, treatment entry occurs with an average of only five CSO sessions. And regardless of whether the resistant individual ever enters treatment, CSOs typically feel more satisfied with their lives and are psychologically healthier.

CRAFT is a program that is based on behavioral principles and cognitive-behavioral techniques. It is an outgrowth of the Community Reinforcement Approach (CRA), a scientifically supported treatment that was designed for substance abusers who already had agreed to seek therapy. The earliest version of CRAFT was developed by Robert Meyers and tested by Sisson and Azrin in the 1980s. During their CRA work with problem drinkers, these researchers/clinicians realized that although a substantial number of drinkers were unwilling to seek treatment, their highly motivated family members could exert a powerful influence on them by altering how they interacted in both drinking and nondrinking situations. In order to capitalize on this critical role, CRAFT was designed so that therapists could teach family members relevant skills, such as how to reward sober behavior and discourage drinking or drug use, to communicate in a positive manner, to employ problem-solving techniques as needed, to take care of their own needs, and to effectively suggest treatment to the substance abuser. Throughout the process, potential domestic violence issues are considered.

Although the "family training" part of Community Reinforcement and Family Training may be obvious at this point, "community reinforcement" may be less so. Within the CRAFT model, this implies that CSOs must change aspects of the "community" at home so that sobriety alone is positively reinforced (rewarded). Additionally, it involves having CSOs reinforce themselves directly by getting reconnected with pleasurable aspects of their extended community that typically have been disrupted as a result of dealing with a loved one's chronic substance abuse problem.

What types of therapists can effectively learn and implement CRAFT? Perhaps the most important point to stress is that one does *not* need to be a chemical dependency counselor or have experience within the addictive behaviors area in order to be a CRAFT therapist, given that the client (the CSO) is *not* the substance abuser. And although there may be some advantage to having a cognitive-behavioral or behavioral orientation when learning CRAFT, this is not absolutely required if a counselor is truly open to experimenting with a new empirically supported program, and proper supervision is available. This book clearly outlines and explains the CRAFT procedures in such a way that solid clinicians from diverse professional backgrounds (e.g., counselor, social worker, psychologist) should be able to learn them. Numerous case examples and therapist–CSO dialogues are provided for illustration purposes throughout.

This clinician-friendly book fills a notable gap in the therapy field, as it offers a successful, scientifically based new program for working with distraught individuals who love a treatment-refusing substance abuser. Importantly, the CRAFT program's prominent emphasis on reinforcement is typically embraced by clinicians and CSOs alike, which in turn fuels a sense of optimism and enthusiasm that has long been missing from work in this difficult problem area.

ACKNOWLEDGMENTS

We would like to acknowledge the support of the National Institute on Alcohol Abuse and Alcoholism and the National Institute on Drug Abuse in funding the studies that form the scientific base of CRAFT. We would also like to thank Bill Miller for his role in securing several of these grants, the entire staff of the Center on Alcoholism, Substance Abuse, and Addictions for their role in executing the projects, and the many family members of substance-abusing individuals who participated in the CRAFT studies. Additionally, we want to thank Jim Nageotte of The Guilford Press for his gentle guidance and support. Finally, we want to thank our good friends Marta Goodrich Dougher, John Gluck, Sarah Erickson, Mark McDaniel, Paul Amrhein, and Liz Nevarez for patiently listening to us gripe about "the book" that seemed to have a life of its own.

CONTENTS

CHAPTER 1

DESCRIPTION OF COMMUNITY REINFORCEMENT AND FAMILY TRAINING

Monica is desperate. She has tried everything humanly possibly to convince her husband that he needs professional help for his drinking, but to no avail. She has begged, screamed, nagged, threatened, cried, and even left him temporarily, but he adamantly refuses to get treatment. Periodically he cuts back for a day or two, but he quickly returns to his same old pattern. Lately he seems like he is under the influence of alcohol all the time. Yet he insists that Monica is making too much of his drinking; that he doesn't really have a problem with alcohol, he just likes to drink. At a substance abuse treatment center, it was suggested she attend an Al-Anon meeting. She was not really comfortable, however, with their directive to lovingly detach herself from her husband. And so Monica feels hopeless once again. Although she debates about leaving her husband on a daily basis, she knows she never will. Still, she cannot just sit back and watch while he slowly destroys himself, their marriage, and their family. But what can she do? To whom can she turn for help?

Community Reinforcement and Family Training (CRAFT) is an empirically based therapy program for the family members or friends of individuals with substance abuse problems who refuse to get treatment. CRAFT-trained therapists work with a "concerned significant other" (CSO), such as Monica, to accomplish three major goals, two of which are focused on the individual who is abusing alcohol or drugs, and a third that is directed toward the CSO. The first goal and ultimate objective is to influence the substance-using individual to seek treatment, but in the interim, the second goal is to reduce that individual's alcohol or drug use. The third goal is to

help the CSO make other positive life changes so that her or his own psychological functioning improves, regardless of whether or not the resistant substance abusing loved one (Identified Patient; IP) enters treatment.

The empirical results of this approach have been impressive.
Depending on the study, CRAFT-trained CSOs have engaged 64–86%
of their resistant alcohol- or drug-abusing loved ones in treatment. In
addition, the CSOs themselves typically report feeling happier about
their lives, regardless of the outcome with their IP. These successful
CSOs have represented a wide variety of CSO–IP relationships, including being the IP's spouse, parent, sibling, or child. Notably, CRAFT is
an efficient program that usually requires relatively few CSO sessions
prior to the IP's engagement in treatment, and CRAFT therapists do
not need an extensive background in the substance abuse field, if they
are supervised adequately.

RATIONALE FOR ENLISTING THE SUPPORT OF CSOs

CRAFT is an outgrowth of the Community Reinforcement Approach
(CRA), a scientifically supported behavioral treatment that is conducted
directly with the substance-abusing individual (e.g., Azrin, 1976; Azrin,
Sisson, Meyers, & Godley, 1982; Hunt & Azrin, 1973; Smith, Meyers, &
Delaney, 1998). In the course of their work with drinkers in the 1970s, the
early Community Reinforcement Approach researchers surmised that the
drinkers' spouses potentially could play a critical role in prompting the
drinkers to begin treatment. In part, this observation was the product of
having witnessed spouses' influence within the Community Reinforcement
Approach program, where they served as disulfiram (i.e., Antabuse) moni-
tors or active partners in marital therapy (Azrin, 1976; Azrin et al., 1982).
The researchers' confidence in CSOs also was based on the observation
that although the individuals with substance abuse problems were commonly uninterested in seeking help (Foote, Szapocznik, Kurtines, Perez-
Vidal, & Hervis, 1985; Institute of Medicine, 1990; Miller & Rollnick, 1991;
Snow, Prochaska, & Rossi, 1992), their family members were highly motivated to support any positive form of change. In fact, they often were the
ones to contact the treatment facility in the first place. Furthermore, since
family members tended to have extensive contact with the substance-abusing individual (Stanton, 1982; Stanton & Heath, 1997), the Community
Reinforcement Approach researchers concluded that CSOs were in an ideal
position to exert considerable influence over drinking decisions (Azrin et
al., 1982; Sisson & Azrin, 1986). In support of these fundamental convic-
tions were the frequent reports of individuals with alcohol and drug problems that their eventual pursuit of treatment was related to pressure from

family and friends (Cunningham, Sobell, Sobell, & Kapur, 1995; Hingson, Mangione, Meyers, & Scotch, 1982; Room, 1987).

One final factor that convinced Community Reinforcement Approach researchers to work with CSOs was concern about the CSOs' well-being. It is firmly established that CSOs' own quality of life suffers in the process of chronically dealing with stressors that are associated with their IP's substance use (Ryan et al., 1997). The stressors typically include violence, verbal aggression, financial problems, marital conflict, disrupted relationships with the children, and social embarrassment (Jacob, Krahn, & Leonard, 1991; O'Farrell & Birchler, 1987; Paolino & McCrady, 1977; Romijn, Platt, Schippers, & Schaap, 1992; Velleman et al., 1993; Zweben, 1986). Since CSOs often respond to these stressors with depression, anxiety, complaints of physical illness, and low self-esteem, it is likely that they would benefit from psychotherapy themselves (Brown, Kokin, Seraganian, & Shields, 1995; Collins, Leonard, & Searles, 1990; Orford & Harwin, 1982; Roberts & Brent, 1992; Ryan et al., 1997; Spear & Mason, 1991).

CSO TREATMENT OPTIONS

A dearth of clinical services for CSOs, coupled with program philosophies that are antithetical to the notion of involving loved ones in the IP engagement process, have been obstacles to CSOs in their efforts to obtain treatment for their IPs. As outlined in Chapter 10, the main traditional intervention for CSOs has been a 12-step program such as Al-Anon (Al-Anon Family Groups, 1984) or Nar-Anon (Narcotics Anonymous, 1993). These CSO-oriented programs advocate loving detachment from the drinker or drug user and an acceptance of the CSO's own inability to control the substance-abusing individual's behavior. Perhaps understandably, these teachings have met with resistance from many CSOs who are unwilling or unable to step aside and remain uninvolved. The second traditional approach, the Johnson Institute Intervention, centers around a "surprise" meeting at which the substance abuser is confronted by loved ones about the alcohol or drug use and all of the problems created by it. The elevated dropout rates associated with this program appear to be driven by CSOs' discomfort with the highly confrontational role expected of them (Barber & Gilbertson, 1997).

Unilateral family therapy (Thomas & Santa, 1982) is a general term for an unusual type of "family" therapy that involves one or more family members *other than* the substance-abusing individual. This nontraditional intervention is based on the belief that CSOs *can* and *should* be active in engaging their loved ones in treatment (Barber & Crisp, 1994; Garrett et al., 1998; Thomas & Ager, 1993). At the same time, CSOs are never viewed as responsible for the IP's substance use. For the most part, unilateral family therapy entails teaching CSOs procedures to help reduce IPs' substance use and increase their motivation to enter treatment. The various unilateral family therapy programs differ in such areas as the extent to which they incorporate confrontational techniques, the precise skills emphasized within their training, and the time-frame for introducing program components. In terms of evaluating this approach, the findings of some unilateral family therapy programs are difficult to interpret, because they lack well-controlled experiments to support their efficacy (Landau et al., 2000; Thomas, Santa, Bronson, & Oyserman, 1987), or they do not exclusively deal with outright treatment refusers as participants (Landau et al., 2000). Furthermore, the majority of these interventions has only been tested in alcohol (as opposed to illicit drug) populations (Barber & Gilbertson, 1996; Thomas & Ager, 1993). Finally, the success rates for IP engagement in these programs have been consistently lower than those generated by CRAFT (Barber & Crisp, 1995; Thomas & Ager, 1993; Thomas et al., 1987).

CRAFT PROGRAM OVERVIEW

CRAFT is a unique type of unilateral family therapy that has received scientific support for working with the CSOs of individuals with both alcohol (Miller, Meyers, & Tonigan, 1999; Sisson & Azrin, 1986) and drug problems (Kirby, Marlowe, Festinger, Garvey, & LaMonaca, 1999; Meyers, Miller, Hill, & Tonigan, 1999; Meyers, Miller, Smith, & Tonigan, 2002; Waldron, Turner, Ozechowski, & Hops, 2003). Based on behavioral principles, it utilizes reinforcement strategies as opposed to confrontational techniques. CSOs receiving the CRAFT treatment in a series of studies (described in Chapter 10) were taught how to rearrange contingencies in the IP's environment, such that clean and sober behavior was reinforced and drinking or drug use was effectively discouraged. The CSOs' new skills were geared toward ultimately influencing IPs to enter treatment. At the same time, an emphasis was placed on enhancing CSOs' satisfaction with their own lives in other specific areas (Meyers, Dominguez, & Smith, 1996; Meyers, Miller, & Smith, 2001; Meyers & Smith, 1995; 1997; Meyers, Smith, & Miller, 1998; Sisson & Azrin, 1986).

The major components of CRAFT as discussed in the remainder of the book are:

1. *Motivational strategies.* Setting positive expectations by describing the CRAFT program, its success, and the potential benefits for the CSO.

2. *Functional analyses of the IP's substance-using behavior.* Outlining the triggers and consequences of the IP's use and developing CSO intervention strategies based on this information, such that the environmental contingencies to encourage and support clean and sober behavior are rearranged.

3. *Domestic violence precautions.* Assessing the potential for violence in the CSO–IP relationship, identifying the triggers for IP aggression, and devising prevention and protection plans.

4. *Communication training.* Examining the CSO's current communication style with the IP, providing a rationale for improving communication, teaching positive communication skills, and rehearsing through the use of role playing.

5. *Positive reinforcement training.* Identifying appropriate small rewards for the IP and instructing the CSO in how to use these to reinforce only clean and sober IP behavior.

6. *Discouragement of using behavior.* Showing the CSO how to introduce "time-outs" from positive reinforcement at IP substance-using times, demonstrating how to allow the natural consequences for using, and teaching a standard problem-solving strategy.

7. *CSO self-reinforcement training.* Exploring the CSO's dissatisfaction in various life areas, developing goals and a plan to address these problems, and assisting the CSO in identifying and "sampling" reinforcers for her- or himself.

8. *Suggestion of treatment to the IP.* Determining the best time and manner for suggesting treatment, preparing the CSO to face a possible refusal, and having arrangements in place at a treatment agency or with a provider to accept the IP for treatment without delay.

THE REQUIREMENTS FOR BEING A COMPETENT CRAFT THERAPIST

What are the preconditions for working as a capable CRAFT therapist? One study indirectly investigated CRAFT therapists' skills by comparing their CSOs' engagement rates. Substantial variability was found; engagement rates across therapists ranged from 50 to 100% (W. Miller et al., 1999). Nonetheless, the *lowest* engagement rate for any CRAFT therapist was better than the *highest* engagement rate for the therapists delivering the other two treatments: Al-Anon and the Johnson Institute Intervention. Conceivably, therapist characteristics were partially responsible for the discrepancies in CRAFT engagement rates, but the critical factors have not been identified. The presupposition, of course, is that in order to be a good CRAFT therapist, the person must first be a good therapist.

This conclusion is based on the authors' experience as clinical supervisors on multiple CRAFT trials, as well as the research that highlights the important role of therapist empathy (Miller, Benefield, & Tonigan, 1993; Miller, Taylor, & West, 1980; Valle, 1981) and the formation of a strong therapeutic alliance in substance abuse treatment outcome (Connors, Carroll, DiClemente, Longabaugh, & Donovan, 1997; Kahn, 1997).

Upon examining the demographics of therapists who have successfully implemented CRAFT in the six outcome studies to date, a diverse group emerges in terms of gender, ethnicity, and age. As far as training and experience, the vast majority of the CRAFT therapists in these studies had master's degrees, and the clinicians in two of the projects had substantial experience (Kirby et al., 1999; Sisson & Azrin, 1986). The therapists in the remaining studies, who were primarily graduate students in clinical psychology doctoral programs, had minimal clinical experience overall and even more limited substance abuse experience. Yet they had received solid academic preparation for substance abuse work and they were closely supervised (Meyers et al., 1999; 2002; W. Miller et al., 1999).

The notion that one does not need to be a chemical dependency counselor in order to be a CRAFT therapist is of considerable importance. A misperception exists among many therapists that one must be a substance abuse "expert" in order to implement CRAFT. The fact that CRAFT therapists actually deal with the *non*-substance-abusing individual, the CSO, should be stressed repeatedly. Otherwise, the countless clinicians who are uncomfortable working with individuals with alcohol or drug problems (Miller & Brown, 1997) may inadvertently eliminate themselves as potential CRAFT therapists. Of course, this is *not* to suggest that having a fundamental understanding of substance abuse and marital or family dysfunction is inconsequential; knowledge of these areas would surely be beneficial for counselors working in the alcohol or drug field in any capacity (O'Farrell & Fals-Stewart, 1999).

Regardless of a therapist's previous experience, the proper training and supervision of CRAFT is a critical issue. For those clinicians who are committed to learning CRAFT, a 2- to 3-day training workshop and a careful reading of this book are standard beginning components. During the early stages of utilizing CRAFT in the workplace, most therapists require supervision from a CRAFT-trained behaviorist or cognitive-behaviorist. Not only is the phenomenon of "drift" (i.e., reverting to one's more familiar mode of conducting therapy) well documented in treatment trials in general (Carroll et al., 2000), but novice cognitive-behavioral therapists sometimes mistakenly believe that they are properly implementing a new program (e.g., CRAFT, CRA) when, in actuality, they are merely applying several isolated procedures without adopting the philosophy and goals that drive the treatment (Meyers & Smith, 1995; Miller & Meyers, 2001).

Limited amounts of general or specialized clinical experience need not constitute an insurmountable impediment to mastering CRAFT. However, interesting challenges have been raised in CRAFT (and CRA) workshops when instructing therapists of certain theoretical orientations. Based on anecdotal evidence, it appears advantageous to have a cognitive-behavioral or behavioral orientation when learning CRAFT. At the same time, it is *not* absolutely necessary to have such an orientation if one is open-minded about new therapeutic approaches. The standard behavioral components of CRAFT (e.g., homework assignments, role plays) are sometimes met with skepticism by therapists from other orientations, but the procedures are not difficult to master if one "buys into" the theoretical foundation. The ease in accomplishing this depends on the individual therapist; some experienced professionals find themselves reluctant to set aside beliefs and procedures that have been part of their career identity since graduate school (Rogers, 1995). A case in point is the reliance upon the use of heavy confrontation. Despite research showing that higher levels of therapist confrontation are associated with poorer substance abuse outcomes (Miller et al., 1993, 1995), some counselors are unwilling to abandon it. These individuals may have difficulty embracing CRAFT, as may those from the subset of avid disease model therapists who exclusively assign the cause of the problem to the drinker or drug user's biological constitution, while completely ignoring the context in which it occurs (Miller, 1986; Miller & Hester, 1995). For counselors who remain interested in learning CRAFT despite these particular ideological or stylistic differences, the supervision issue becomes even more significant.

SUITABLE CSO CANDIDATES FOR CRAFT

At this point, research cannot predict who will be a successful CRAFT client. Clinical experience based on involvement with the CRAFT projects has demonstrated that if an IP left the CSO (e.g., moved out of state), the chances of engagement naturally dropped. Also, periodically it became obvious that a CSO did not have a clear commitment to getting the IP into treatment, and instead was interested solely in obtaining therapy for her- or himself. Neither of these courses of events was apparent at the time of the Intake. Perhaps a better way to broach the question of suitable CSO candidates is to describe the selection parameters for the CSOs used in the various CRAFT trials. Certainly there is no guarantee that future clients with these qualities will be successful, or that those without them will not be, but it is a reasonable place to start. Among the first factors to consider are aspects of the CSO–IP relationship. To begin with, the studies primarily enlisted CSOs who were first-degree relatives (i.e., parents, siblings, children) or romantic partners (i.e., spouses, girlfriends, boyfriends) of IPs. Although there was an occasional exception (e.g., a close friend), this more distant type of CSO–IP relationship has not been fully tested. A related issue is whether an interested CSO has sufficient contact with the IP to afford ample opportunity to influence his or her behavior. One of the studies required that the CSO and IP be living together (W. Miller et al., 1999), but the others simply required that the CSO have contact with the IP at a minimum of about 3 days per week. Therefore, CSOs who have infrequent contact with their IP may not be appropriate candidates. Importantly, a history of serious domestic violence between the CSO and IP or any recent violence were grounds for exclusion from all but two of the studies (Kirby et al., 1999; Sisson & Azrin, 1986), indicating that CRAFT has not been adequately tested with such a population.

With regard to CSO descriptors, it is critical that a CSO be willing to participate fully in CRAFT. A fair number of CSOs who inquired about the CRAFT studies erroneously believed that a therapist would take complete responsibility for the engagement process. As described in Chapter 10, the CSOs in these studies were a highly diverse group in terms of ethnicity, gender, and sexual orientation. Furthermore, they ranged in age from 18 to 81. The characteristics of interested CSOs who were excluded from the studies should also be considered, as it is unknown whether such individuals would be good candidates for CRAFT. Ineligible CSOs were those who had substance abuse problems themselves or otherwise impaired behavior, were under 18 years of age, or had less than a sixth-grade reading level.

A cautionary note appears in order: Although a summary of the inclusion/exclusion criteria for the CRAFT studies and an overview of the wide range of participants' characteristics may be informative, the results from these controlled studies may be somewhat different from those obtained with highly heterogeneous populations under less stringently monitored conditions.

FINDING CSOs AND MAKING TREATMENT ACCESSIBLE

Therapists who are *not* working within a substance abuse treatment agency, and thereby are not regularly receiving calls from CSOs, may be uncertain where to find them. Given what we know about the emotional distress experienced by the CSOs of substance abusers (Jacob et al., 1991; O'Farrell & Birchler, 1987; Romijn et al., 1992; Velleman et al., 1993), conceivably a fair number of CSOs are already part of the mental health system. Nevertheless, we cannot assume that CSOs receiving treatment for depression or anxiety have actually discussed the family substance abuse problem with their therapist. Consequently, when conducting a standard social or family history with a client, it is generally worthwhile to inquire briefly about drinking or drug problems in the home (Ryan et al., 1997). And since research suggests that nondrinking family members in alcoholic households attend health care facilities significantly more frequently than do members of nonalcoholic families (Holder & Blase, 1986), physicians might also be well advised to raise the issue of family substance abuse problems during office visits with certain habitual patients.

One complicating factor is that most distraught CSOs probably do *not* seek help directly from a therapist or even indirectly from a physician. Interestingly, a 20-year survey discovered that 40% of Americans seek help from a clergy member when they are struggling with personal problems (Veroff, Kulks, & Douvan, 1981). Since the types of issues commonly presented to clergy are in the same category of problems experienced by CSOs (Larson et al., 1988), it would be reasonable either to inform the clergy about the availability of programs such as CRAFT, or to train pastoral counselors to implement these programs themselves. As discussed in Chapter 4, CSOs of substance-abusing IPs are familiar victims of domestic violence and consequently may be located at domestic violence shelters or hospital emergency rooms (see Smith, Laframboise, & Bittinger, 2002). Staff at these agencies could be trained to screen for signs of substance-abusing IPs in the household (in particular, see "Assessment of Violence" in Chapter 4, pp. 81–83), with the intent of referring the CSOs to CRAFT therapists.

Depending on the level of determination to reach distressed CSOs, one could "advertise" CRAFT programs. This could readily be accomplished via the distribution of pamphlets at any of the sites already mentioned (e.g., hospitals, domestic violence shelters), through public service announcements, or by providing information in the types of classes that might draw these CSOs, such as courses on substance abuse or domestic violence and trauma (Smith et al., 2002). The legal and social service systems also provide opportunities to locate CSOs in need of assistance, since child welfare workers often are involved in family cases in which parental substance abuse is a major concern (Hohman & Butt, 2001).

There are an unlimited number of reasonable places in which to locate CSOs in need of services. If they are found outside of the mental health system, suggestions for CRAFT treatment must be made with the CSO's mental health insurance coverage in mind. Practitioners sometimes express concern that the cost of CSOs' sessions will not be eligible for insurance reimbursement, because CSOs are not the individuals with the substance abuse diagnosis. In actuality, standard mental health coverage should not be an issue for most insured CSOs, because the majority of them can rightfully be given a psychiatric diagnosis (see "Rationale for

Enlisting the Support of CSOs" earlier in this chapter, pp. 2–3). Further-more, progressive companies sometimes view this IP "pretreatment" as an allowable expense, since getting the alcohol- or drug-dependent family member into treatment sooner, as opposed to later (or not at all), is a long-term fiscal savings to them in the medical arena (Landau et al., 2000). When CSOs have limited finances or no mental health insurance, affordable options for accessing CRAFT-trained therapists eventually might be found at various agencies that offer sliding-fee payment plans (e.g., university doctoral training clinics, community mental health clin-ics). The CRAFT program is also now available in a new book designed specifically for CSOs, entitled *Get Your Loved One Sober: Alternatives to Nagging, Pleading and Threatening* (Meyers & Wolfe, 2004). However, it is recommended that CSOs who are using this book still receive guidance from a professionally trained counselor.

SUMMARY

Ambivalence and lack of motivation to seek treatment are extremely com-mon in individuals with alcohol or drug problems. CRAFT is a scientifi-cally supported intervention that engages these treatment-refusing indi-viduals by working through concerned family members or friends. In a series of studies, CRAFT-trained CSOs were able to influence these resis-tant substance abusers to enter treatment in 64–86% of the cases, and in a relatively brief period of time. This success was demonstrated across vari-ous types of CSO relationships with IPs (e.g., spouse, parent) and for mul-tiple drugs of abuse (e.g., alcohol, cocaine, marijuana). Furthermore, CRAFT-trained CSOs typically felt better about themselves after treat-ment, regardless of whether or not their IP entered therapy. Finally, an individual need not be a chemical dependency "expert" to become a com-petent CRAFT therapist. The specific components of the CRAFT pro-gram and detailed instructions for implementing them follow in the remaining clinical chapters of this book. The final chapter supplies the research evidence for CRAFT.

CHAPTER 2

BUILDING AND SUSTAINING MOTIVATION OF CONCERNED SIGNIFICANT OTHERS

This chapter describes how to initiate treatment with a CSO, and importantly, how to proceed in a manner that capitalizes on her or his motivation. It begins with a discussion of assessment and confidentiality issues as they apply to this unusual population, and then proposes ways to maximize the utility of the information gathered about the presenting problem. Key motivational suggestions are woven throughout the chapter, including a recommended therapeutic style of interacting, as well as specific strategies designed to help your client (i.e., the CSO) remain optimistic and engaged in treatment. The chapter also explains how to introduce CRAFT's premises, goals, and procedures, and how to discuss the CSO's role and responsibilities as a participant in the program. Since a large array of topics is covered in the introductory session, an outline of the main components is provided in Table 2.1.

REVIEWING STANDARD ASSESSMENT MATERIAL

In some work environments it is standard practice for clients to have already completed an assessment battery prior to seeing their therapist. If this is the case, be sure to take time to review this wealth of information before your first session. Not only does this save the CSO from having to repeat so much of the historical information, it also enables you to formulate ideas immediately about possible treatment strategies, based on the idiosyncrasies of the case. Furthermore, it provides an opportunity dur-

TABLE 2.1. OUTLINE OF TOPICS COVERED IN INTRODUCTORY SESSION

- Review assessment material (pp. 11–14).
- Address confidentiality issue (pp. 14–15).
- Ask CSO to describe IP's problem briefly (pp. 15–17).
- Ask CSO to describe past attempts to influence IP's use (pp. 17–18).
- Set positive expectations (pp. 20–23 and Table 2.2).
- Describe potential benefits to CSO (pp. 23–25).
- Identify CSO's reinforcers (pp. 25–27).
- Explain CRAFT's basic premises (Table 2.3).
- Explain CRAFT's 3 goals (pp. 32–35).
- Give overview of CRAFT's procedures (Table 2.4).
- Review CSO's responsibilities (pp. 37–38).

In the process, did you remember to:
- Verbally reinforce the CSO whenever appropriate? (pp. 12, 18–20, 27)
- Instill a sense of optimism? (pp. 14, 20)
- Move toward solutions instead of "staying stuck" on problems? (pp. 15–16)
- Use a nonjudgmental, nonconfrontational, empathic style? (pp. 18–20)
- Deliver the message that the CSO is not responsible for the IP's problem? (pp. 19, 28)
- Identify the source(s) of the CSO's current motivation for treatment and the CSO's reinforcers in general? (pp. 15–17, 25–27, 35)

---

ing the initial session to praise your client for taking the time to fill out the questionnaires. Such opportunities are important aspects of treatment, because the proper use of verbal reinforcement requires demonstration, as do all behavioral strategies. Although this demonstration typically occurs in the context of a role-played interaction between a therapist and client, it is preferable to supplement this rehearsal with real-life modeling when occasions present themselves. Techniques that you demonstrated naturally in your interactions with a CSO would not necessarily be labeled as a "technique" for the client initially.

In the event that you do not have a standard assessment battery but would like to adopt one for CSOs, an option is to select instruments from among those administered in the majority of the CRAFT studies. Obviously the full research set would not be needed for clinical purposes, and so some suggestions are listed below. One instrument, the Relationship Happiness Scale, is included here (Figure 2.1, end of chapter) because it is a standard component of the CRAFT and CRA programs. Also listed are

Thomas et al.'s two unilateral family therapy spouse inventories, and a few supplementary instruments that appear worth considering. These measures focus on the CSO's level of functioning and the status of the relationship between the CSO and the substance abuser (IP). Estimates of the substance use itself are collected later (see Chapter 3). In addition to the questionnaires' names and sources, the number of items for each and an approximate administration time are included:

CSO functioning

1. Beck Depression Inventory (Beck, Steer, & Garbin, 1988); 21 items, 5 minutes.
2. State–Trait Anxiety Inventory (Spielberger, Gorsuch, Lushene, Vagg, & Jacobs, 1983); 40 items, 8 minutes.
3. State–Trait Anger Expression Inventory (Spielberger, 1988); 44 items, 10 minutes.
4. Physical Symptoms (Moos, Cronkite, Billings, & Finney, 1987); 26 items, 5 minutes.
5. Rosenberg Self-Esteem Scale (Rosenberg, 1965); 10 items, 5 minutes.
6. Social Support Questionnaire—Short-Form Revised (Sarason, Sarason, Shearin, & Pierce, 1987); 6 double items, 10 minutes.
7. Social Functioning and Resources section of the Health and Daily Living Form (Moos et al., 1987); 69 items, 15 minutes.

CSO–IP relationship

1. Dyadic Adjustment Scale (Busby, Crane, Larson, & Christensen, 1995; Spanier, 1976; suitable for intimate couples only); 32 items, 10 minutes.
2. Relationship Happiness Scale (Azrin, Naster, & Jones, 1973); 10 items, 5 minutes (see Figure 2.1).
3. Conflict Tactics Scales (Straus, 1979); 19 items, 8 minutes.
4. Areas of Change Questionnaire (Jacob & Seilhamer, 1985); 34 items, 10 minutes
5. Family Environment Scale (Moos & Moos, 1986); 90 items, 15 minutes.
6. Spouse Sobriety Influence Inventory (Thomas, Yoshioka, & Ager, 1994a); 52 items, 15 minutes.
7. Spouse Enabling Inventory (Thomas, Yoshioka, & Ager, 1994b); 47 items, 15 minutes.

What should you be looking for in the initial assessment material? Many purposes can be served by assessments. As noted, one is to determine the client's baseline level of emotional functioning, and a second is to evaluate the status of the CSO's relationship with the IP. If you are

interested in monitoring the client's ongoing progress, later you can compare this information against midtreatment evaluations using the same
instruments. Baseline functioning can also be contrasted with posttreatment levels as a measure of final improvement. A comprehensive assessment should also offer insight into the question of possible domestic violence (Chapter 4), the pattern and function of the IP's substance use
(Chapter 3), and previous therapy attempts (see "CSO's Past Attempts to
Address the IP's Use" in this chapter, pp. 17–18).

In line with standard clinical practice, you should also spend time
examining the stated presenting problem. If formal assessment instruments have been administered, they will contain much of the relevant
information, but valuable details must be probed in the first session. The
information you are seeking to elicit as part of the CRAFT protocol is
unique, in that you are interested in speculating about both the behavior
of the client seeking treatment currently (i.e., the CSO) as well as the
loved one who is not (i.e., the IP). Specifically, you want to determine *all*
the reasons why a particular CSO might be motivated to change her or his
own behavior in the quest to ultimately influence someone else's problem
behavior. The techniques for accomplishing this goal are presented later
in this chapter and in Chapter 3. This information is critical in treatment
when devising strategies for altering longstanding patterns of interaction
between the CSO and the IP.

The most important objectives to accomplish in the first session are
to provide cause for optimism and to instill in the client a sense that you
understand the situation at hand. As you prepare to meet the CSO,
remind yourself that throughout the process of explaining CRAFT, you
should remain upbeat, positive, supportive, motivational, and empathic,
while focusing on the specific issues that brought the CSO to therapy.

CONFIDENTIALITY ISSUES

Whereas it always is important to discuss confidentiality issues with clients, the ramifications of failing to do so may be even more pronounced
with CSOs. Why? A fair number of CSOs do not initially tell substance-
abusing loved ones that they are in treatment. In some cases, the CSO's
silence is due to fear of the IP's reaction (e.g., violence, ridicule); in other
cases, the clients simply want to explore CRAFT on their own before sharing any details of the experience. Regardless, some CSOs may not want
the therapist or staff to call their homes or send any mail. It may take
weeks before CSOs are ready to discuss their therapy involvement with the
substance user, and occasionally clients *never* reveal it. In these situations
a guarantee of confidentiality is essential, because otherwise you could

inadvertently put a CSO in harm's way. Of course, if it becomes apparent that abuse is ongoing, you may need to take other actions (outlined in Chapter 4).

Taking precautions to maintain confidentiality does not imply that it will be impossible to contact these CSOs in the event of an emergency. Sometimes clients are comfortable having you call their home as long as you do not reveal your affiliation with a therapy clinic. Also, CSOs can be asked to give the number of a family member or friend (other than the IP) who can serve as a contact person. If the CSO cannot think of a person who could serve as a contact, then you would immediately devote some therapy time to discussing the rationale for having such a confidant, as well as the steps for identifying and obtaining one (refer to Chapter 4).

CSO'S DESCRIPTION OF THE IP'S PROBLEM

Early in the first CRAFT session, give the CSO the opportunity to describe the substance use problem and its repercussions. Let the client talk for a short time without interruption. In addition to supplying an overview of the problem and its severity for you, it will serve a rapport-building function. Listen for family, financial, social, child-rearing, physical, and occupational difficulties. These problems may have negatively affected not only the CSO and the substance user, but also the children, extended family members, friends, and coworkers. For example, perhaps the CSO's entire family no longer gets invited to festivities at friends' houses, as a result of the IP's unacceptable behavior during previous get-togethers. The CSO's description of the negative outcomes of the IP's use provides a further explanation as to why the CSO is seeking therapy now, and possibly may offer preliminary insight into the IP's desires and needs as well. Then ask questions to fill in any missing basic details about the substance use, including the preferred substance, how much and how often it is used, and mode of administration (e.g., smoked, snorted). The circumstances under which the substance use occurs are addressed later in the process, using a task called a functional analysis (Chapter 3).

Without much encouragement, most CSOs are very willing to discuss the many problems created by their IP's substance use. In fact, you will likely have trouble refocusing CSOs who otherwise would monopolize the entire session (and subsequent ones) with exacting accounts of the numerous times their substance-abusing loved one has harmed him- or herself and those he or she supposedly cherishes. Your job as a CRAFT therapist is to respond with empathy, but then to switch gears rather swiftly so that *solutions* to problems become the emphasis. Explain that rehashing problems alone cannot change anything, whereas new strategic action *can*. Assure

CSOs that they will have more time to discuss additional issues during future therapy sessions. Get the necessary information and then gently move the client into a problem-solving mode (outlined in Chapter 7, "Problem-Solving Procedure," pp. 187–191). Help CSOs recognize that the sooner you begin to address these issues, the sooner you will move toward the cardinal goal of influencing the substance user to enter treatment.

An example of a conversation between a therapist and a CSO at such a point in the first session follows. Assume the CSO has already spent a solid 10 minutes describing the problems created by her brother's use, as well as the deep hurt it has caused her. The therapist has processed the anger and hurt briefly with her and now attempts to take the next step:

THERAPIST: Thank you, Loren. I think I have a good idea as to why you're seeking help right now. You've outlined several very upsetting problems that have resulted from your brother's smoking and drinking.

CSO: Oh, that's *nothing*. I haven't told you half of what's gone on. The other day Roberto forged a signature on a doctor's excuse so he wouldn't get into trouble for missing work again. Do you believe that?! And last week he told his boss he was late because he had to drive me to the airport. He had a hangover. That's why he was late! It's one thing after another. I could kill him!

THERAPIST: Those certainly sound like upsetting things. I'm not surprised you're angry and frustrated. And as we discussed a few minutes ago, you're probably also really sad underneath it all. We'll get back to all of these feelings again soon. But for now, let's move ahead and talk about some of the ways you've already tried to get Roberto into treatment.

CSO: Last month he was bragging to my kids about how he always manages 3-day weekends . . . even when they're not official holidays. Why is he telling them that? That's nothing to brag about! And then he has the nerve to ask me for money! Maybe he should try showing up for work.

THERAPIST: Loren, he certainly has done a lot of things to upset you and your family. There's no doubt about that. I bet you could easily spend several sessions just telling me all of the "horrible" things he's done over the years that have hurt you deeply. But I think it's time to get to work. It's really in your best interest to focus now on the things this program has to offer that can actually help you *change* the situation for the better, like getting him into treatment.

CSO: But I thought I was supposed to talk about my feelings in therapy.

THERAPIST: You *definitely* are. And we've only just started to do that today.

We'll talk more about your feelings throughout—especially some of the ones that you've hinted may be hidden under the anger. Remember how I asked what you were feeling besides anger, and you said maybe you were feeling some sadness?

CSO: I *am* sad. I hate to see my brother so messed up.

THERAPIST: And that's why you're here. You care about him. We'll definitely talk about your sadness and all your other feelings more. But I think it's important to get a plan of action in place, so that we can work on starting to make positive changes. I'd like to at least get a jump on the change process right now . . . before you leave today.

CSO: That makes sense. OK. What should we do next?

Although CSOs usually have no trouble telling you about the problems caused by their loved one's substance abuse, they commonly have difficulty talking about their resultant feelings. Or, as illustrated in the dialogue above, perhaps only one predominant feeling is expressed, such as anger. Less accessible ones, such as sadness, guilt, and hopelessness, are often not mentioned without prompting. So it may be worthwhile to ask the question, "Besides feeling _____ [angry, guilty] as you think about the problems caused by your _____ [brother's, husband's, etc.] substance use, what else do you feel?" This discussion allows clients to get in touch with the fact that they still care about the IP, which in turn moves them beyond the surface feelings that may be acting as roadblocks to strides toward change. Furthermore, the exploration of feelings lets CSOs experience, early in the therapeutic process, CRAFT's reliance on a compassionate, positive, motivational style. Even though CRAFT is a structured behavioral treatment, it places great value on CSOs feeling comfortable and open about expressing their emotions.

CSO'S PAST ATTEMPTS TO ADDRESS THE IP'S USE

Ask CSOs to describe their own previous attempts to solve the substance abuse problem, including any attempts to persuade the IP to enter treatment. Note that although some of their failed attempts may be based on strategies that sound moderately similar to certain CRAFT procedures, with probing it usually becomes apparent that the strategies were neither carried out properly nor consistently. However, it is not necessary to explore this area now. *Do* make a note of it, so that later in the session when you are describing the CRAFT procedures, you can comment on the differences between what you will be asking the CSO to do and how she or he has executed somewhat related procedures in the past.

For the moment it is helpful to explain more generally that without expert advice and guidance, the client may have been spinning her or his wheels during previous attempts to address the problem. Describe how many CSOs try the same tactics repeatedly, thinking that sheer effort and perseverance will surely effect change. When things do not work out, the frustrated individuals try even harder by doing more of the same thing. But trying harder with the same unproductive strategy does not suddenly work. Still, be sure to praise the CSO for any attempts, regardless of whether they ever worked, pointing out how it demonstrates love and concern for the IP. Tell the client that you will be teaching a new program for addressing the substance abuse problem, one which is radically different, in all probability, from anything she or he has undertaken previously. Support the CSO's willingness to experiment with new ways of interacting with the loved one—ways that do not entail yelling, crying, threatening, or nagging. Inform all CSOs that CRAFT helps them take charge of their part in the relationship *without* putting responsibility for the substance user on their shoulders.

THERAPIST'S STYLE OF INTERACTING

It would be a mistake to assume that in order to be a good behavior therapist, you need only be directive and follow a set of procedures. As noted in Chapter 1, in order to be a good CRAFT therapist, you first need to be a good clinician. Critical qualities of a good clinician include being empathic, nonjudgmental, genuine, and warm (Beck, Rush, Shaw, & Emery, 1979; Goldfried, 1982; Rogers, 1957; Valle, 1981; Weiner, 1975). Not only are these qualities necessary in terms of conveying respect and enhancing communication within the therapeutic relationship, but they also increase the chance that the client will attend therapy sessions, comply with homework assignments, take suggested risks, communicate honestly, and achieve a better treatment outcome (Connors et al., 1997; Kahn, 1997; Miller et al., 1980, 1993; Valle, 1981). One method of conveying this recommended positive and accepting attitude, and thereby strengthening the therapeutic bond, is the appropriate use of verbal reinforcement. CRAFT therapists rely heavily on verbal reinforcement, in part, because it is an integral component of any behavioral approach (Spiegler & Guevremont, 2003). Additionally, many CSOs have been abused verbally and physically and are in desperate need of supportive responses. You may be the only person who is unconditionally and reliably kind to them.

CRAFT is a motivational approach. Consequently, you should avoid arguments and deflect any defensiveness by making supportive, empathic, or understanding statements. Above all, steer clear of confrontation. Confrontation has proven ineffective when utilized by therapists with substance abusers (Miller et al., 1993, 1995) and when used by CSOs within the Johnson Institute Intervention (Liepman, Nirenberg, & Begin, 1989; W. Miller et al., 1999; see Chapter 10). The notable success of motivational procedures within the substance abuse arena further supports the adoption of a motivational style (Brown & Miller, 1993; Miller, Wilbourne, & Hettema, 2003; Rollnick, Bell, & Heather, 1992; Senft, Polen, Freeborn, & Hollis, 1995). Given that one of your goals is to become the CSO's ally, a motivational approach should work to strengthen that perception and the resulting therapeutic bond.

What does a supportive and nonjudgmental style sound like in a CRAFT program? Examples of commonly used statements during the first session are:

- "I'm not going to ask you to do anything that you don't want to do. This program is here to meet *your* needs."
- "I'm sure we could all second-guess a lot of the decisions we've made in our lives. What's important is that you're here now."
- "It sounds like you've gone out of your way, again and again, to try to make things work in your family."
- "In this program, *you're* in charge of where we go and when."

One of the most important occasions in which a nonjudgmental, empathic style is clearly the only acceptable approach is when a CSO blames her- or himself for the IP's problems. This self-blame may be expressed as guilt over what should have been done differently over the years or in "if only" terms: *if only* she or he were a better _____ (wife, husband, mother, friend), the IP would not still resort to drug use. A major task throughout CRAFT is to clarify that the CSO is *not* responsible for the substance abuser's behavior. Still, let the CSO express these feelings about participating, unintentionally or otherwise, in the substance abuse predicament. Respond with statements such as:

- "Most people would have done the same things you did in those situations."
- "We've all made mistakes in our lives. The important thing is how we learn from them and move on."
- "You were doing what you thought was best for your family at the time."

Once CSOs understand that you are not going to judge them and that their responses appeared logical, given the circumstances, they often are willing to give up *a little* of the self-blame for the problem. In turn, this diminished burden leaves them more receptive to the idea of learning new skills that would allow them to take control over their lives. Importantly, they feel both relieved and energized.

Keep encouraging and reinforcing the CSO at every opportunity. Acknowledge what a painstaking, endless job it is to cope with a loved one's drinking or drug use, and how doing so, most certainly, has required acts of great courage at times. Discuss how the client's efforts and sacrifices have kept the family together and the household functioning. Then explain that together, the two of you will make the most of the CSO's dedication to, and knowledge of, the substance-using partner, so that better strategies can be adopted for influencing him or her.

SETTING POSITIVE EXPECTATIONS

CSOs begin treatment with widely varying degrees of emotional functioning and an assortment of coping styles. In terms of treatment expectations, at one extreme are those who present themselves as determined to succeed and convinced that they will. At the other extreme are depressed, anxious, and skeptical CSOs. Regardless, your job is to help CSOs stay focused on, and committed to, the change process. So, in addition to offering empathy and support, it is important to take a directive stance while instilling optimism. CSOs need to believe that they will be able to take charge of their lives and find happiness again. As noted, part of this process involves acknowledging the myriad of problems CSOs have suffered, and affirming that, although they are not the cause of the problems, they can be part of the solution. This line of thinking begins the process of restoring self-esteem and lays the foundation for the development of self-efficacy.

The vast majority of CSOs are reasonably motivated and prepared to work at the point of entering treatment, so in these cases, your job is to harness and guide this motivation, and later address any signs of waning commitment. However, as noted previously, occasionally CSOs enter a CRAFT program with the mistaken belief that the therapist will assume full responsibility for getting their loved one into treatment. Since these CSOs anticipate playing only a minimal role in engaging their IP, they are taken aback at the notion of their active—and crucial—participation. This unsettled feeling is compounded by their built-up frustration and anger with the substance abuser. Lack of enthusiasm for the role of critical player in the change process is addressed by introducing the topics described below, and by reviewing the specific reasons why the CSO is the most logical choice for a change agent (outlined in "CRAFT's Basic Premises" in this chapter, pp. 27–33).

Regardless of the CSO's level of optimism or motivation at the onset, you should still try to enhance her or his positive expectations regarding the likelihood of engaging the IP into treatment. One way to establish this positive expectancy is by expressing your familiarity with the types of problems that the CSO is describing; you can refer to other similar CSO situations with which you have dealt, in general and brief terms. This shows that you understand CSOs' problems and have experience working with such individuals. The result is increased client confidence in your ability to manage her or his particular case. There are secondary benefits to having this discussion as well. For instance, it lets CSOs know that they are not alone with their problem; that many others have found themselves in similar difficult circumstances. This realization is important because commonly it is the precursor for CSOs to start to believe that the problems created by the substance use are not their fault.

In addition to enhancing expectations by establishing your credibility of having worked with CSOs, you should also discuss the positive therapy outcomes experienced by CRAFT clients. In essence, you are making the point that therapy has worked for other CSOs, and so it can work for them as well. As a CRAFT therapist you have the advantage of being able to describe a program that consistently has had positive outcomes in clinical trials. As outlined in Chapter 10, there have been six CRAFT trials: two with adult drinkers, three with adult drug abusers, and one with adolescent drug abusers. All have shown positive outcomes. In approximately 7 out of 10 cases, the treatment-refusing substance user *does* enter treatment after a loved one is trained in CRAFT procedures. Furthermore, it does not matter whether the CSO is a spouse, parent, sibling, or close friend of the substance user; each can be successful. The type of drug of abuse is also inconsequential. Additionally, many IPs have already decreased their use substantially by the time they enter treatment. Finally, the CRAFT program has been shown to reduce depression, anxiety, anger, physical symptoms, and other psychosocial problems suffered by the CSO (Kirby et al., 1999; Meyers et al., 1999, 2002; W. Miller et al., 1999; Sisson & Azrin, 1986). These improvements are usually found regardless of whether the CSOs engage their substance user into treatment. Informing your clients that they are likely to benefit in similar ways can be highly motivational. Table 2.2 summarizes the main points to present to clients about CRAFT's scientific support.

The following is a suggested conversation you might have when introducing the scientifically proven success of CRAFT to a CSO:

THERAPIST: I'd like to take a few minutes to discuss the track record of the type of therapy I've mentioned we'll be using. In a way, we're both lucky to be part of a therapy process that's proven to be extremely effective in helping people with the type of problem you've described. We've discovered that when people, such as yourself, are

TABLE 2.2. CRAFT's Scientific Support

1. CSOs are successful at getting their treatment-refusing loved ones with substance abuse problems into treatment *nearly 7 out of 10 times.*

2. Success is evident across a *variety of* CSO–IP *relationships* (e.g., spouses, parent and child, siblings, friends) and for many types of abusive *drugs* (e.g., alcohol, marijuana, methamphetamine).

3. *Regardless* of whether the IP enters treatment, most *CSOs feel better* themselves (e.g., less anxiety, depression, anger, physical concerns).

trained in CRAFT procedures, they're successful at getting their treatment-refusing loved one into treatment almost 70% of the time. *Nearly 7 out of 10 people are successful.* And from our conversation so far, I can say that I think *you* can be successful, too, if we keep working together and stay focused.

CSO: Sounds great. But at the same time I can't help but wonder if I'm going to be one of the 3 out of 10 who aren't successful. What if I can't do it right?

THERAPIST: I appreciate you sharing your concerns. Therapy seems to work best when people are not afraid to say what's on their mind and how they're feeling. As far as your question, we don't know for sure in advance when CRAFT isn't going to work. Not surprisingly, though, we've noticed a problem in situations in which the contact ends between the substance abuser and the treatment-seeking loved one. This loss of contact may happen because the substance-abusing individual leaves town, or the healthy family member, who's already in treatment, moves out. Or, occasionally, we get people who are mostly interested in getting therapy for themselves, and who use this program as an opportunity to do so. In those cases we sometimes discover that the person was never really invested in getting the substance user into treatment.

CSO: Oh, so being successful doesn't have a lot to do with whether a person can do the therapy the right way?

THERAPIST: I'm convinced that you can learn what's necessary by working together with me. I should mention that we've taught the program to all types of folks: spouses, parents, sisters, friends. And the type of drug being used doesn't make much difference either. It *will* require hard work and a commitment on your part. I will give you plenty of assignments to do at home that will be very important, because they'll allow you to put into practice the things we plan and rehearse during our sessions. I know it's a lot, but if we work together as a team, I think you can be successful. What do you think?

CSO: Well, I'm certainly willing to give it my best shot.

THERAPIST: Glad to hear it. You really *can't* lose, because concerned family members such as yourself usually end up feeling better about themselves—less depressed and anxious—even if their loved one never enters treatment. Does that make any sense?

CSO: I think so. Maybe they just get on with their lives somehow.

THERAPIST: You're right, they do, and their lives are enriched by participating in CRAFT. We teach folks how to take better care of their own needs as part of this program, and usually it affects many parts of their lives in a positive way. Do you have any questions about what we've talked about so far?

As shown in this sample conversation, the therapist presents the outcome of the CRAFT studies in lay terms, which also serves as a preview of the three goals of CRAFT. The therapist uses an opportunity to verbally reinforce the client for being open about sharing concerns. In response to the client's fear of being one of the ones whose therapy is not successful, the therapist conveys anecdotal findings that ongoing contact between a CSO and IP is an essential ingredient, as is the CSO's genuine interest in treatment engagement for the IP. The therapist reassures the client that the techniques *can* be learned, but also introduces the notion that commitment and hard work (e.g., completing homework assignments) will be a big part of that. The therapist then asks for further reactions before moving on.

DESCRIBING POTENTIAL BENEFITS FOR CSOs

Another method for motivating CSOs is to discuss the potential treatment benefits. You have already broached this topic if you have covered the empirical success of CRAFT. Still, it is helpful to further describe the benefits that are likely to be gained, even if the IP never enters treatment. Inform CSOs that as they change their own lives, the substance user may change in response. If the substance user does *not* change, clients can still enhance their own satisfaction if they follow through with treatment and give the process a chance to reduce the negative psychosocial effects. Assuming you have introduced the fact that CRAFT-trained CSOs tend to become more psychologically healthy, remind them that depression, anxiety, anger, and physical complaints frequently diminish, whereas self-esteem increases. How does this improvement happen? A variety of positive changes occur all at once when individuals take charge of their lives. A number of contributing factors are discussed in the following material.

The reduction of the potential for domestic violence can be a significant benefit of CSOs' involvement in CRAFT. However, if violence is an apparent current concern, dealing with the issue takes precedence, including determining whether the CSO is even an appropriate candidate for CRAFT at this time. If further investigation reveals it is reasonable to proceed with the CSO, explain that since violent outbursts are often associated with substance abuse (Greenfeld, 1998; Kyriacou et al., 1999), the probability of such episodes should be lessened if the IP reduces drinking or illicit drug use. Regardless, the potential for aggressive behavior should drop, because CSOs are taught methods for recognizing early triggers for violence and for responding in a safer manner. With this said, if this is your first reference to domestic violence with a client, it is useful to add that all CRAFT procedures are introduced with safety as a primary concern, and that any newly acquired skill should be used only if there appears to be no chance for a violent reaction from the substance abuser (see Chapter 4 for a complete description of issues related to violence).

Explain to CSOs that another advantage of CRAFT is learning skills that are helpful in numerous areas of their lives, not just in dealing with the substance user. For instance, some CSOs use their newly acquired communication skills with other family members or with colleagues at work, and they see payoffs in the form of improved relationships. Others regularly utilize CRAFT problem-solving skills to deal with everyday hassles. CRAFT also teaches clients how to make their social and recreational lives more of a priority. When CSOs apply these skills, they typically increase their social activities and outlets and, in the course of which, make more friends. As a result, CSOs find themselves enjoying their expanded social support systems.

Another benefit of CSO treatment is that it identifies ways to reduce the distress of other family members. In some cases CSOs' chief motivator for entering treatment is the welfare of their children. Clients learn how to assist children and other family members who are exhibiting signs of growing concern about the substance user's behavior. Helping individuals take action to deal with the source of the family anguish is an integral part of CRAFT. Sometimes family distress is best reduced by learning when and how to create physical distance from the IP. At other times non-substance-abusing family members decide that the best course of action is to join the CSO for CRAFT sessions, so that they can participate in the process directly. Periodically, CSOs discover that their new-found strength, self-esteem, and support allow them to make serious decisions about whether they want to remain in the relationship with their substance-abusing spouse.

In regard to the specific alcohol- or drug-related benefits that manifest themselves while *only the CSO* is in treatment: Tell CSOs that many drinkers in the alcohol studies had reduced their consumption considerably prior to even starting therapy. In all probability this improvement was due to the implementation of various CRAFT procedures by CSOs at home. So highlight the fact that IPs who remain adamantly opposed to treatment conceivably could *still* reduce their substance use as a result of CRAFT—and as discussed below, substantially decreased substance use can have far-reaching implications for the CSO.

The final phase of the discussion regarding potential treatment benefits should focus on additional advantages to the CSO *if the IP enters treatment*. Assuming that treatment attendance means that the IP is also in the process of decreasing his or her use, you could mention that CSOs frequently experience a host of positive changes at this time, such as fewer family arguments, improved financial stability, and an increased number of enjoyable social activities. If children are involved, mention that these changes produce better parental role models for them. If the CSO and IP are an intimate couple, then improved emotional and sexual satisfaction often result. As noted in the next section, it is critical to determine which factors are most important to each CSO, so that you can emphasize those benefits and make a note to refer back to them, as needed. Most of these case-specific benefits will come directly from the CRAFT Functional Analysis for a Loved One's Drinking/Using Behavior (see Chapter 3).

Inform CSOs that one final way they may profit if their IP begins treatment is by being invited to participate in couples counseling, a component of many alcohol and drug treatment programs. This opportunity is noteworthy for two reasons: (1) couples gain access to a setting in which they can safely address general relationship satisfaction directly; and (2) behavioral couples therapy has proven to be one of the more effective treatments for substance users (Epstein & McCrady, 1998; Fals-Stewart, O'Farrell, & Birchler, 2001; Fals-Stewart et al., 2000; O'Farrell & Fals-Stewart, 1999, 2000; Winters, Fals-Stewart, O'Farrell, Birchler, & Kelley, 2002; Stanton & Shadish, 1997).

IDENTIFYING THE CSOs' REINFORCERS

A practice that goes hand in hand with describing potential benefits of the CRAFT program (and overlaps somewhat with it) is the identification of a CSO's idiosyncratic reinforcers. Although the topic of reinforcers is discussed at length in later chapters, it is necessary to establish a basic understanding of reinforcers/rewards at this point. In brief, a positive reinforcer is anything that increases the behavior it follows. In other words, it is something of value to the individual that influences her or him to respond a certain way in order to obtain that "reward." In a relationship in which there is a treatment-refusing substance abuser, one obvious reinforcer for the CSO is the IP's cessation of drug or alcohol abuse. The prospect of reaching that reward is what motivates most CSOs to seek CRAFT treatment in the first place. Recognizable progress toward that goal serves as an ongoing incentive for CSOs to continue attending sessions and to tackle homework assignments outside of sessions.

In your initial conversations with CSOs, watch for additional signs of potential reinforcers (aside from the obvious ones of getting the IP to enter treatment and decrease use). Many of these reinforcers are not readily apparent, unless you are in the habit of looking for them. A straightforward example of this point is the CSO who speaks sadly about not being able to take the last few courses she needs to complete her degree program. She states that her husband (the IP) cannot be counted on as a reliable babysitter due to his heavy drinking, and consequently she cannot attend evening classes. You would label the obtainment of her degree as a reinforcer for the CSO, because it appears to be important to her and would, in all probability, motivate her to work diligently in therapy in order to lay the foundation for acquiring it. In other words, the CSO might make learning and implementing the CRAFT procedures a top priority, not only because she wants her husband to enter treatment and reduce his drinking, but because if he *does*, he could then become the reliable babysitter she needs to free her for her evening classes. This search for reinforcers essentially is a quest to find reasons why the CSO, and eventually the IP, are willing to change their behavior.

The identification of a CSO's sources of reinforcement and motivation begins at the first session, often by asking why she or he is seeking treatment at this time. In addition to describing the IP's drinking or drug problem, a CSO always talks about the problems created by the use. These reported problems can provide insight into things of value (i.e., reinforcers) *lost* as a result of the excessive substance use. As the client describes the problems, listen closely to discover possible reinforcers. For instance, a CSO may make the following comment:

> "I can't stand how much Lamont argues with our daughter. I remember when they used to be really close. Now all they do is fight and get on each other's nerves. And I know it's not just because she's a teenager. I've seen him be real nice to her when he's not high."

This statement may indicate that the quality of the relationship between the CSO's husband and daughter is very important to her, and consequently it could be used to motivate the client to make behavioral changes. For instance, she could be trained in communication skills (Chapter 5) and then asked to explain to the IP her concerns about his deteriorating relationship with their daughter. Or the CSO might be encouraged to plan simple but pleasant family activities for times when the IP is not using (Chapter 6), so that the positive aspects of the father–daughter relationship may, once again, be realized. These actions are only preliminary steps, given that the father–daughter relationship has the best chance of becoming healthy if the IP enters treatment.

Another example of a possible reinforcer is revealed in the following CSO's statement:

"If I had enough money to pay our bills, I wouldn't worry so much. I just can't get caught up. And he's no help. He's not working right now."

Based on this information, you would surmise that money is a current reinforcer. The substance-abusing loved one is unemployed, and the CSO is worried about financial matters. With this reinforcer in mind, explain to her that the IP's employment problem can be addressed once he begins treatment. In this way, the CSO can anticipate eventually obtaining a series of reinforcers that build upon each other as a result of her IP getting into treatment: his reduced substance use first, less money spent on alcohol/drugs as a result, then employment for him, and ultimately greater financial stability for the family. You could also refer back to this incentive during her treatment if she grew discouraged or were not complying with homework assignments.

You must become proficient at finding and using unique CSO reinforcers, because they are the backbone of the treatment process. As noted, many of these reinforcers automatically become obvious once the CRAFT functional analysis is completed (described in Chapter 3). The liberal use of a universal reinforcer, such as praise, was already mentioned as another important component of CRAFT. This reinforcement can take the form of applauding a client for finishing an assessment battery, or acknowledging a CSO's devotion to her family that is evidenced by her efforts to seek help. Verbal reinforcement establishes an upbeat and positive tone and models an important skill that will be taught formally in subsequent sessions.

CRAFT'S BASIC PREMISES

When providing an overview of the CRAFT program to CSOs, tell them it is designed for family members or friends who are invested in obtaining treatment for a treatment-refusing substance abuser. Mention how many other available programs think that CSOs should detach themselves from the individual who drinks or uses drugs, because it is believed that the substance abuser alone can correct the problem. Explain that the CRAFT program is different: It views CSOs as crucial collaborators in engaging resistant loved ones into treatment. In part, this conclusion is based on substance abusers' reports that their decision to pursue treatment often was prompted by the direct influence of CSOs, or CSOs acting in concert with courts, employee assistance programs, or other informal social networks (Cunningham et al., 1995; Hingson et al., 1982; Room, 1987). Discuss how the few other programs that utilize CSO involvement in IP engagement believe that family members must use confrontational techniques. Explain that CRAFT steers clear of confrontation.

Acknowledge that CSOs have a vast amount of information about the drinker or drug user's behavior. This knowledge, in fact, often motivates CSOs to enter treatment in the first place, as they hope to learn how to cope with or change that problematic behavior. Furthermore, CSOs typically have substantial contact with the IP (Stanton, 1982; Stanton & Heath, 1997)—a critical factor, given the behavioral techniques that are utilized in CRAFT. Finally, CSOs who seek treatment for a loved one usually are motivated and willing to work hard to promote positive changes, because they are concerned about the IP *and* because CSOs themselves stand to benefit in multiple ways from IP treatment engagement.

Reiterate to CSOs that the CRAFT program is designed to help them take control of their lives. The process begins by asking the CSO to examine the problems created by the substance user *and her or his behavior in reaction to those problems*. Properly managing the discussion that ensues is a challenge; namely, delivering the sometimes confusing and upsetting message that although CSOs are *not* responsible for the substance abuse problem, their own behavior may inadvertently make it easier for the person to continue using at times. Without belaboring the point, state that most people would respond in ways similar to them because they are natural reactions of people who care. Add that these automatic CSO responses can be changed through CRAFT training so that they instead support clean, sober IP behavior. Although the topic of the client's role in the maintenance of the substance-using behavior is one that some therapists would rather avoid, it should be raised in the initial session because it is part of the rationale for focusing on the CSO's behavior.

Explain to CSOs that behavior change is predicated on psychological learning principles. People do not change their behavior without a reason, and substance users are no exception. In other words, CRAFT teaches clients how to reward their IP's sober, positive behaviors, and how to withdraw rewards on occasions when the IP is using. CRAFT therapists work with CSOs to identify appropriate behaviors on which to concentrate, and suitable consequences to enforce.

In the segment that follows, the therapist introduces the principle of reinforcement as it pertains to the IP's behavior, and provides examples. In the course of doing so, she gently broaches the issue of how the CSO may have been unintentionally helping to maintain the IP's substance use. She then explains how this problematic behavior can be addressed through the program.

THERAPIST: One of the main premises of CRAFT is that we should focus on rewarding people when they are doing something right, as opposed to punishing them when they are doing something wrong.

It's like that old saying, "You can catch more flies with honey than with vinegar." In other words, as much as possible, we want to reward, or reinforce, your husband for certain positive behaviors, such as coming home sober or spending time with your children when he is sober. Jaime, I imagine that you're already rewarding some of Vernon's behaviors. Can you give me some examples?

CSO: I never really thought of it as a "reward," but since you mentioned giving him something when he comes home . . . I guess I reward him by letting him read to the kids, instead of me doing it, as long as he's home by about 8:00. He always stops at a friend's house for a few drinks after work, and sometimes he doesn't get home 'til 10:00. I feel like I can't keep the kids up after 8:00. But they have such a great time when he horses around with them in the evening. I hate it when they all miss out. When Vernon is late, he begs me to let him go wake them up so that he can play with them a little. Sometimes if he asks me real nice, I let him. Maybe that's a reward too.

THERAPIST: Letting your husband play with the children definitely sounds like a reward for him. I can tell that you really know what Vernon likes. That will help us tremendously here in your program.

Note: Here the therapist praises the client for possessing the valuable skill of knowing what her husband, the IP, truly finds rewarding. The therapist also should be making a mental note of the client's unsuccessful attempts to limit her rewarding of her husband *only* to when he arrives home on time. Since the reinforcement of appropriate behavior is a principal component of CRAFT, it will be necessary to explain later how CRAFT's reinforcement procedures are different from those already tried by the CSO. An obvious place to start would be the client's failure to follow through with a planned contingency, thereby leading to the inconsistent delivery of rewards.

THERAPIST: Jaime, one of the things we'll do in CRAFT, besides identify possible rewards, is look at the *timing* of the rewards you give. Let me ask you, what kind of shape is your husband in at 10:00? Or at 8:00, for that matter?

CSO: Actually, he's pretty toasted no matter what time he gets home. Why?

THERAPIST: Well, what do you think about rewarding him when he's had a lot to drink?

CSO: But I'm not rewarding him for drinking a lot, I'm rewarding him for coming home on time . . . sort of. Or maybe I'm rewarding him for talking sweet to me. Why? What should I be doing?

THERAPIST: This is something we'll obviously need to look at more closely later. But from what you've told me, I'd have to wonder if it feels *to him* like you're indirectly supporting his decision to come home late ... and drunk, even though you absolutely have no intention of doing so.

CSO: How could I be doing that? I don't want to support it. I hate it!

THERAPIST: Maybe "support" is too strong a word here. It would be more accurate to say that there are probably things you could do differently when he arrives home "toasted" that would show less *tolerance* of his drinking. Do you know what I mean?

CSO: Hmm. Maybe. I guess I do "tolerate" it, even though I hate it. I've given up trying to talk to him about it.

Note: The therapist introduces the concept of timing, as it pertains to the delivery of a reward. By doing so she also links the IP's late arrival home with his excessive drinking, so that the series of behaviors being rewarded become more obvious. The therapist should again take note of a reported ineffectual CSO behavior that approximates a CRAFT procedure: the discussion of the drinking problem with the IP. Since you eventually will be asking the CSO to engage in such a conversation, you should plan to explain then the reasons why the experience should prove more successful than her previous conversations on the topic. For example, you could state that she will receive extensive communication training before initiating the discussion and that she should do so only when the timing appears optimal (discussed in Chapters 5 and 6).

THERAPIST: I can understand your frustration. Here's the problem, though. When we tolerate somebody's behavior, it makes it a little easier for that person to keep doing that same behavior. I think we all tolerate things in others that we don't really like, and a certain amount of that kind of behavior is healthy. But if we're tolerating excessive drinking, we're probably not doing specific things to oppose it. So it makes sense to question whether tolerating Vernon's drinking is your best option. Of course, there are lots of other considerations that we'll have to get to, such as what you've already tried, and which new behaviors would be safe and comfortable for you to try next.

Note: The therapist settles on the word "tolerates" to describe the client's reactions to the alcohol use, since the CSO seems to agree with that description without being unduly upset in the process. The therapist also normalizes the CSO's reaction to her husband's drinking. Finally, the need to be safe is mentioned, a theme that will be repeated many times.

CSO: What *should* I be doing when he comes home late and drunk?

THERAPIST: We'll need to take some time to figure that out, once I know you and your situation better. It depends on a lot of factors. For instance, maybe it would be reasonable for you to let Vernon know in advance, *at a time when he's sober,* that you'll have the kids ready for bed and their books all laid out for him as long as he's home on time. But you'll probably also add that you're not going to give in to his request to get the kids up the next time he comes home late after drinking all evening. And then it would be very important to follow through with this and *not* give in, no matter how sweetly he talks to you. You seem to have much of this plan in mind already. I can see why it's difficult to actually carry it out at the time. For instance, you mentioned that it's hard to see the kids miss out on any opportunity to play with their dad.

CSO: It is. But I know it's not good for them to be woken up all the time, especially to see their daddy drunk. OK. I think I can do this. It doesn't sound so bad.

THERAPIST: Good. But remember, I'm just tossing out ideas here. We haven't decided on a plan yet, so don't go home and try this! We've got to wait until we feel the time is right.

Note: The therapist provides an example of a new CSO reaction to the husband's late arrival home after a night of drinking, but cautions the client not to enact the behavior yet. Not only is the therapist concerned about safety, but she has inadequate information to decide on the most suitable plan. The therapist also takes another opportunity to compliment the CSO (for her plan), and acknowledges the common difficulty of following through on a preset course of action.

THERAPIST: So CRAFT training will involve determining the ideal times and ways to reward your husband's appropriate behavior and to hold back on rewards when, for example, he's late and drunk. I think you can guess that a big part of CRAFT entails you carrying out these "assignments" at home. That's where the real changes need to take place.

CSO: It makes sense.

THERAPIST: Eventually, it will be important to *make sure* Vernon knows how much you approve of certain behaviors. At that point CRAFT will also involve communication training so that you could tell him, for example, that it's great to have him home early so he can spend time with you and the kids. As far as withholding rewards when he comes home drunk, you might be taught to simply leave the room, or as I mentioned before, to ignore his requests to get the children out of bed. Once we've had time to practice communication techniques, you might explain your actions to your husband on the spot. You may want to say, "Vernon, I love you, but you're drinking again, and

I'm not going to be part of it. I'm going upstairs to watch TV. Please do not wake the children. They love seeing you, but it's not good for them to be woken up at night. " The right combination of praise and resolve should pique your husband's curiosity and may even prompt him to change his behavior in response to your new stance. Well, what do you think?

CSO: It sounds like it's worth a try.

The therapist provided a relevant illustration of reinforcement principles (i.e., giving and withdrawing reinforcement), but cautioned the client not to change any behavior prematurely. Full consideration must always be given to the "big picture" before finalizing any plan, including the potential for threatening reactions by the IP. Importantly, the therapist introduced the notion that they will need to examine the CSO's behavior for any possible, unintentional demonstrations of support of the IP's substance use. In addition, the therapist discussed the role of homework assignments and verbally reinforced the CSO whenever suitable opportunities presented themselves. Finally, the therapist mentally noted several occasions of failed attempts by the CSO to change her husband's behavior; these could be reintroduced and commented on at an appropriate time in future sessions.

The main premises of CRAFT that should be covered in your first session are outlined in Table 2.3.

THREE MAIN GOALS OF CRAFT

An integral component of the first session is the introduction of the three major goals of the CRAFT program. These goals are numbered for organizational purposes only, not necessarily in order of importance: (1) decrease the IP's substance use; (2) get the substance user to enter treatment; and (3) increase the CSO's own happiness, independent of whether the IP enters treatment.

DECREASE THE IP'S SUBSTANCE USE

In presenting the goal of decreasing the IP's substance use, explain to CSOs that the CRAFT program may lead to sobriety in very different ways from other treatments with which they are probably familiar. Importantly, CRAFT's distinctive methods have had better results when compared with other more commonly used programs, such as Al-Anon and the Johnson Institute Intervention. Although ultimately CRAFT aims to

TABLE 2.3. BASIC PREMISES OF CRAFT

1. The program is designed for CSOs who want to *engage a treatment-refusing substance abuser* into treatment.

2. It is different from other CSO programs because it promotes *active, positive participation* in engaging the IP into treatment, as opposed to detachment or confrontation.

3. CSOs are considered *ideal collaborators* in the treatment engagement process because they have a great deal of *knowledge* about the IP's behavior and are likely to be successful at influencing it due to their frequent *contact* with the IP and their high level of personal *motivation*.

4. CRAFT initially involves examining the problems created by the substance use and the *CSOs' typical reaction* to them (which inadvertently supports the use at times).

5. Behavioral *learning principles* (e.g., giving and withholding positive *reinforcement*) form the basis of CRAFT.

6. *Relevant examples* of some of these learning principles in action include [fill in for your client].

---

get an IP to enter treatment, a preliminary objective is to influence the IP to cut back on the using behavior. If the IP does so, there is a greater chance that he or she will seek professional help. But in the event that the IP never starts treatment, this goal ensures that the CSO will have at least learned techniques to support decreased substance use.

Explain that the process begins by CSOs changing old behavior patterns into new, nonenabling, appropriate, supportive behaviors. Caution CSOs not to be surprised, however, if the IP temporarily *increases* the maladaptive behavior in response to the changes. Reassure the CSO that the IP eventually is likely to reduce the drinking or drug use, *if* the CSO *consistently* executes her or his new behavior toward the IP. Provide an example to illustrate your point. Take the case of the wife who traditionally criticizes her husband (the IP) when he comes home under the influence of alcohol. Assume the wife is trained to forego the criticism and to respond, instead, by saying, "I can see you've decided to drink tonight. You probably remember us talking about how I don't like to be with you when you're drinking, and how I planned to leave for the night if you did. So I'm heading over to my mother's. I'll see you in the morning." Although the wife's response does not directly prompt the husband to enter treatment, he is more apt to reconsider his actions before drinking the next time (or before drinking as much). His alcohol use may actually increase initially as he tests out the ramifications of his behavior within this new system, or perhaps as he expresses his anger passive-aggressively. But the drinking is likely to diminish if the CSO correctly and consistently follows through on her new learned response. Or the husband may start asking questions about his wife's new reaction to his drinking. Either way, he is primed to sample treatment.

At this point CSOs sometimes ask whether treatment engagement efforts are still necessary if the IP has significantly cut back the drinking or drug use. Although special circumstances might alter your response, the standard reply includes the following reasons why engagement attempts normally should not be abandoned:

- Moderate, ongoing use is often a source of continued concern for CSOs because they fear usage will escalate again, and, in fact, it *is* extremely difficult for many previously heavier users to indefinitely maintain a low level of alcohol or drug use (as opposed to abstaining) (Hester, 2003).
- Many of the problems associated with the substance use are often still present, even though the substance use may have decreased.
- If things are improved as a result of the IP's lowered level of use, conceivably they would get even better once the IP begins treatment and starts working on problems other than solely the substance abuse.
- The use of illicit drugs in any amount still carries legal consequences.
- CSOs frequently feel as if they are shouldering a tremendous burden alone if the IP does not have a therapist.

GET THE SUBSTANCE USER TO ENTER TREATMENT

Not only is treatment engagement a major goal of CRAFT, for some CSOs this is really their *only* goal. As noted, CRAFT has been successful in influencing the resistant IP to enter treatment almost 70% of the time (W. Miller et al., 1999; Meyers et al., 2002). You should explain how the process of achieving this task varies with every CSO and IP, and how therefore it will take time to discover the strategies indicated for their particular case. Let CSOs know that there are many steps prior to asking the substance user to enter formal treatment. Only after discussing various components of the procedure at length and practicing the scenario repeatedly in the context of a supportive role play, complete with feedback, will the time be right for making the request. Tell CSOs that waiting for the optimal time to suggest treatment is essential for success.

Provide an example of how the invitation to enter treatment might unfold. For instance, state that the CSO (the husband) tells the substance user (the wife) that he is in treatment because he loves her and is trying to get help to make their relationship healthier. The CSO adds that he would like her to join him in treatment, or at least to come in and meet his therapist. Clarify that this request would only occur after the husband had received training in communication, had participated in an extensive number of role plays, had anticipated and resolved foreseeable problems, and had determined the best time to raise the subject. Point out that the IP's substance use is often not even mentioned as part of the treatment invitation.

INCREASE THE CSO'S OWN HAPPINESS INDEPENDENT OF WHETHER THE IP ENTERS TREATMENT

State that you will help CSOs learn how to take better care of themselves. This care may entail scheduling enjoyable events for homework, such as visiting family and friends, going to the movies, hiking, taking gardening classes, exercising, or just getting out and having fun. As a CRAFT therapist, you will teach CSOs how to find satisfaction in life independent of the substance user. In part, this differentiation will allow substance users the space to think about whether they want to participate in any pleasurable alcohol- and drug-free family activities, and to ponder the possibly sobering reality that family life can go on without them. Furthermore, this segment of CRAFT gives CSOs the message that they are important individuals who deserve to be happy, and that the happiness does not need to be driven by the IP's status.

All three goals should be mentioned in the first session. Depending on the sequence of the topics addressed, sometimes this occurs relatively early in the session. For instance, it would be natural to touch upon the goals in the process of describing CRAFT's scientific support, or when explaining the concept of CSO reinforcers. In these cases the goals would not necessarily have to be presented again. Still, some CSOs may require a review of certain goals, and others may want time to dwell on issues relevant to one goal over another. You can always allow for that time and provide complete information later or in the next session. Be aware of each client's needs; clients should participate in the program at their own speed.

CRAFT PROCEDURES

Explain to CSOs that CRAFT is a menu-driven approach. In other words, not every component of CRAFT is used with every client. One size does not fit all! The decision regarding which components to use depends primarily on the individual CSO's needs *and* her or his willingness to try the procedure. Furthermore, let clients know that although they will be given clear guidance, they do not have to do anything they do not want to do. This message tends to reassure anxious CSOs, who sometimes are apprehensive about unknown therapy expectations. These procedures, however, are not intended to be used like a shopping list; instead, they should be introduced in whatever order and at whatever pace makes the most sense clinically for each client. For instance, a particular procedure might take a full session with one CSO, but only 5 minutes with a different CSO. In sum, depending on the client, you will use different combinations of procedures, or the same procedures but at different times, or the same procedures but of varying durations. You should feel comfortable altering the process; do not stay wedded to a specific formula. Be flexible enough to meet the idiosyncratic needs of the CSO while incorporating the parts of CRAFT that appear germane, and while keeping within the CRAFT philosophy.

Explain to CSOs that CRAFT is skills-based and that, consequently, a major thrust of the program is to teach new skills, including *how* and *when* to use them. As an example, ask your clients to describe their current CSO–IP communication style. Whether it consists primarily of blaming and yelling or no communication at all, tell clients you will train them to state their views calmly but assertively (Chapter 5). Breaking the cycle of negative communication is a first step toward a more positive relationship overall, as well as being a prerequisite for effectively inviting the IP to enter treatment. You might also ask CSOs whether every day seems to bring on more and more insurmountable problems, and if, at this point, they believe that no matter what they attempt to change, they will fail. Inform clients that you will teach them techniques for effectively breaking down and solving problems of a wide variety (Chapter 7).

Remind CSOs that some of the skills they will learn are geared *directly* toward influencing the IP's use. CSOs will be asked to change their behavior in specific ways so that sober behavior is rewarded and substance-using behavior is ignored or discouraged. It is preferable to provide a brief illustration of this principle, even if you already have done so, because CSOs frequently do not fully understand what is meant by this statement. A common example would be a wife (the CSO) who usually shouts at her husband (the IP) and makes accusations when he is drinking. Due to her unresolved anger, she then either stays away from him or criticizes him when he is sober. The wife would be taught to reward her husband by giving him something he values (e.g., a pleasant time together, a dinner treat, a hug) when he is *not* drinking, and to withdraw reinforcement (e.g., leave his presence) when he is using alcohol. Be sure to inquire about the CSOs' reaction to this information regarding changing their own behavior.

Remind CSOs that one of the three goals of CRAFT focuses on the enhancement of their own happiness. Discuss how over the years of living with a substance user, many CSOs spend less and less time with family and friends. Embarrassment, guilt, and fear tend to keep them from participating in outside activities, as they become caught up in the pretense of keeping the family looking "normal." Tell your clients that they will learn skills that eventually will allow them to feel comfortable rekindling some of their old supportive relationships. Spending time and talking with a close friend or relative can help CSOs in numerous ways, not the least of which is to provide moral support for attempting to get the substance user to accept treatment. Once CSOs experience the relief of renewed support, they might ask if it would be acceptable to have a confidant(e) accompany them to therapy, particularly if they believe that IP engagement is more likely to occur with the help of another CRAFT-trained loved one. In most cases you would welcome the opportunity to involve a member of the CSO's support network. Inform all CSOs that in addition to engagement and social-support-building skills, many other types of skills can be taught to CSOs, if desired, such as methods for obtaining a new job (see Meyers & Smith, 1995, pp. 121–126).

Since the majority of CSOs are primarily interested in the specifics related to influencing the IP to enter treatment, it is imperative to touch upon this issue directly in the first session. Explain that they must learn certain skills in order to maximize their chance of success, and that the timing of the treatment request is critical as well. In a word, they must be patient initially. Knowing precisely *when* and *how* they should approach the substance user to discuss treatment entry is extremely important.

Table 2.4 summarizes the main points to address when presenting an overview of the CRAFT procedures.

CSO RESPONSIBILITIES AS PART OF CRAFT

Describe the CRAFT program as a very active process for CSOs. This "activity" takes the form of role plays and other skills-training exercises during sessions and homework assignments between sessions. From the outset you should stress the importance of clients' responsibility to comply with assigned tasks. Tell them that the skills they will be learning, like most skills, will require consistent practice. Efficiency alone might necessitate practice outside of sessions, but homework is also important as a means of rehearsing new skills in the real world. Reassure CSOs that eventually they will reap the benefits of their practice, as the enacted skills pave the way to successful outcomes in their lives.

Another responsibility of CSOs is to make their own safety a priority. Obviously you will share this responsibility in your coverage of domestic violence issues. Still, the CSOs know better than anyone else what they risk in their home life. As mentioned earlier, a fair number of clients enter treatment without the substance user's knowledge, and a subset requests that the therapist *not* contact them at home. Not surprisingly, the

TABLE 2.4. OVERVIEW OF CRAFT PROCEDURES

1. CRAFT is a *menu-driven* program whose components and procedures are selected on the basis of an individual CSO's needs and desires.

2. CRAFT is a *skills-based* program that teaches general skills (e.g., communication, problem-solving) designed to be useful in *multiple arenas* of a person's life.

3. Most of these skills also are used to promote *changes in the IP's substance use* and eventually to *successfully influence the IP to enter treatment*.

4. CRAFT includes skills to help *reintroduce happiness into CSOs' lives*, regardless of the IP's outcome.

5. Although the foundation is laid early for inviting an IP to enter treatment, it is critical to *wait for the optimal time*.

---

reason behind such a request usually involves safety concerns. Interestingly, the opposite occurs more often: Many CSOs immediately want to invite the substance user to enter treatment, even before the CSOs are trained and ready to properly anticipate and handle the assortment of possible scenarios. As a CRAFT therapist, you will learn to finesse a balance between encouraging CSOs to move forward, while simultaneously advising them to do so slowly, strategically, and under your guidance.

Another responsibility of most CSOs is to support the substance user once that individual enters treatment, such as by participating in relationship counseling. Many programs for the substance abuser, including the Community Reinforcement Approach, consider behavioral couples therapy to be an integral part of the treatment (Azrin et al., 1973; Epstein & McCrady, 1998; Fals-Stewart et al., 1996, 2001; O'Farrell & Fals-Stewart, 2000; Meyers & Smith, 1995). In essence, getting the IP to seek treatment is just the beginning of the process for many CSOs.

SUMMARY

This chapter describes the issues typically addressed and the procedures utilized in an initial session with CSOs. As noted, the first session is an introduction to CRAFT, with the objective of encouraging CSOs and "hooking" them into the program, while building their confidence. Additionally this session affords therapists the opportunity to gain preliminary insight into each CSO's idiosyncratic reinforcers and the function of the IP's use. Lastly, the first session serves to provide basic information about what CSOs can expect as clients in a CRAFT program, so that they can make an informed decision about whether or not they want to proceed.

FIGURE 2.1. **RELATIONSHIP HAPPINESS SCALE**

This scale is intended to estimate your *current* happiness with your relationship with your loved one in each of the 10 areas listed below. Ask yourself the following question as you rate each area:

How happy am I today with my loved one in this area?

Circle one of the numbers (1–10) beside each area. Numbers toward the left indicate various degrees of unhappiness, and numbers toward the right reflect various levels of happiness. In other words, state exactly how you feel today about that particular relationship area, using the numerical scale (1–10).

Remember: Try to exclude all feelings of yesterday and concentrate only on your feelings *today* in each of the areas. Also try not to allow one category to influence the results of the other categories.

	Completely Unhappy						**Completely Happy**			
Drinking/Drug Use	1	2	3	4	5	6	7	8	9	10
Household Responsibilities	1	2	3	4	5	6	7	8	9	10
Raising the Children	1	2	3	4	5	6	7	8	9	10
Social Activities	1	2	3	4	5	6	7	8	9	10
Money Management	1	2	3	4	5	6	7	8	9	10
Communication	1	2	3	4	5	6	7	8	9	10
Sex and Affection	1	2	3	4	5	6	7	8	9	10
Job or School	1	2	3	4	5	6	7	8	9	10
Emotional Support	1	2	3	4	5	6	7	8	9	10
General Happiness	1	2	3	4	5	6	7	8	9	10

Name: _____   Date: _____

FUNCTIONAL ANALYSIS OF A PROBLEM BEHAVIOR

One major objective of the CRAFT program, as noted, is to teach CSOs to change their behavior toward the IP, so that, in turn, the IP alters his or her behavior in response. In order to be in a position to guide the CSO's behavior change, you need to have a complete picture of the context in which the IP's problematic behavior occurs. In other words, both you and the CSO must be able to identify the antecedents or "triggers" of the behavior, as well as its short- and long-term consequences.

Although many behaviorists and cognitive-behaviorists learn how to use a procedure called a "functional analysis" to outline target behaviors, most of them do not routinely incorporate it into their practice. This is *not* the case for community reinforcement therapists, however, because functional analyses are an integral part of the overall Community Reinforcement Approach (CRA) program (Meyers & Smith, 1995; Chapter 2). The CRAFT program utilizes them as well. In line with the format offered as part of the Community Reinforcement Approach, two different types of functional analyses are used. The first type addresses a behavior that is being targeted to decrease, such as substance use, and the second type focuses on prosocial behaviors that are targeted to increase. An unusual "twist" is needed to modify functional analyses to suit the CRAFT program, because it is the CSO who actually completes these functional analyses of the (treatment-refusing) IP's behavior.

OBJECTIVES OF THE FUNCTIONAL ANALYSIS

A functional analysis is a framework for understanding the factors that influence the occurrence of a particular behavior. Behavioral theory recognizes that behavior does not occur in a vacuum; rather, there are identifiable antecedents that set the stage for it. The behavior is maintained over time because of the positive consequences experienced by the individual when he or she engages in that behavior. The functional analysis is used to gather this assessment information so that ultimately strategies can be devised to influence the occurrence of the behavior, either by attempting to decrease it (a problem behavior) or increase it (a healthy behavior). For a problem behavior, the premise is that in addition to the short-lived positive consequences that are experienced, there are negative consequences for it as well. However, the IP may not acknowledge the association between the negative consequences and the substance use, or the negative consequences may not be powerful enough to compete with the positive consequences at this point. Regardless, these negative consequences are worth examining as part of the functional analysis, because they may provide insight into reasons why the IP might be willing to consider altering the behavior eventually.

DESCRIBING THE FUNCTIONAL ANALYSIS OF A PROBLEM BEHAVIOR TO THE CSO

The CRAFT functional analysis of a *problem* behavior (i.e., substance abuse) typically is conducted as a semistructured interview with the CSO, near the end of the first session or the beginning of the second. On rare occasions, you may elect to send a client home with a form called the CRAFT Functional Analysis of a Loved One's Drinking/Using Behavior (Figure 3.1, end of chapter) to get started on during the week, but only after you have explained the rationale and provided a few examples. In such a scenario, you would discuss the form and its implications in extensive detail with the client at the next session. More commonly, the functional analysis is conducted with your assistance.

The rationale for having the CSO complete a functional analysis of the IP's problem behavior starts with a reminder about one of the major goals of the CRAFT program: to influence the IP's substance use behavior by changing the CSO's own behavior toward the IP. Although ultimately the objective is to influence the IP to enter treatment, in the meantime it is important to interact with the IP in such a way that the IP's drinking/using is more apt to decrease. This reduction in use not only benefits the IP and the CSO–IP relationship; there also appears to be a correlation between a reduction in IP use and the acceptance of treatment (W. Miller et al., 1999; Sisson & Azrin, 1986). Perhaps these somewhat healthier individuals are simply able to make healthier decisions (i.e., to seek treatment). Another possibility is that IPs who have decreased their substance use in response to the CSO's CRAFT procedures may be more open to the idea of receiving professional assistance in cases when they know it consists of the type of intervention they have already experienced as helpful.

As you proceed with setting the stage for the functional analysis, explain that in these preliminary phases of therapy the CSO should only be assisting in gathering information and should refrain from changing any behaviors prematurely. It is necessary to proceed cautiously, given that an assessment of the potential for domestic violence is yet to be conducted. Also state that although ideally it would be the *IP* completing the functional analysis, obviously that is not an option due to the IP's refusal to see a therapist. Nevertheless, the client has much to offer in this exercise, given her or his wealth of knowledge about the IP's use and related behaviors. Furthermore, explain that because of her or his extensive contact with the IP the CSO is the natural choice in terms of altering behavior toward the IP, which is one of the intended outgrowths of the exercise. Mention that the functional analysis exercise will demonstrate that the episodes are actually more predictable than the CSO probably realizes, and that with predictability often comes a sense of optimism, direction, and control for the CSO.

In continuing your explanation of the rationale for conducting the functional analysis, next give an overview of the segments of the analysis itself and describe their purpose. For example, state that you will ask the CSO about the people, places, and things that typically are associated with the IP's use, in order to formulate ideas about how the CSO might intervene at those times to decrease the behavior. Then describe how the functional analysis is an efficient tool with which to monitor any alterations in the amount or type of use. Finally, mention that the consequences of the IP's use will be explored, beginning with the short-term positive consequences experienced by the IP that appear to be maintaining the problem behavior. Explain that this information will be used to have the CSO find and encourage healthier ways for the IP to obtain similar positive consequences. Then add that the less immediate negative consequences for the IP's use will be outlined as well, so that they may be offered as part of the rationale when appealing to the IP to make some major behavioral changes. Table 3.1 summarizes the rationale for, and description of, the CRAFT functional analysis of a problem behavior.

GETTING STARTED: PROBLEM BEHAVIOR OVERVIEW

In beginning the functional analysis, inform the client that it is common for CSOs to not know the answers to some of the questions asked about their IP's use; this lack of knowledge is *not* considered a problem. The CSO will be able to provide plenty of useful information, despite the fact

TABLE 3.1. CRAFT FUNCTIONAL ANALYSIS OF A LOVED ONE'S DRINKING/USING BEHAVIOR: RATIONALE AND DESCRIPTION

1. The goal is to alter the IP's substance use by *changing how the CSO interacts* with the IP.

2. *Reduced use* of alcohol or drugs will be *healthier* for the IP and the CSO–IP relationship, and will increase the chance that the *IP enters treatment*.

3. The current focus is on *gathering information*; for safety purposes there should be no changes in CSO behavior yet.

4. The CSO is an ideal person to complete the functional analysis for the IP and act upon the findings, due to the *CSO's knowledge* about the IP's use and the amount of CSO–IP *contact*.

5. In completing the functional analysis, the CSO will see that the substance use episodes are more *predictable* than realized, and with this new information often comes a clear sense of direction and optimism for the CSO.

6. A functional analysis outlines the *triggers* for the IP's use, thereby stimulating ideas about when and how the CSO might intervene at those high-risk times.

7. A functional analysis provides an estimate of the *amount of current use*, so that progress can be monitored over time.

8. A functional analysis identifies the short-term *positive consequences* of the use as experienced by the IP, thereby pinpointing the IP's *reinforcers*, which need to be accessed in healthier ways.

9. It also identifies the *negative consequences* of the use, which may then be pointed out when appealing to the IP to change his or her problem behavior.

that some gaps will appear. Let the CSO know that you will jot down responses on a functional analysis form during the interview. Show the form to the CSO (Figure 3.1), and state that you will be giving her or him a form to follow as a guide, once a preliminary overview is obtained.

Start the actual functional analysis by first asking the CSO to think of and describe a common drinking/using episode for the IP. Tell the CSO that since it would be unrealistic to describe *all* of the pertinent substance-abusing situations, your plan is to use this representative episode to gain general information about the IP's typical drinking/using environment. Some clients immediately start providing the details of an episode, whereas others are uncertain as to what constitutes an *episode* or whether any of the episodes they have in mind are truly "common." Inform the uncertain CSOs that an *episode* is simply an occasion on which the IP has used the substance of concern. An episode is considered *common* if there is a discernible pattern of use that occurs on a fairly regular basis. But tell the CSO that this pattern need not be identical each time in order to be considered a good example of a common episode; it would just need to share certain basic characteristics, such as when and where it took place. Nevertheless, some CSOs initially insist that there is no pattern to their IP's use, and consequently they do not know how to select an episode. In this instance it may be helpful to ask the CSO whether, for example, the IP uses in a particular manner most weekdays and then a different way on weekends. You can then ask the CSO to select the weekday or weekend pattern, depending on which one occurs more frequently or which one carries the potential for the most severe consequences. Usually this type of categorization anchors the construct sufficiently so that the exercise can proceed. In the event that it does not, you may simply ask the CSO to describe the most recent episode, as it is likely to be a fairly representative one.

While the CSO is providing an overview of a common IP drinking/using episode, jot down the details in the appropriate section of the functional analysis form. Given the usual manner in which these stories unfold, plan on skipping back and forth on the form. The gaps will be filled in during the more formal part of the semistructured interview, which is next. The benefit of simply allowing the client to describe the episode more generally first is that it precludes the realistic risk of the functional analysis exercise appearing too mechanical. With this risk in mind, it is also *not* necessary for you to proceed with the formal part of the functional analysis interview in the order in which questions are outlined on the form, if it seems reasonable to follow up on the CSO's comments in some other manner. Regardless, the general sequence of events outlined on the form for the behavior—namely, starting with triggers and ending with consequences—is reviewed after the information is collected.

The dialogue presented below is a sample session between a CRAFT therapist and a female CSO at a time when they are ready to do a functional analysis of the CSO's husband's cocaine use. Assume that the rationale for a functional analysis of the IP's problem behavior has already been given, along with an explanation of the process. The conversation begins with the therapist asking for a general description of a common using episode:

THERAPIST: Now that we've talked about the purpose of the exercise called a "functional analysis," I'd like to go ahead and do one. Remember that we'll be outlining a "typical" using episode—one that happens fairly often. So which typical cocaine episode would you like to outline for Chris?

CSO: As far as I know, he only uses cocaine on the weekends: either Friday or Saturday night.

THERAPIST: Do we need to narrow it down to either Friday or Saturday night, or are the circumstances pretty similar for both nights?

Note: The therapist is trying to select an episode that occurs regularly, but is also hoping to outline it in a way that the findings will generalize to other somewhat similar episodes.

CSO: Chris does coke with the same bunch of people he hangs out with at the bar. So in that way, I could describe a weekend episode that would hold for either Friday or Saturday night.

THERAPIST: Let's use it, then. If we run into problems because the behavior doesn't actually fit for both nights, we can easily change it at that point. So, Natasha, let's start by you simply describing to me what you know about Chris's weekend cocaine episodes. Don't worry about following the order listed on that chart I showed you. Just go ahead and describe it in your own way first.

Note: The therapist does not want to introduce any unnecessary structure at this point. By allowing the CSO to tell the story in her own words, many of the details will be obtained anyway, and the process will not be experienced as so perfunctory. With this concern in mind, the CSO is not yet given a functional analysis chart to follow.

CSO: OK. I think I'll describe what happened last Friday, since it was the same old thing again. Chris had promised to be home from work by 7:00, because we were going to stay home and order a pizza for dinner. We like the shows that are on TV Friday nights, so sometimes we plan to do that. So I didn't buy anything to make for dinner, but you know, I knew enough *not* to order the pizza until he got home. We've been through this too many times before.

THERAPIST: So you found yourself in a familiar situation. I take it he didn't make it home on time?

CSO: No. He didn't get home until 2 A.M. He started drinking after work at 6:00, so that's a long evening. At least he called me to let me know he was OK, but that wasn't until around 11:00. But I knew long before then he wasn't coming home.

THERAPIST: That's interesting that he called, though.

CSO: We had a huge argument about it a few weeks ago. I told him I couldn't stand not knowing if he was OK.

THERAPIST: So it sounds like, in some situations, he responds to your needs when you specifically ask him to. That's a good sign.

Note: The therapist uses this opportunity to comment on the CSO's ability to get what she wants from her husband, at times, by asking for it. This fact reinforces the notion that she will be able to influence his behavior again in the future.

CSO: I suppose. I had to practically threaten him, though.

THERAPIST: Well, hopefully we can find a more comfortable way for you to influence his behavior in the future. So what happened once he got home?

Note: The therapist could stop the narrative and begin focusing on the triggers for the episode, but instead she encourages the CSO to finish telling the story in a conversational manner first. The therapist also could probe for the CSO's feelings (e.g., anger, frustration) in that situation, but doing so would divert the conversation away from the objective of the functional analysis. The CSO's feelings will be addressed later.

CSO: I was half asleep on the couch when he came in. I think I said something about him never keeping his word, and about him choosing his friends over me again. Then I just went to bed. He followed me, but he didn't say anything. I could tell he was high, though.

THERAPIST: And the next morning?

CSO: Well, he knew I was upset, so when he finally got out of bed at around 10:30 he asked me if I wanted to go see a movie that afternoon. Oh, and he asked me if I wanted to go out and get some brunch.

THERAPIST: And what did you do?

CSO: I told him I'd tell him later, that I didn't want to talk to him yet. But he knows that I don't like to wreck our weekend by being mad at him. He knows that I always give in. I figure that I might as well spend time with him while I can. Anyway, I turned right around and said "yes."

At the conclusion of a CSO's overview of a common using episode, the therapist typically has obtained valuable information about the consequences of the IP's substance use, at least in terms of how the CSO handles it. This particular case is no exception, since the CSO reported that although she was extremely upset with her husband for returning home high at 2 A.M., she nevertheless allowed him to "make it up" to her by spending time with him the next day. Other than the wife being annoyed with her husband for a few hours, she presented no immediate negative repercussions for his unacceptable behavior. Eventually, information such as this would be used when planning how the CSO should respond differently to future episodes.

Discovering some of the consequences of the use is not the only worthwhile information obtained in the overview. Therapists also learn something about the environmental factors (i.e., people, places, or times) that are associated with the use. Although the details about the IP's internal state (i.e., thoughts, feelings) are not normally offered by the CSO until the therapist specifically probes later in the functional analysis, it is not unusual for some of the *CSO's* feelings to become apparent at this early point in the interview. In this sample case the CSO viewed *herself* as responsible for spoiling the weekend if she did not go along with her husband's plans the next day. The issue of responsibility for the problem is introduced in the first CRAFT session and then revisited, when clinically indicated, throughout the program. The therapist in this scenario opted to continue with the functional analysis rather than address the CSO's feelings at that moment.

GUIDING THE CSO IN IDENTIFYING TRIGGERS OF THE IP'S USE

Once the CSO has provided a general description of the IP's problem behavior, you should determine which of the missing pieces of the functional analysis need to be completed. Typically, details about the antecedents (i.e., triggers) for the use are scanty. Triggers are the "high-risk" environmental factors, such as people, places, and other "occasions," that set the stage for the IP's substance use. Triggers are also the internal factors: the IP's thoughts and feelings that seem to precede the onset of the use. In most cases it is worthwhile to spend considerable time inquiring about antecedents, in part, because doing so helps the CSO realize that the problem behavior is influenced by reasonably predictable external and internal factors. As noted previously, with this realization often comes a sense of direction and optimism. Furthermore, a fairly predictable behavior offers many options when planning behavioral changes the CSO can make during these high-risk times that should work to influence the IP's decision to use in the first place. Each of these points should be reviewed with the CSO.

To gather more information on triggers, specifically ask the client to describe the events that led up to the IP's substance use for the already selected common episode. It is usually easier to begin with the *external* (environmental) triggers (Figure 3.1, column 1). You should substitute the appropriate choice for person (he or she) and behavior (drinking or using) when posing the following questions:

1. "*Who* is your loved one usually with when drinking/using?" Many individuals who abuse substances have regular friends or relatives with whom they tend to use. Often the CSO is aware of these individuals and is able to answer the question with confidence. If the CSO has difficulty responding because the IP tends to use with many different individuals on many different occasions, remind the CSO that you are focusing on

just one common episode. Alternatively, if the CSO knows that the IP always uses with the same group of individuals but does not know them by name, assure the CSO that names are unimportant and simply collect some descriptive information about them. At other times CSOs state that they have no idea with whom their IP associates when using. In this case you should tell the CSO that details about other external factors for the episode can prove to be equally helpful. And if the CSO reports that the IP uses alone, you should note this point and proceed to the next question.

2. "*Where* does he/she usually drink/use?" In many cases the CSO is able to report a specific location in response to this query, such as "the bar on the way home from work," "the restroom at the factory," "the company van," or "the garage." Again, if the CSO has difficulty providing this information, do your best to guide the process while always taking care to verbally reinforce the CSO for any degree of detail provided. Importantly, keep in mind that the purpose is to obtain sufficient information about the episode so that triggers can be examined as potential points for intervention.

3. "*When* does he/she usually drink/use?" If not already known for the episode in question, clarify which times of the day and days of the week the IP is more likely to abuse the substance of choice. If the behavior does not take place every week, then the frequency of occurrence should be recorded as well. The response for this external antecedent often is straightforward, since it is linked with the questions about people and places that have already been answered. Nevertheless it is still worthwhile to inquire, because you are attempting to pull together a complete picture of the IP's high-risk environment.

Once the external triggers have been identified, ask the CSO to explain, in her or his own words, why it is important to be cognizant of these factors. This step ensures that the CSO is aware of the purpose of the exercise. Then introduce the notion of *internal* triggers (Figure 3.1, column 2). Explain that individuals often experience familiar thoughts (e.g., "I can't handle this anymore," "I deserve a treat") and feelings (e.g., anger, anxiety) prior to drinking or using. State that you understand it may be difficult for the CSO to try to put a label on the IP's thoughts and feelings, but that you are only asking the CSO to come up with a logical guess. Remind the CSO that your goal is to eventually help her or him find a way to intervene, so that the IP becomes more apt to respond to these internal triggers in a healthier manner.

The responses that CSOs are capable of giving regarding the internal triggers vary tremendously. Some clients insist that their IP's decision to use seems to come from "out of nowhere," and consequently they feel clueless about their IP's thoughts. In these cases you might mention that even the IPs themselves are often unaware of this connection in the beginning, and so it is natural for the CSO to assume that one does not exist. Encourage the CSO to offer an informed opinion about possible internal triggers, based on what she or he *does* know about the IP's episode, in general. With this said, specifically ask the CSO:

1. "What do you think your loved one is *thinking* about right before drinking/using?" Encourage the CSO to proceed slowly at this point and to simply do the best she or he can on a task where achieving 100% accuracy is neither possible nor necessary. In addition, mention that the objective for the CSO is *not* to attempt to mind read but to realize that there *is* a pattern to the substance use. In other words, you are challenging the notion that the use just comes from "out of nowhere"; that a decision is reached in response to somewhat predictable antecedent thoughts. If the CSO still has trouble getting started, you may decide to illustrate with a few common examples. For instance, you could report that some CSOs believe their IPs are thinking along the lines of, "It's too much—I give up" or "I need to take the edge off" right before they use. You would explain that these thoughts suggest that the IP is trying to escape feelings of frustration, anxiety, or perhaps anger. Other CSOs say that their IPs probably are thinking more along the lines of "It's time to celebrate" or "I can't wait to feel that high again"—which suggest an interest in rewarding themselves through the positive sensations they associate with substance use. You should briefly inform the CSO that one of the first areas of focus will be relying on the CSO to help the IP find healthier ways to obtain some of these desired outcomes.

2. "What do you think he/she is usually *feeling* right before drinking/using?" This question about the IP's feelings follows naturally from the question about the IP's thoughts. As noted above, one can often surmise the underlying emotional state from the content of the thoughts. But in some cases the CSO has been unable to infer any of the IP's thoughts and, consequently, may have great difficulty imagining the associated emotions as well. In such situations you may want to focus the CSO on the IP's observable behavior, since conjecture about the associated feelings may then be easier. For instance, you might ask the client if her husband (the IP) ever clenches his fists or jaw prior to using. If so, one might wonder if anger were an internal emotional trigger for him. Or if the CSO reports that her husband appears fidgety and paces shortly before using, question whether these behaviors might be indicators of anxiety, anxiety that might also be contributing to the substance use. In either case, remind her that she knows her husband better than anyone else and that any information is helpful.

The dialogue between the CRAFT therapist and the CSO introduced earlier continues. The therapist has already heard an overview of the cocaine-using episode and so proceeds to fill in the gaps on the functional analysis chart, beginning with the triggers.

THERAPIST: OK, Natasha. Thanks for giving me that description of a typical episode. Now I'd like to ask you a few specific questions so that we can fill in some missing pieces. Here, I'm going to give you a copy of the CRAFT Functional Analysis of a Loved One's Using Behavior. I've already filled in parts of my copy, and I'll share that with you as we go along.

Note: The therapist hands the CSO a copy of the form (Figure 3.1). Alternatively, the therapist could outline the episode on a board. Figure 3.2, end of chapter, is a sample functional analysis completed for this CSO.

THERAPIST: Let's start with the triggers for Chris's cocaine use—the things that seem to lead up to it, or the things that always seem to be there each time he has a weekend episode. You can see that the first two columns of the form are divided into external and internal triggers. And notice that I've already filled in a number of the items, based on what you've just told me. For example, as far as external triggers, I know that Chris hangs out with the same bunch of people from the bar. And the episode we're focusing on now occurs on Friday nights. But I bet you can give me a few more details. Let's see . . . as far as *who* Chris uses with, who exactly are these folks from the bar? Are they also people he works with? What else can you tell me about them?

CSO: I know that he doesn't work with them. He's told me that he doesn't want people at work to know about his "private life," as he puts it. He says it's none of their business. So he always goes to a bar that's not near where he works. He's mentioned some of the people by name. Do you need to know that?

THERAPIST: Not necessarily, but we may as well add their names if you know them, because it will make it easier to talk about the episode.

CSO: Sure. They're all guys. There's Phil, Doc, and Steve. Those are the main ones he mentions. But I don't think Steve goes to Doc's every week. I heard Chris say something about Steve skipping out and going home more lately because they have new twins.

THERAPIST: I'm going to add that information here on the chart. So he uses with guys not associated with work: Phil, Doc, and Steve. Good. Now the second question asks *where* he typically uses. You said he meets up with the guys in a bar.

CSO: Yes, their favorite place is called Red's Filling Station ... or just Red's.

THERAPIST: I'm going to write that in, because that's where the episode starts, but do you know if that's where he actually uses the cocaine?

CSO: I know he doesn't do the coke there. He's told me that they go over to Doc's place. I know Doc is divorced and lives alone, so he can get away with it.

THERAPIST: I'm going to add that under question 2 then. Now for question 3: We already said this episode is for Friday nights. But getting back to one of our original issues, is it sounding like this will pretty much apply to Saturday nights too?

CSO: I don't think they start at Red's on Saturdays, but I know they end up at Doc's.

THERAPIST: Then let's keep Saturday a separate episode. I bet a lot of the same triggers and consequences will still apply, but since we're just trying our first functional analysis, it's better to keep it simple. Also, it sounds like there *are* some unique triggers for Friday night that occur early in the chain of events.

CSO: Yes, I guess so, if you count Red's.

Note: The therapist limits the functional analysis to Friday evening episodes because it has unique triggers, at least in terms of the setting for the drinking. Early triggers are critical to focus on, because it often is easier for a CSO to influence an IP's behavior if the CSO intervenes early in the chain of events that sets the stage for the substance use.

THERAPIST: Natasha, let's see if we can add anything about these triggers that's specific to Chris's decision to leave Red's and go to Doc's to use cocaine. Actually, we only really need more information about *when* he uses cocaine, because you already said that he drinks and uses with the same people, and that he leaves the bar and goes to Doc's. So that takes care of the *who* and *where* items. He starts drinking on Friday nights right after work. Do you know what time he typically leaves Red's to go to Doc's place?

CSO: It's pretty late; well, *I* think it's late. When he calls me to say he's OK, it's always from the bar. I can tell by the noise in the background. Like I said, this week it was around 11:00. I get the feeling he calls right before he's leaving. Sometimes I hear one of his friends telling him to hurry up so they can go.

THERAPIST: Good detective work! So he probably leaves for Doc's around 11 P.M. All right. But let me just ask you: Does Chris ever go to Red's *without* ending up at Doc's snorting coke afterward?

CSO: Sometimes, especially if it's in the middle of the week. And it's even with the same guys. As far as Fridays, I'd say he ends up at Doc's three or four times a month, mostly three.

THERAPIST: I wonder if his decision to go to Doc's and use cocaine is due to *how much* he's been drinking? Maybe he only ends up using cocaine when he's had a fair amount to drink.

CSO: Boy, I'm not sure. I know he's stayed out drinking past 11:00 P.M. at times, without using coke. I think it has more to do with knowing it's the weekend and he doesn't have to work the next day. He thinks he can "celebrate." Oh . . . but maybe he drinks more first as part of that celebration.

THERAPIST: Well, we can get back to that. Let's look at this from a slightly different angle. Do you know what's different about the one Friday night each month when Chris *doesn't* go to Doc's after being at Red's?

CSO: I think sometimes it's because he has a commitment early the next morning. But at other times, I don't have a clue what it's about.

THERAPIST: That's helpful though. OK, let's go ahead and look at the second column on the form, the one that asks for *internal* triggers. These might actually help us see what else is different about those times at Red's Filling Station when Chris decides to go to Doc's. Do you remember when we talked about internal triggers?

CSO: I don't remember exactly what they were. I think it had something to do with stuff going on inside him.

THERAPIST: That's right. Internal triggers are your husband's thoughts and feelings that seem to lead up to his cocaine use. And this is a good time to mention again that I understand you'll just be making an educated guess here; that you certainly wouldn't be expected to know your husband's thoughts and feelings for sure.

CSO: Hmmm. It will definitely have to be a guess, because I'm not even there. But like I said, he talks about celebrating. I don't know what he's celebrating exactly; the end of a stressful week, I guess. He *does* have a stressful job. He's a manager. And I'm scared to death that he's going to end up losing his job because of drugs. (*Starts to cry.*) He told me once that he worries about it, too.

THERAPIST: (*Waits a moment.*) I imagine that you have a lot of stress from worrying about him, whether it has to do with his job or something else. But, you know, it's actually a good sign if he's worried about his job too, because it shows that he has some sense of the seriousness of his drug habit, and that his job is important to him. This information will be useful to us later.

Note: The therapist is always watchful for signs of an IP's reinforcers, such as a job, since reinforcers are helpful to refer to later in treatment, when encouraging the IP to make some behavior changes.

THERAPIST: OK. We're focusing specifically on those triggers for Chris's cocaine use that are somewhat *different from* his drinking triggers, because apparently his drinking at Red's doesn't always lead to cocaine use. So, in other words, we don't only want to figure out the reasons he goes to drink after work. Now you just mentioned that Chris likes to "celebrate" the weekend. What do you think he's saying to himself about the upcoming weekend that might influence his decision to go to Doc's?

Note: Although the drinking episode certainly sets the stage for the cocaine use on Friday nights, drinking at this bar is not always an antecedent for snorting cocaine. Consequently, the therapist instead attempts to uncover specific triggers that influence the husband's decision to leave the bar and to go to his friend's house. The issue of the amount of alcohol the IP has had to drink on those different occasions will be revisited eventually, to determine whether it plays a role.

CSO: He's probably thinking, "I earned this celebration."

THERAPIST: Good. What else can you say about Chris's thoughts or feelings right as he's deciding to go to Doc's? I'm assuming that making the decision to go to Doc's is the same as deciding to use coke. Would that be a fair assumption? Does he ever go to Doc's, as far as you know, and *not* use coke?

CSO: I don't think so. He never seems to go there to just drink more or hang out. He wouldn't want to bother driving there and risk getting a DWI [drinking while intoxicated] if there wasn't a big payoff.

THERAPIST: So he worries about getting a DWI? That's useful to know, because maybe it will become important enough to him that he might even be willing to change his drinking behavior. It's similar to the job idea; maybe being able to hang on to his job will be the incentive for Chris to stop using coke.

Note: The therapist again labels and comments on something of value to the IP. It may be useful to consider this reinforcer later, when the CSO is discussing with the IP reasons for him to reduce his substance use. But, as stated previously, the therapist does not focus specifically on the negative consequences of alcohol (e.g., fear of a DWI), because alcohol is not the target substance at the moment, and it would only serve to complicate the picture unnecessarily. Of course, given that the IP appears to be drinking a considerable amount regularly, this behavior conceivably will become a target in the IP's own treatment. In terms of the relevant cocaine triggers, the therapist decides to focus on the point in the evening when Chris decides whether to go to Doc's, since this decision appears to be pivotal in relation to his use of cocaine.

THERAPIST: OK, since Chris's decision to go to Doc's is the same thing as Chris deciding to use coke, it's reasonable to focus on that decision point. What do you think . . . can you imagine what Chris might be thinking or feeling around 11:00 P.M. when he and his friends at the bar decide to go to Doc's?

CSO: That's a tough one. He's always telling me that he had no intention of ending up at Doc's.

THERAPIST: I imagine he's being honest when he tells you that. And yet, since it keeps happening, I bet we can find some common triggers for it that are quite separate from his intentions.

CSO: Let me see. I don't know if this is what you mean, but a couple of times he's called me to say he's on his way home, and I've heard one of his buddies . . . I think it was Phil . . . calling him a "wus," and yelling that *his* wife doesn't keep track of *him* like that.

THERAPIST: And how do you think Chris would feel if Phil said that to him?

CSO: I don't know. Maybe pressured. And embarrassed.

THERAPIST: Embarrassed?

CSO: Yes, embarrassed because he's married to someone who keeps close tabs on him. Embarrassed by me, I guess. (*Starts to cry again.*)

THERAPIST: Isn't it possible that he gets embarrassed when his friend picks on him, but that it doesn't necessarily mean he's embarrassed by you? In fact, a lot of people would interpret your behavior as a sign of caring. Didn't you say that Chris's other friend, Steve, doesn't go to Doc's sometimes because of new twins? I would imagine that Steve's wife had some role in that change. So maybe it's not a problem with you being unreasonable.

CSO: Yes, I guess you're right. Somehow I always end up feeling like I'm doing something wrong, though.

THERAPIST: I can see why you feel that way right now, but isn't there a part of you that knows you are doing your best to save your relationship; that you're "keeping tabs" on Chris out of love for him?

CSO: Yes. I just need to remind myself of that now and then.

Note: The therapist takes a moment away from the structured functional analysis to discuss the client's feelings and concerns. The therapist also makes a mental note of the fact that one of Chris's friends from the bar *does* go home to his family periodically without using cocaine first. Possibly part of the strategy developed with the CSO will be to suggest that she and Chris spend more time with Steve and his wife.

THERAPIST: Let's see, we were trying to come up with some thoughts and feelings that Chris might have when he's making the decision to go to Doc's instead of home. Based on what you've overheard Phil saying to him, ribbing him, you're guessing that Chris might feel embarrassed and pressured. That makes sense, because in order to save face he'd feel like he had to go with them. I'm putting these feelings on the list of triggers. What would you imagine are some of the thoughts he's having while he's feeling embarrassed and pressured?

CSO: He's probably wishing Phil would stop being so loud. I know that embarrasses him. Oh, but you asked about thoughts. Maybe he's thinking that the easiest way to shut Phil up is to agree to go to Doc's. I don't know. I'm just sort of making this up.

THERAPIST: You're making it up, but you're basing it on things you know about your husband and his friends. So it's an "educated" guess, which is all we really need. I'm going to add this thought about shutting Phil up to the chart. How about other thoughts or feelings he might be experiencing at the time? Picture Chris in that situation. He's been at the bar for almost 5 hours now. He's had a fair amount to drink. He knows he was supposed to be home hours ago, and he's just told you he's on his way. But his friends are pressuring him to go to Doc's, just like he does every week. He thinks about what's waiting for him at Doc's.

Note: The therapist introduces some brief imagery to assist the client in generating additional possible internal triggers for her husband.

CSO: I imagine he's talking himself into going with his friends. Like I said before, he likes to celebrate the weekend. And he likes getting high, so I'm sure it doesn't take much encouragement. I bet he's happy as he thinks about it. And he's probably happy to be part of that "special" invited group that goes to Doc's. I don't know. Maybe he's also telling himself that I'll be mad, but that I'll get over it, like I always do. And he's probably thinking that he'll make it up to me somehow. So although he's feeling guilty at first, I bet he's pleased with himself for coming up with good reasons to go. Oh, and I like what you said before about him "saving face" by going. That sounds like Chris.

THERAPIST: You're describing a small battle that goes on inside him, which is probably an accurate reflection of what he's thinking and feeling. So these internal triggers that point him in the direction of deciding to go to Doc's are rationalizations about how you'll get over it and how he'll make it up to you. Plus, since Chris can "save face" with his friends by giving in to them, it probably makes him feel more in control or more powerful by going with them. How about I add these to our list as well?

In identifying IPs' triggers for substance use, both the CSOs and the therapists usually learn a great deal *in addition to* the specific antecedents. For example, CSOs discover that they know a lot about the pattern of their IP's using behavior, and that it is more predictable than previously believed. Therapists commonly detect several of the IP's reinforcers in the course of the discussion, which later become useful when IP motivators for change are the focus of a session. Ideas for healthier social activities sometimes become evident as well, as when Natasha mentioned that one of Chris's friends did not always use cocaine. The case also illustrates that, at times, it becomes apparent to both the CSO and the therapist that one of the probable triggers for illicit drug use is heavy drinking. Although a reduction in drinking may be the healthiest action for the IP, *and* an act that is required in order to halt the cocaine use, this possible aspect has not been determined yet. The issue could be addressed by the IP's therapist once the husband has entered treatment.

OUTLINING THE DRINKING/USING BEHAVIOR

The next part of the CRAFT Functional Analysis of a Loved One's Drinking/Using Behavior entails gathering information about the substance abuse in terms of quantity and frequency. This information is collected for two reasons: first, so that the CSO can clearly see the direct connection between the triggers and the substance use, and second, so that changes in the amount of abused substances can be tracked over time. Frequently the client is unaware of the actual quantity of alcohol or illicit drugs used, particularly if the CSO is not physically with the IP at those times. Nevertheless, an attempt should be made to obtain an estimate of the use, so that the CSO will have at least some point of comparison for determining whether the use seems to be increasing or decreasing.

The dialogue between the therapist and Natasha continues. As noted, in this fairly common scenario, illicit drug use often follows a period of drinking. The therapist will inquire about both types of substance use, in part because the best place for the CSO to intervene is not yet known. Also, since drinking at the bar is one of the main triggers for the cocaine use and consequently a possible point of intervention, it would be useful to know precisely how much alcohol is being consumed so that the IP's state of mind at a critical decision point for him can be considered. The alcohol-related responses will be placed in brackets, since alcohol is not the target substance.

THERAPIST: Let's move on to a description of the substance-abusing behavior itself, which is in the third column here. We should look at your husband's cocaine use first, since that's the main drug we're focusing on. But I also think you should try to estimate the amount he drinks, since we may eventually decide to take a closer look at that. A lot of people only use some type of illegal drug after they've had a lot to drink. If that seems to be the case with Chris, we may end up trying to get him to cut back on the drinking—or down the road, his own therapist might. Does that make sense?

CSO: I'm not sure *what* makes sense about his drug use anymore. But like I said, he does seem to only use coke after he's been drinking.

THERAPIST: Fair enough. Back to Friday nights at Red's. As you can see, the third column asks how much a person uses. I've already filled in some of it. As far as the cocaine goes, you said that this week he went to Doc's house around 11:00, and then got home around 2:00. Is that a pretty typical Friday night? Oh, and does it take very long to drive to Doc's? We'll need to subtract that out if it's substantial.

CSO: It takes him around 15 minutes to get there. And I'd say that's a pretty typical amount of time for him, give or take an hour.

THERAPIST: Once we subtract a total of 30 minutes travel time, it would make it 2½ hours of cocaine use. Now that doesn't mean he's actually snorting coke the whole time, just that he's in the setting where he uses for that long. So that's item 3. Can you guess how much coke he uses?

CSO: I really don't have any idea.

THERAPIST: Don't worry about it. Most people don't know. Now I'm going to ask these same questions for his drinking. But I'm putting the responses in brackets, since it's not the main substance of interest for us. OK. I've already filled in item 3, because you said he drank at the bar from a little after 6:00 until 11:00 usually. Oh . . . unless he continues to drink at Doc's?

CSO: I don't think so. Not much, anyway.

THERAPIST: I'll keep it at 5 hours then. What does he usually drink at Red's? And how much?

CSO: I know he usually starts off with a shot of something: tequila or whiskey. And then he drinks beer the rest of the night. But I guess sometimes he has another shot or two, if it's a special occasion. He says he likes to stay with beer so that he doesn't have trouble driving home. But if you ask me, I think he could get picked up for the amount of beer he drinks.

THERAPIST: Can you guess how many beers he has during those 5 hours?

CSO: Hmmmm. I don't know. Maybe a little more than one an hour. When I've seen him drinking, I've noticed that he starts out fast but then slows down some. And he always drinks a bunch of soda, too, when he's out.

THERAPIST: So your estimate of a little more than one an hour is probably right. That would make it about six or seven beers, total. I'm assuming that we're talking about either bottles or the standard draft size. They're not the big 16-ounce ones, are they?

CSO: No, he likes bottled beer in the regular-size bottles.

THERAPIST: And I'll list the one shot of tequila or whiskey, since that's normal for him. OK. So what do you think as you look at the amount he drinks most Friday nights?

CSO: It seems like an awful lot. Don't you think so?

THERAPIST: It *is* worth looking at more. But in some ways it's a good sign, because it suggests that he makes the decision to use cocaine when his judgment is impaired. One option would be to work on influencing him to drink less, so he'll be less likely to make the decision to go to Doc's.

In the course of collecting basic information about quantity and frequency of substance use, remember that it is not critical to know exactly how much an IP is using. An estimate of the degree of use is sufficient in terms of tracking changes over time or in response to different procedures attempted. It is more important for the client to see the strong connection between the triggers and the problem behavior. Also note that a variety of other issues get raised or clarified when simple quantity/frequency data are being obtained. In the current scenario it became apparent that although the CSO was interested in focusing on her husband's cocaine use, the husband was also drinking a fairly large amount of alcohol. The therapist used the opportunity to conduct a reality check of the CSO's view of her husband's drinking. Importantly, not only did the therapist respond in a nonjudgmental manner when asked her opinion of the IP's drinking, but she also framed it as a positive sign regarding the circumstances under which the IP makes the decision to use cocaine.

IDENTIFYING THE SHORT-TERM POSITIVE CONSEQUENCES EXPERIENCED BY THE IP WHEN ABUSING SUBSTANCES

Although therapists sometimes feel uncomfortable raising the issue of positive consequences associated with substance use, you should assume that IPs experience (and are aware that they experience) at least some immediate rewards for abusing substances or they would cease to engage in that behavior. For instance, the IP might turn to drugs as an escape from everyday hassles, as a self-confidence booster when socializing, as a way to dull emotional pain, or to be accepted by friends. It is necessary to discuss the topic openly with the CSO, because the details contain crucial information about the factors that are maintaining the substance-using behavior. Eventually the IP will be taught healthier ways to obtain some of the rewards, so that drugs and alcohol are not the only choices. In the meantime, with your guidance, the CSO might be able to influence the IP to select one of these healthier options. As outlined in Chapter 6, you would also train the client to reinforce the IP whenever he or she chooses a positive alternative over substance use.

The dialogue between the CSO and her therapist continues. They are now focusing on the fourth column of the CRAFT functional analysis chart. Notice that since cocaine is the target substance, the therapist spends time discussing the positive consequences of drinking only if it seems helpful in sorting out the IP's cocaine-related reinforcers. More details related to the rewards associated with drinking can easily be added later, if necessary.

THERAPIST: When I first explained the general purpose of doing a functional analysis of Chris's using behavior, I mentioned that part of it involves looking at what he would consider the benefits of his cocaine use; *you* know . . . the "rewards" he gets out of it. Does it seem odd to think of his substance use as having "rewards"?

CSO: Well, I'm sure it feels that way to him.

THERAPIST: Good. I'm glad you can see it that way. Some wives have trouble making that connection. But you've got it; it's how *he* views it, not how you do.

Note: The therapist checks with the client on this issue, because oftentimes CSOs have difficulty seeing beyond their *own* view of the consequences of the substance use; namely, negative ones. Had Natasha responded in such a manner, the therapist could proceed instead to the negative consequences of the use, so that the CSO would be assured that these were not being ignored; the positive consequences could be covered last.

THERAPIST: Again, I've already filled in the answers to some of these questions based on the overview you gave me up front. I'm going to concentrate only on the cocaine use, since that's the drug we're targeting. But I may try to contrast the positive consequences of the cocaine use with the positive ones for alcohol at one point, simply so we can see what the cocaine offers Chris above and beyond what the alcohol provides. Let's go ahead and run down each of these questions. Just do the best you can. Item 1 asks, "What do you think Chris likes about using coke with his buddies?"

CSO: I think it's just more of the same thing he gets out of drinking with them; he likes hanging out with them—which is why I can't figure out why he can't just leave it at the drinking. Why does he have to make it worse?

THERAPIST: That's part of what we're trying to sort out here. To help answer that question, it would be great if we could figure out what he gets out of the cocaine use that he doesn't already get from drinking. Any ideas?

CSO: Hmmm. He really seems to like these guys; maybe it's because they're so different from his other friends . . . like from work. He says they're kinda "crazy." Oh . . . but I guess that still doesn't explain why he can't just drink with them.

THERAPIST: Maybe it does, though. If these guys routinely go to Doc's every Friday, maybe Chris thinks he needs to go with them in order to feel like he's one of them? You said before that they pressure him to go when he announces that he's going home. So if he gives in and goes with them, the "reward" he gets is feeling like he belongs. Actually, part of this is really the answer to item 5, which asks about pleasurable feelings. I'll go ahead and jot it down there.

Note: It is common and natural to move back and forth within a column while gathering specific information. This fluidity is another way to guard against allowing the procedure to become too mechanical.

CSO: If we're talking about pleasurable feelings, you'd better add that he likes the feeling of getting high. He's told me that a million times.

THERAPIST: Good. How about item 2 now: What does Chris like about using *at Doc's,* specifically?

CSO: I think he feels safe there. Nobody's going to find them. And as he's told me, nobody's there to bother him.

THERAPIST: Good. And 3: What is it about using cocaine on Friday nights that he likes? We've sort of addressed this question already.

CSO: Yes, like I said before, he likes to "celebrate" the weekend, and the coke routine makes Friday night extra special. I think he feels cheated if he misses out. I remember one Friday recently when he skipped Doc's because he had some early morning appointment. He moped around the entire next morning. He even called Phil to see what he'd missed! Can you imagine? It's not like he doesn't know what goes on there week after week!

THERAPIST: True, but it supports our hunch that he gets something extra out of going to Doc's, even though he's already spent *hours* with the same guys in the bar.

CSO: I don't know. Maybe it makes him feel special, like the guys really like him. He's told me more than once that not everybody gets invited to Doc's. I guess I was supposed to be impressed by that. And like I said, these friends are very different from his work friends. I get the feeling that they remind Chris of the kids he used to hang around with in high school. He used to get into quite a bit of trouble with them, but he always refers to those times as the "good old days."

THERAPIST: That's interesting. So somehow this particular scenario might be bringing back fond memories of the fun he used to have with his friends in high school. I'll put that under Item 1 as well.

CSO: Yes. I could ask him, to be sure.

THERAPIST: That's not a bad idea, but let's wait on it for now. A minute ago you said that Chris recently left the bar one Friday night without going to Doc's. So occasionally he *is* able to come home instead.

Note: The therapist first cautions the wife to proceed slowly while they are still gathering information. Posing questions to the husband about his cocaine use should be rehearsed in advance during a session, once specific communication skills have been taught. The therapist next highlights the fact that the IP apparently *has* been successful in the recent past at choosing to avoid using cocaine. The therapist will refer back to this point in future sessions, when the discussion about influencing the IP's behavior is introduced, since the factors that allowed him to make a healthier decision may need to be called upon again.

THERAPIST: Natasha, it's almost like Chris lives a separate life on the side, like when he was a teenager getting into trouble and enjoying himself. What do you think?

CSO: I think he should grow up! And why wouldn't he get enough of that from drinking all night in a bar? That's closer to what he used to do as a teenager.

THERAPIST: Good question. Well, the cocaine use is illegal, so that makes it more "dangerous." Maybe that's part of the thrill that he connects with high school. And like you said, he feels special because he gets invited to join the group that goes to Doc's. Lots of people are in the bar each Friday, but only a few go to snort coke together.

CSO: So how's he going to feel "special" without doing that?

THERAPIST: Another good question. Our job is to come up with some ideas about that. For example, maybe Chris could spend more social time with the one friend from the bar who doesn't always go and use coke—Steve. But we're getting ahead of ourselves. That all comes later. Don't worry about it for now.

Note: Although the client is asking a reasonable question, the therapist decides to address it only briefly, and then to finish gathering functional analysis data. Generating healthier ways for the IP to access the short-term positive consequences associated with substance use is an entire procedure of its own.

THERAPIST: We addressed most of the questions about short-term positive consequences of Chris's cocaine use, with the exception of some of the thoughts he might be having while he's doing it. Think about the positive feelings you've identified, because they'll give you ideas about his thoughts. Can you come up with some?

CSO: He's probably thinking about how much fun he's having. I wonder if he's feeling guilty, though.

THERAPIST: Let's save the guilt for now. We only want to consider *positive* experiences at this point.

CSO: Oh, that's right—positive thoughts. (*Pauses.*) I bet he's thinking about how great it is to be part of the group. Do you know what I mean?

THERAPIST: I do. And I bet you're right on target. Great job. Now let's go back and see if anything else comes to mind, as you contrast his reaction to cocaine with his reaction to alcohol.

CSO: Everything is pretty much the same, except he probably doesn't feel quite as special while they're all at the bar still. And it probably isn't quite as exciting to him. Oh, I've heard him say that he's not stressed out when he's high.

THERAPIST: Good. So the cocaine also offers him the additional benefits of feeling special with these friends, feeling excitement, and not being stressed. I don't have these last two things in column 4 yet.

Determining *why* an IP abuses substances is not an endpoint in itself. Once you recognize the reinforcing value of the substance for a particular IP, the foundation is in place for helping the CSO consider alternative, healthier ways for the IP to achieve similar results. This latter exercise frequently occurs in the next session. But just as was the case with the other segments of the functional analysis already completed, the *primary* purpose of this series of questions is not their *only* purpose, as other therapeutic opportunities often arise. For example, in the current scenario the therapist reinforced Natasha for her insight and comments, which in turn strengthened the therapeutic relationship and encouraged Natasha to speak up again. The therapist also pointed out that the IP had, on at least one recent occasion, been successful at making the decision not to use cocaine, even though he had been drinking at the time. This piece of information offers hope to Natasha that Chris could make such a decision again *and* gives the therapist ideas regarding ways to influence the IP's using behavior.

IDENTIFYING THE LONG-TERM NEGATIVE CONSEQUENCES OF SUBSTANCE USE EXPERIENCED BY THE IP

In the final segment of the CRAFT functional analysis of a problem behavior, the CSO outlines the various long-term negative consequences of the substance use experienced by the IP. The consequences are labeled *long-term* to contrast them with the positive rewards experienced directly from the substance use that tend to be immediate and relatively brief in duration. The major purpose of this task is to determine which of the IP's *reinforcers* (e.g., his job, marriage) have been adversely affected as a result of the substance use. If the reinforcer involves the CSO, conceivably the damage could be repaired eventually, as part of a contingency set up by the CSO in exchange for clean and sober IP behavior. Certainly repair will not be possible to arrange for every lost reinforcer. Some of the negative consequences, such as compromised health, are the result of chronic and heavy use, and are not affected by the CSO's best negotiations with the IP. Still, they may be important to keep in mind as long-term reinforcers, which the IP and CSO can work toward achieving together. A second function of formally outlining the negative consequences of the IP's use is to allow the CSO the opportunity to react emotionally to the unpleasant substance-related circumstances with which she or he is so familiar. Many clients have already expressed their distraught feelings about their IP's use by this point in the session, but for those who have not, this portion of the exercise encourages such an expression.

In describing this final column of the functional analysis, you should mention that the client might recognize certain negative consequences of the IP's use that the IP does not seem to be aware of, or admit. As far as this exercise, it is perfectly acceptable to include these CSO-identified consequences, since the information may prove to be helpful later, when the CSO approaches the IP with specific reasons to alter the using behavior. But given that it is also useful to know with which of the negative consequences the IP would agree, you should decide upon some way to mark them, such as with an asterisk. In most cases, it is easier for the CSO to negotiate a behavior change when the IP agrees that something of value has been lost or is threatened due to the substance abuse.

The final portion of the dialogue between Natasha and her therapist follows. The therapist has already made a few notations in the fifth column, based on information that was mentioned in the course of doing the first four columns. She begins by explaining the notion of negative consequences and using these examples.

THERAPIST: How are you holding up, Natasha? We're almost done with this exercise.

CSO: I'm fine. The more we work on stuff, the closer I feel like we're getting to being able to do something about Chris's problem.

THERAPIST: That's a good attitude. OK. We're going to finish up this functional analysis by listing the negative things that have happened to Chris as a result of his cocaine use. We'll only contrast these consequences with the negative consequences of drinking if it helps clarify issues. Now these negative things can either be things that only *you* recognize, or ones that Chris would agree with too. I'll give you some ideas by going down a couple of categories, but first I want to show you that I've already written in a few items here, based on comments you made before. As far as his cocaine use, I've listed under the "job" category that he's afraid that people at work will find out about his private life, and that he might lose his job. Right? I think you said Chris made a point of not "celebrating" with people that he worked with, for that very reason.

CSO: Yes, that's right. But he can't be *that* worried or he'd stop.

THERAPIST: Maybe so. A lot of times it takes more than just "worry" for people to change their behavior, though. Now since Chris has actually made this remark about his job, we can assume that he agrees with this particular negative consequence. So I'll put a star next to it. I would guess that you'd say there are negative consequences of his use in the interpersonal area, so why don't we do that one next. *Are* there interpersonal problems that result from his cocaine use?

CSO: Well, *I* sure think there are. Actually, he'd say there were too, but maybe for different reasons.

THERAPIST: Go ahead and tell me what *you* think are the negative interpersonal consequences first then. And again, let's try to focus on just the cocaine, if possible.

Note: The therapist encourages the CSO to think of negative consequences of her husband's cocaine use regardless of whether he would agree. His opinion can be identified later.

CSO: His cocaine use has really strained our relationship. It seems like I'm always worrying about him getting caught or hurt. I start to get nervous as I think about the weekend coming up. And it doesn't help that he's so moody. I think he feels sick or hungover or something. So that puts a strain on things between us, too.

THERAPIST: That makes perfect sense. Let me add that to the chart under "Interpersonal." Is there some part of this that Chris would agree with, or were you thinking he'd describe the consequences differently?

CSO: He'd probably agree that I'm more nervous and worried since he's started using coke. But he'd just say that it was *my* problem.

THERAPIST: But even though he says it's your problem, would he agree that his use and your worrying about it have put a strain on your relationship?

CSO: I'm not sure. I know he wouldn't admit that his mood on the weekends has hurt anything.

THERAPIST: Maybe not. And yet you mentioned before that you were able to get him to start calling when he was out late. I would guess that your relationship means a lot to him, and that he accepts some of the responsibility for the strain, or he wouldn't have agreed and followed through. What was that about?

Note: The therapist again takes the opportunity to identify one of the IP's reinforcers: the marital relationship.

CSO: I said that I couldn't take it much more; that I was going to start "disappearing" on Friday nights too, if I didn't at least hear from him. But I'm sure he thinks the problem has been solved now that he calls me at 11:00. I'm still not happy, though.

THERAPIST: Well we can add that you're still unhappy with him for staying out so late and using. That's an interpersonal problem, whether or not he agrees with it. But from what you're describing, I'd say that he knows he's at least contributed to the strain on your marriage by his use.

CSO: You may be right. Go ahead and star it.

THERAPIST: Let's look at some of these other categories. Has Chris experienced any physical problems from using cocaine? You mentioned him being sick on Saturdays?

CSO: But I don't know how much of his sick behavior the next day is from the drinking and how much is from the coke.

THERAPIST: One way to figure it out is to picture what he's like the day after he's just been drinking, and compare that to a day after he's been both drinking and snorting. This gives you an idea of what the additional effects of the cocaine are. Or we can base our conclusion on what we know, in general, about the effects of cocaine. I'd guess that the day after using coke, he'd be feeling the opposite of how coke makes him feel: physically tired, and maybe his appetite would be bigger than usual. Any nausea and headaches would probably be from alcohol. When you said Chris acted sick the next day, what symptoms were you referring to?

CSO: Well, he definitely seems tired, even though he sleeps in. Sometimes he seems hungrier than usual, unless he's feeling nauseous from the drinking. And he acts irritable if he thinks he can get away with it.

THERAPIST: Irritable. Let's put that down in the next category, under emotional consequences. You did mention him being moody before. And while I'm thinking about it: Would Chris agree that coke makes him feel tired, hungry, and irritable the next day?

CSO: Tired and hungry, yes. Irritable, no.

THERAPIST: Then I'll just star the first two. Can you think of any other emotional consequences of his cocaine use?

CSO: *I* have a lot of emotional consequences from his use! Does that count? (*Laughs sadly.*)

THERAPIST: Your feelings definitely "count," which is why you're here. But I think I'd like to keep *your* emotional consequences under the interpersonal category, since they certainly would affect your relationship with Chris. Natasha, before we do any more of this exercise, how about we take a few minutes to talk about your feelings?

Note: The therapist acknowledges that the CSO's feelings are important and then offers her the opportunity to express them.

CSO: If it's OK with you, I don't really feel like getting into that right now. It wears me out. Let's just go on to the next category.

THERAPIST: Fair enough. This isn't a one-time offer anyway. (*Smiles.*) So, are there any emotional consequences that possibly are not an immediate effect of the cocaine wearing off, but ones that may have appeared over time? Is he different emotionally than he used to be before he started using?

CSO: He seems to get down on himself more. He doesn't directly tie it to the coke, but I've noticed that he criticizes himself in other areas, like, for not being able to get stuff done. And when he's not irritable, he seems more down. Maybe he's depressed. I'm not sure.

THERAPIST: I'll add that he gets down on himself for his inability to follow through with his plans, and that he seems down. How about legal problems? Has anything negative in the legal arena happened as a result of his cocaine use?

CSO: Not yet, but he worries about it. He's afraid that he'll get caught and end up in jail. And that's part of why he's worried about losing his job.

THERAPIST: I'll put his fear down then. We've already covered the job category. How about financial consequences from his use?

CSO: Well, I'm sure there are, but he hides it from me. When I ask about it, he always says he doesn't pay much for the coke because his friends give him a good deal. Still, I can't help but think of all the other things we could be doing with that money.

THERAPIST: I'll add it, then. We don't need to know the amount. The final category is a general one, "Other." It's a place to put any other negative consequence of Chris's cocaine use that doesn't fit in the above categories. What do you think?

CSO: You may think this is weird, but I heard on the news last week that cocaine might harm a man's sperm. We were planning on having children someday, and now I'm worried that maybe we won't be able to because of his stupid habit. (*Cries briefly.*) Of course, I wouldn't go ahead and try to get pregnant with things going the way they are.

THERAPIST: You have a valid concern, but hopefully one that won't end up being an issue in the long run. I'll add it to the column of negative consequences. And would Chris agree that any of these last few consequences are the result of his use?

CSO: Not really. Well, he looked worried when I told him the sperm story, so maybe that one.

Listing the negative consequences of an IP's use is an exercise that elicits a wide range of emotions. On the one hand, CSOs welcome the opportunity to tell someone all of the upsetting and painful things that have happened to themselves and their families as a result of the substance abuse. But at the same time, developing a comprehensive list of the negative consequences and seeing them in black and white can be a difficult experience for clients. So it is very important, after the final column has been generated, to take time with the CSOs to determine how they are handling the exercise. The summary step of the CRAFT functional analysis exercise is helpful in this regard, because it offers direction and hope for change.

SUMMARY OF THE FUNCTIONAL ANALYSIS: CONNECTING THE DOTS

Upon completion of the functional analysis you should quiz the CSO. The emergent picture should demonstrate the CSO's solid understanding of the context that frames the IP's substance-abusing behavior for at least the one episode under discussion. Praise the CSO for her or his hard work, and then offer a few illustrations of how this information will be utilized to guide the formulation of the intervention with the CSO. This interchange reinforces the notion that the functional analysis was *not* simply an empty exercise, but one that supplied important details about the problem behavior that will shape the entire intervention process. In addition, check in to see how the CSO is handling the discussion, in general. Natasha's therapist conducts the summary in the dialogue below.

THERAPIST: Let's step back a minute now and see if we can make some sense of all this information. Triggers first. So, Natasha, if I were to ask you now what kinds of things seem to lead up to Chris's cocaine use on Friday nights, what would you say?

CSO: I'd say, hanging out with three particular friends and drinking at a bar—drinking a lot—and then deciding, with his buddies' help, to continue the celebration at Doc's.

THERAPIST: Good. And what did we figure out was different about these guys that plays a part in Chris deciding to use with them?

CSO: That they are *not* coworkers of his, so he doesn't have to worry about people from work, including his boss, finding out about his drug habit.

THERAPIST: Exactly. And since some of these external triggers will apply to Saturday night episodes as well, we'll talk later about how we might use some of this same information in planning a strategy for Saturdays, too. Now, what about some of the things going on inside Chris at the time he makes the decision to use? Feel free to look at the chart, if you need to. Remember, we said that making the decision to go to Doc's was really the same thing as Chris deciding to use cocaine.

CSO: Right. At the time he's deciding about Doc's, he's probably feeling happy as he thinks about getting his "hard-earned celebration," and how he's part of a special group of guys. Oh . . . and here it also says that he's thinking he can "save face" by going, and that he figures he can make it up to me anyway. Hmmmm. That's interesting. It hadn't really registered that he might actually be saying that to himself at the time he makes the decision to go. Makes me wonder if I'm doing the right thing by pretty much letting him get away with it the next day.

THERAPIST: One of the reasons why we do a functional analysis is so that we can take a look at the way you *are* currently handling some of your inter-actions with your husband to see if maybe we can come up with some-thing more effective. And, remember, the main reason why we are looking at possibly changing *your* behavior is because it's the best way we have right now to influence *his* behavior. It would be a different story if *Chris* was the person sitting in front of me now, instead of you.

Note: The therapist uses this opportunity to gently agree that perhaps the CSO's behavior toward the IP after he has used might be worth examin-ing. The fact that the CSO came to this realization in the course of doing the functional analysis is an added benefit of the procedure. Note that the therapist is careful about not blaming the client for her typical pattern of responding.

THERAPIST: Natasha, I can see that you're going to do a great job in the CRAFT program. You already have identified one behavior of yours that maybe we should consider working on a bit. But don't do any-thing new yet! As I've said before, we need to carefully consider potentially problematic reactions of your husband first. I know we haven't talked much about actual interventions, but just in looking at these triggers, can you see any other possible place to influence Chris's decision to use coke?

CSO: That's a tough one, because I'm not even there when he makes the decision. Once he's had a lot to drink, it's really hard to do much of anything.

THERAPIST: That's definitely the case if we're thinking about changing your behavior on Friday nights. But another option is to let him know your plan ahead of time. For instance, on a Thursday night you might say that you're not going to go to a movie with him on Saturday if he's been out using on Friday night. Or you could take the preferred positive approach and tell him what you *will* do with him if he doesn't use coke. You mentioned that he sometimes comes home on Friday nights without going to Red's because he has an early Saturday morning commitment. Maybe we'll have you plan an enjoyable early Saturday morning activity with him. If you tell him about it in advance, he might just come home straight from Red's so that he can get up for the activity the next day.

CSO: You know, we both used to love going to the flea market the first thing Saturday morning. We haven't done that in ages.

THERAPIST: We'll figure out the best way to change your behavior in order to get fun, healthy activities, like flea markets, back into your lives again. OK. Let's go ahead and review the consequences of his use; first the positive ones. We already did that, to some extent, when we imagined his thoughts in anticipation of using. So how would you fill in the blank, "Chris keeps using cocaine because . . . "? Look at the chart, if you'd like.

CSO: He uses coke because it reminds him of those "dangerous" high school days. He likes hanging out with these "wild" guys and doing crazy things. It makes him feel special.

THERAPIST: Good. And you asked before if there were some way he could feel special without using cocaine. That's part of what we'll be trying to come up with . . . some ideas for him, and some incentives for him to try those ideas instead of using. But it would really help if we could also come up with ideas of ways he could let loose and hang out with "wild" guys without engaging in such risky behavior. As I said before, based on what you told me about Steve choosing to go home instead of going to Doc's occasionally, I'm thinking that Steve might be the best option for an alternative activity, especially if his wife is involved, too. Finally, how about the negatives—the good things he's lost or the damage that has been caused by his use? Just give me a few.

CSO: That's easy. Our relationship is strained, and we both worry a lot, especially about him getting caught and losing his job. And he's irritable.

THERAPIST: Some of these things would change naturally if he stopped using, but in the meantime, we'll start by focusing on ways to take some of these negatives away at those times that he's *not* using. We have the most control over your relationship—at least, your part in it— so we'll probably start there by having you do things to enhance the relationship for both of you, but *only* when he's not drunk, high, or hungover. This is where an activity like the flea market might fit in. We'll talk a lot more about this later.

As noted, the purpose of the functional analysis summary is to present a framework for a common episode, and to suggest a few directions in which the therapy will be moving so that the CSO has a clearer picture of what the CRAFT program will entail. Furthermore, by having the client respond to questions about triggers and consequences, instead of you simply reviewing all the information, you can determine whether the CSO fully understands the purpose of the exercise. It is not necessary to cover each point raised in the interview, however. Finally, it is not uncommon for CSOs to have insight into their own role in maintaining the problem behavior in the course of doing the functional analysis—which, in turn, makes that particular point of intervention easy to describe and implement later. Nevertheless, if the topic of her or his role in maintaining the alcohol or drug use did not get raised by the CSO during the functional analysis, you should inquire about it.

CSOs commonly report at their next session that in thinking about the functional analysis exercise during the week, they remembered new information (e.g., triggers, positive consequences) that could be useful. Add these details to their chart, discuss their implications, and compliment the CSOs for continuing their therapeutic work at home.

COMMON ISSUES ENCOUNTERED IN CONDUCTING THE CRAFT FUNCTIONAL ANALYSIS

In the dialogue presented throughout this chapter, various fairly common issues were raised in the course of describing and conducting the sample functional analysis exercise. These and other relevant issues are reviewed briefly below.

1. Therapists conducting functional analyses for the first time run the risk of moving through the exercise in too mechanical a style. It is important to gather details, but not in a manner that sacrifices empathy and support. You can guard against this error by (a) first asking the CSOs for an overview in their own words and filling in the appropriate sections on the chart as they are talking; (b) using open-ended questions whenever possible; (c) not being overly compulsive about filling in every blank if the process becomes too time consuming; and (d) not necessarily conducting the interview in the outlined order if the conversation flows more naturally another way. Experienced CRAFT therapists can conduct entire functional analyses comfortably without referring to the form at all.

2. You will need to make decisions about whether the "common episode" of use selected by the CSO is suitable. Ideally, this regularly occur-

ring episode should contain elements (e.g., triggers, consequences) that generalize to other episodes, so that multiple functional analyses are not required. If an appropriate common episode is still limited in its generalizability, you may decide to give a homework assignment of filling out a functional analysis form for another type of episode.

3. At times polysubstance abuse is apparent, and you must determine whether to conduct separate functional analyses for the different drugs, or whether to outline unique triggers and/or consequences within the same exercise. The basic rule is to minimize the number of functional analyses, while, at the same time, being careful not to allow any one functional analysis to become too complicated. If the drugs are used as part of the same episode but with one serving as the trigger for the other (as was the case for Chris, for whom alcohol was one of the main triggers for cocaine use), then you would simply treat the "triggering" drug as an antecedent to the second drug. In other words, refer briefly to the triggering drug in columns 1 and 3 (i.e., external triggers and the using behavior). Sometimes it is useful to try to distinguish between the positive consequences offered by the two drugs, so that the reinforcement value of the target drug is evident. If the drugs are used in separate episodes, check briefly to see if any of the triggers or consequences are the same for both. With sufficient overlap, it may be possible to generalize and work from the one formal functional analysis. On average, one or two functional analyses for the IP's substance-abusing behavior are conducted initially for each CSO.

4. Many therapeutic opportunities present themselves in the course of the functional analysis exercise, for which you should be prepared to respond. For example, there are often opportunities (a) to encourage the CSO to express her or his feelings about the IP's problem and to respond in a supportive manner; (b) to verbally reinforce the CSO for helpful comments or simply for participating fully in the process; (c) to point out to the CSO that she or he is *not* responsible for the IP's problem behavior; (d) to note certain behaviors of the CSO that might be suitable candidates for modifying in an effort to positively influence the IP's behavior; (e) to identify IP reinforcers for future reference; and (f) to point out the past success of the IP in occasionally avoiding substance use, or the CSO in obtaining requests from the IP, thereby instilling optimism and confidence.

SUMMARY

This chapter presents a CRAFT functional analysis of an IP's substance-abusing behavior. It will become apparent, however, that this basic format can be used to outline the context of other problem behaviors, such as domestic violence episodes (Chapter 4), as well as healthy behaviors (Chapter 6). Once the rationale for the functional analysis is fully understood and the exercise has been conducted comprehensively at least once, many clients are able to identify and refer to triggers and consequences appropriately without having to rely on filling out more charts. Typically, IPs who enter behavioral treatment programs complete their own functional analyses.

FIGURE 3.1.   CRAFT FUNCTIONAL ANALYSIS OF A LOVED ONE'S DRINKING/USING BEHAVIOR

External Triggers	Internal Triggers	Drinking/Using Behavior	Short-Term Positive Consequences	Long-Term Negative Consequences
1. *Who* is your loved one usually with when drinking/using?	1. What do you think your loved one is *thinking* about right before drinking/using?	1. *What* does your loved one usually drink/use?	1. What do you think your loved one likes about drinking/using [*with whom*]?	1. What do you think are the negative results of your loved one's drinking/using in each of these areas (* the ones he/she would agree with): a. Interpersonal: b. Physical:
2. *Where* does he/she usually drink/use?	2. What do you think he/she is usually *feeling* right before drinking/using?	2. *How much* does he/she usually drink/use?	2. What do you think he/she likes about drinking/using [*where*]? 3. What do you think he/she likes about drinking/using [*when*]?	c. Emotional:

3. *When* does he/she usually drink/use?

3. Over *how long* a period of time does he/she usually drink/use?

4. What pleasant *thoughts* do you think he/she has while drinking/using?

5. What pleasant *feelings* do you think he/she has while drinking/using?

d. Legal:

e. Job:

f. Financial:

g. Other:

FIGURE 3.2. CRAFT FUNCTIONAL ANALYSIS OF A LOVED ONE'S DRINKING/USING BEHAVIOR: COMPLETED

External Triggers	Internal Triggers	Drinking/Using Behavior	Short-Term Positive Consequences	Long-Term Negative Consequences
1. *Who* is your loved one usually with when drinking/using? Friends (not coworkers) Phil, Doc, Steve	1. What do you think your loved one is *thinking* about right before drinking/using? I earned this celebration. If I go it will shut Phil up. Natasha will be mad, but I'll make it up to her tomorrow. I'll save face if I go.	1. *What* does your loved one usually drink/use? [Tequila/whiskey] [Beer] Cocaine	1. What do you think your loved one likes about drinking/using [*with whom*]? They're "crazy"; different from coworkers. Fond memories of "good old" high school days. 2. What do you think he/she likes about drinking/using [*where*]? Feels safe there. Nobody will bother them.	1. What do you think are the negative results of your loved one's drinking/using in each of these areas (* the ones he/she would agree with): a. Interpersonal: *Strained marriage** (from me worrying* and his moods). I'm unhappy. b. Physical:
2. *Where* does he/she usually drink/use? Doc's place [starts drinking at Red's Filling Station, though]	2. What do you think he/she is usually *feeling* right before drinking/using? Pressured, embarrassed Happy in anticipation of using Happy that he's part of that special group In control, powerful	2. *How much* does he/she usually drink/use? [t/w: a shot] [Beer: 6–7 12-oz bottles] Cocaine: ?	3. What do you think he/she likes about drinking/using [*when*]? Likes to celebrate the weekend. Pleasant routine (feels cheated if he doesn't go). Makes him feel special.	He's tired,* hungry* c. Emotional: He's irritable. Criticizes himself for not getting stuff done. He's down (depressed?)

3. *When* does he/she usually drink/use?

After 11:00 on Friday nights [after drinking since 6:00]; 3–4 x/mo.

3. Over *how long* a period of time does he/she usually drink/use?

[Alcohol: 5 hrs.]
Cocaine: 2½ hrs.

4. What pleasant *thoughts* do you think he/she has while drinking/using?

This is fun.

It's great to be part of this group.

5. What pleasant *feelings* do you think he/she has while drinking/using?

Feeling like he "belongs"

Getting high

Feels special; the guys really like him.

Excitement

Not stressed

d. Legal:

He's afraid he'll get caught and end up in jail.*

e. Job:

He's afraid people will find out and he'll lose his job.*

f. Financial:

Money spent on coke.

g. Other:

*Sperm damaged?**

CHAPTER 4

DOMESTIC VIOLENCE
PRECAUTIONS

We have included a chapter on domestic violence because it often co-occurs with drinking or drug use (Greenfeld, 1998; Lipsey, Wilson, Cohen, & Derzon, 1997; O'Farrell & Murphy, 2002; White & Chen, 2002). A particular concern of therapists when implementing CRAFT is that an already high-risk situation in the home may become even riskier when a CSO makes changes that sometimes are intentionally meant to be viewed by the IP as "undesirable." Faced with the unappealing alternatives, many CSOs favor proceeding with CRAFT nonetheless. However, because some victimized clients who are feeling desperate may be inappropriately placing themselves in harm's way by participating in a CRAFT program, clinicians must assist them in their decision making. Accordingly, this chapter provides an overview of how to assess risk of CSO–IP violence, and how to effectively work with suitable clients to develop safety plans.

It is essential to understand that this chapter is merely an outline of a method for addressing the substance abuse–domestic violence link; it is not a comprehensive tutorial on the topic. Hence, if you are inexperienced in dealing with these precarious situations, you might consider obtaining supplemental domestic violence training prior to beginning CRAFT, particularly if you believe that your caseload warrants it. You should also be aware that the majority of the studies conducted on CRAFT *excluded* CSOs who reported at Intake that their IPs had engaged in acts of domestic violence or criminal assault in the previous 2 years, or if their IPs had ever shown any *severe* violent behavior (e.g., use of a weapon, infliction of injuries leading to hospitalization). Although it became clear, well into the treatment phase, that a number of active participants had recent histories of abuse after all, this was not tantamount to conducting controlled trials that recruited victims of domestic violence.

Thus, the question of whether it is safe to use CRAFT to treat CSOs involved in some level of ongoing physical abuse has not been adequately tested. Ultimately, the decision whether to proceed with CRAFT must be left to your own clinical judgment, based on the individual case details and the available alternatives for the CSO.

SUBSTANCE ABUSE AND DOMESTIC VIOLENCE

The relationship between intimate partner violence and substance use is well documented (Leonard, 2000). According to the National Crime Victimization Survey, in approximately two-thirds of the cases of former or current intimate partner violence, the abuser had been drinking (Greenfeld, 1998). In two multisite studies of women brought to emergency rooms with injuries resulting from domestic violence, the perpetrators were four to five times as likely to have used illicit drugs than were the male partners of a nonviolent comparison group (Grisso et al., 1999; Kyriacou et al., 1999). Among men seeking alcohol treatment, more than half of their female partners reported experiencing domestic violence in the previous year (Gondolf & Foster, 1991; Stith, Crossman, & Bischof, 1991). Other treatment researchers detected an abuse rate that was four to six times higher for alcoholic than for nonalcoholic men (O'Farrell & Murphy, 1995). Although it cannot be concluded that alcohol or drug use *causes* intimate partner violence (Caetano, Schafer, & Cunradi, 2001), many studies that controlled for multiple high-risk factors reported an association between substance abuse and violence (see Lipsey et al., 1997; White & Chen, 2002).

When domestic violence is discovered in a relationship, it might be natural to assume that the only reasonable course of action for the victim would be to leave the relationship. At some level this response would address the problem of a substance-abusing IP simultaneously. However, even though victims sometimes *do* leave the relationship at the time of the physical abuse, it is common for them to return to the abusive household multiple times (Sullivan, Basta, Tan, & Davidson, 1992), and for months or even years to pass before they do leave (Berlinger, 2001). Given this unsettling outcome, it is understandable that many therapists are not only anxious to intervene, but that they prefer using a treatment that has a solid track record for dealing with at least one risk factor in the violence equation: the substance abuse. Another consideration of therapists is the finding that the children in these violent households pay a high price (Graham-Bermann & Brescoll, 2000), beginning with neglect or abuse (Children of Alcoholics Foundation, 1996). Furthermore, repeatedly witnessing parental aggression has been associated with more behavioral problems in children (Emery, Fincham, & Cummings, 1992), and with the children developing alcohol problems as adults (Caetano, Field, & Scott, 2003; Chermack, Stoltenberg, & Fuller, 2000). In brief, a convincing case can be proffered for using CRAFT with a subset of the CSOs of abusive IPs, but knowing when to decide *against* proceeding with CRAFT is of great consequence.

ASSESSMENT OF SOCIAL SUPPORT SYSTEM

One significant but sometimes overlooked component of a comprehensive domestic violence assessment is the extent to which clients have an outside support network available to them in the event of a crisis. You may prefer to inquire about this network directly. On those occasions when CSOs report having no reliable emergency support system available to them, you should discuss the appropriate public agencies located in the community (see "Temporary Refuge" in this chapter, p. 103). You will address the absence of a support system as a larger clinical issue later in the program, since developing meaningful contacts, aside from the IP, is a vital element of CRAFT. For CSOs who already have a support network, assess whether these supporters are easily accessible and whether the CSOs are truly comfortable turning to them for help. In determining the latter, inquire whether the CSOs have ever discussed the abuse with the individuals in question. If they have done so, ask if a specific plan for seeking aid from these friends in the time of a crisis at home is in place. If obstacles to enacting the plan become apparent, introduce the problem-solving procedure described in Chapter 7 (pp. 187–191) to resolve the issue. For those CSOs who have never revealed the domestic violence to anyone, explore the reasons as well as their feelings about doing so now. If they are interested in sharing this aspect of their lives, have them select a confidant(e) and role-play the conversation while providing guidance and encouragement.

Administering a brief paper-and-pencil questionnaire on social support issues, as a prelude to a discussion of the topic, can be an efficient method for gathering details. Depending on the self-report measure used, not only can you identify the options available for outside assistance in a potential abuse situation, but also the overall degree of emotional support for CSOs as they begin their efforts to implement CRAFT procedures. As mentioned in Chapter 2, the Social Support Questionnaire (Short-Form Revised; Sarason et al., 1987) is one judicious choice, because it quickly assesses clients' perceived support and their satisfaction with it. Another clinically useful instrument noted was the Social Functioning and Resources section of the Health and Daily Living Form (Moos et al., 1987), which evaluates social support using several different formats. For instance, one section pointedly asks how many people are available in times of trouble, whereas another inquires about the number of times in the last month an individual has congregated with family members or friends (e.g., to have a long talk, attend an athletic event or a meeting of an organization, etc.). Depending on the results obtained, you would proceed in one of the manners outlined in the previous paragraph.

ASSESSMENT OF VIOLENCE

When attempting to predict the potential for violence in a relationship, evaluation methods rely heavily on the reported history of violence, including the frequency and severity of past episodes. As with the assessment of social support, you may gather this information through a paper-and-pencil instrument, direct interview questions, or a combination of the two. Screening protocols for identifying potential female victims have been developed for use by health care practitioners (see Centers for Disease Control and Prevention, 1994; Council on Scientific Affairs, 1992; Joint Commission on Accreditation of Healthcare Organizations, 1992). Published, standardized measures are also an option. An example is the popular Conflict Tactics Scales (Straus, 1979), which cover both physical and verbal aggression as well as lifetime and recent episodes for a couple. Violence is then categorized as mild, moderate, or severe. As noted in Chapter 2, this short questionnaire can easily be included in a basic Intake battery. Other standardized measures of domestic violence are available, but since most are designed for the perpetrator to complete, they would require modification for use with CSOs (Otto & Borum, 1998). Whatever the instrument of choice, it should not entirely supplant the need to inquire specifically about current or probable violence. Be sure to include questions about any problems anticipated if the IP learns about the CSO's participation in the CRAFT program, and any consequences thereof.

Some therapists review the results of an abuse questionnaire with CSOs as a way to introduce the discomforting topic of violence. Whereas some individuals are reluctant to describe their experiences as a victim (Abbott, Johnson, Koziol-McLain, & Lowenstein, 1995; Acierno, Resnick, & Kilpatrick, 1997; Miller & Downs, 2000; Schornstein, 1997), others are honestly uncertain as to what constitutes violent IP behavior. Regarding the latter, items from a measure such as the Conflict Tactics Scales can be used to illustrate the various forms of violence. Widely accepted definitions of violence can be provided as well. For instance, although distinct categorizations by level of severity of physical violence vary, examples of physical violence, in general, include pushing, grabbing, shoving, slapping, hitting, punching, kicking, biting, choking, cutting, beating up, hitting with a hard object, threatening or injuring with a weapon, or forcing sexual contact (Chermack et al., 2000; Miller, Wilsnack, & Cunradi, 2000; O'Farrell & Murphy, 2002; White & Chen, 2002).

Given the aforementioned reluctance of CSOs to candidly discuss their victimization, it is imperative to remain keenly observant of any potential signs of abuse, including physical injuries (and contradictory or evasive explanations of them), pronounced depressed or anxious mood, suicidal talk, and pregnancy complications (Levin & Greene, 2000). A frank discussion of IP aggression is necessary nonetheless, and so you need a style of broaching the topic that makes it relatively easy for CSOs to listen and participate. A range of sample invitations to discuss abusive IP behavior follows (Meyers et al., 1996, pp. 270–271):

- "The whole topic of domestic violence is a tough one for most people to talk about, but it's a critical discussion for us to have, given some of the changes in your behavior toward your loved one that we'll be considering."
- "One of the things we've learned about relationships in which somebody drinks heavily, is that it's fairly common to see abuse of a loved one when the drinker is intoxicated. Has that ever happened in your home?"
- "I know this isn't the easiest thing to talk about, but I'm wondering if you can describe any times that your husband just seemed to 'fly off the handle' and ended up hurting you?"
- "Most people don't like to talk about any violence in a relationship with someone they love, and yet, we know it happens. Have there been times when your wife got really aggressive with you and maybe even caused bodily harm?"
- "Does your husband have trouble controlling his temper? What happens when he loses it?"
- "Are you afraid that your brother might hurt you?"
- "What do you think your husband would do if he found out that you were coming to therapy to discuss his drinking? Would you or the children be in any physical danger?"

If your evaluation reveals a history of violence between the CSO and IP, you must assess the current level of risk before deciding how to proceed. Although the list of questions below is not intended to be exhaustive, it includes some of the commonly asked ones (O'Farrell & Murphy, 2002):

- "Has severe violence ever occurred?"
- "How long has it been since the last incident?"
- "Have there been recent threats of serious violence?"

- "Were the police called?"
- "Were weapons used?"
- "Did you require medical attention?"

Occasionally the probability of violence may seem too likely and the outcome too severe to risk continuing with the CRAFT program. The situation might require that you refer the individual to a community agency that specializes in providing resources for victims of domestic violence (Levin & Greene, 2000). You could also provide national Hotline information, such as that outlined extensively in the Substance Abuse and Mental Health Services Administration (SAMHSA) Desk Reference (Levin & Greene, 2000). Legal avenues may need to be explored as well. The specifics for all of these options are outlined later in this chapter. Furthermore, in such cases, you might also opt to provide standard treatment instead of CRAFT for these CSOs. In the event that you decide it is reasonably safe to proceed with CRAFT (or any other therapy), it is imperative to teach clients how to take precautions that minimize any potential for violence, and to help them develop an explicit protection plan (O'Farrell & Murphy, 2002). The remainder of this chapter is devoted to these topics.

A FUNCTIONAL ANALYSIS OF VIOLENT IP BEHAVIOR: RATIONALE AND PROBLEM BEHAVIOR OVERVIEW

In developing a safe plan for proceeding, one fundamental requirement is that at-risk individuals are able to recognize the precursors to violence. There are various methods for ascertaining this information (e.g., Levin & Greene, 2000); the principal CRAFT procedure is a functional analysis. In brief, a functional analysis of violent IP behavior outlines the factors that trigger the violence and the consequences of it. Special attention is paid to CSOs' roles in the interaction, since altering the CSOs' behavior could impact the "normal" negative outcome. As with all functional analyses of problem behaviors, the main purpose is to decrease the behavior. In the case of domestic violence, the CSOs' safety is a top priority.

Your approach to a functional analysis of violent IP behavior toward the CSO depends on whether you already have completed a functional analysis of the IP's substance use, as described in Chapter 3. If you have, you can move rather quickly through the process. Instead of explaining the rationale and procedure again, see if the client can extrapolate this information based on the earlier CRAFT functional analysis exercise. Assist in a supportive manner, as needed. If you have not yet introduced a CRAFT functional analysis of a problem behavior, refer to Chapter 3 for a detailed explanation of its objectives and format, as well as presentation suggestions, examples of clinical applications, and common problems encountered by therapists. The rationale and description you present to CSOs should include the points listed in Table 4.1. These points reflect slight modifications of the summary points outlined in Chapter 3 for substance-abusing behavior.

Once you have covered the rationale and description for this type of functional analysis, ask clients to describe a common violent IP episode that involved them. If there are several distinct types of episodes from which to choose, have CSOs first focus on the one that presented the greatest physical danger. Although the episode will be, in all probability, a time when the IP was under the influence of alcohol or drugs, this condition is not a requirement in terms of the functional analysis. As the CSOs are providing an overview, record the relevant information on a CRAFT Functional Analysis of a Loved One's Violent Behavior chart (Figure 4.1, end of chapter). As with all functional analyses, fill in the missing details by

TABLE 4.1. CRAFT FUNCTIONAL ANALYSIS OF A LOVED ONE'S VIOLENT BEHAVIOR: RATIONALE AND DESCRIPTION

1. The ultimate goal is to *eliminate the IP's violent behavior* toward the CSO.

2. The *cessation of domestic violence* will be *healthy* for the CSO–IP relationship overall, and it will *increase opportunities for inviting the IP* to treatment.

3. The first step is *gathering information* with which to formulate a safety plan immediately following.

4. The CSO is an ideal person to complete this functional analysis, due to the *CSO's direct involvement* with the IP during the episodes.

5. In completing the functional analysis, the CSO will see that the violent episodes are more *predictable* than she or he realized.

6. The functional analysis outlines the *antecedents* for the IP's violence, thereby providing ideas regarding *when* and *how* the CSO might behave differently in order to protect her- or himself at those high-risk times.

7. The functional analysis provides an estimate of the *frequency and severity* of the current violence, so that progress can be monitored over time.

8. The functional analysis identifies the short-term *positive consequences* of the violence, as experienced by the IP, thereby pinpointing certain IP *reinforcers* that need to be accessed in healthier ways.

9. It also identifies the *negative consequences* of the domestic violence, which may then be incorporated into a plan when attempting to get the IP to change the problem behavior.

going back and asking pertinent questions, while taking care to avoid being overly compulsive and thereby appearing "mechanical" during the process.

In glancing over this functional analysis chart, you will observe that it differs slightly from the one for substance use. In column 1, External Triggers, a question was added that inquires specifically about the CSO's behavior right before the violence begins. This point was included because the CSO's behavior, however innocuous, often *is* a trigger (or even an excuse) for abuse. When CSOs' behavior is a salient trigger for the violent episodes, it is preferable that they arrive at this realization on their own. It is difficult for CSOs to receive this type of information from a therapist (or anyone else) without feeling as if they are being blamed. Completing the functional analysis chart helps CSOs recognize this pattern. You will also note a new section on "red flags" at the bottom of the second column. This was simply a convenient location for recording critical information about any previously unmentioned *antecedents* to the violence. Unlike during some substance-abusing episodes, the CSO is *always* present for these domestic violence episodes and, consequently, can observe other precursors. And given the need to respond quickly, at times, in order to avoid IP aggression, it was essential to document these links in the chain of events, along with the others. Several questions were dropped from the (problem) Behavior and Short-Term Positive Consequences columns, because they were less relevant for this particular behavior.

A FUNCTIONAL ANALYSIS OF VIOLENT IP BEHAVIOR: DESCRIBING THE TRIGGERS AND THE VIOLENCE

An illustration of a CRAFT therapist and a CSO doing a functional analysis of the IP's (husband's) violent behavior follows. Assume that the therapist has previously conducted a functional analysis with this client in the substance abuse area and therefore is relying heavily on the CSO to provide the rationale for using the procedure in the current examination of violent behavior. The dialogue begins after the therapist has just asked the CSO to supply an overview of a common (or the most dangerous) violent IP episode that involves the CSO:

CSO: I guess I'll tell you about the type that has me the most worried, because it seems to happen so quickly. It also happens a lot. There's always trouble when he's late for dinner. I just can't seem to tell when he's going to slap or shove me. Sometimes he just yells, and if I'm lucky, he ignores me altogether. But he's always nasty when he's late, because it means he's stopped and gotten plenty to drink on the way home. What else do you want to know?

THERAPIST: We'll get to the missing details in a minute, but first I want to go back to something very important you said: "He's always nasty when he's late." It sounds like you can already predict when he's going to be nasty, right? And he gets physical *some* of the times that he's nasty. So getting home late is a high-risk time. But we'll still have to narrow it down to signs that he's also going to get physical, because he doesn't get violent *every* time he's late. Of course, the safest alternative is to steer clear of him *whenever* he comes home late, but this might not be practical in your situation.

CSO: No, I can't do that. Not with the kids. It would be too disruptive. It happens too often.

THERAPIST: That's what I thought. We're getting ahead of ourselves anyway. Julia, let's go back and talk about the triggers for Justin's violence. Can you tell me a little more about the times he's late? What happens *before* he gets physical?

Note: The therapist decides to gather more information about triggers in a conversational fashion first, rather than moving directly to the functional analysis form and asking the specific questions. The latter will be done next, if it appears useful. A reminder: It is not necessary to complete the chart in the order in which the items appear.

CSO: It's hard to say what happens right before he gets rough, because I really try to ignore him when he's late. But to tell you the truth, I'm not very good at that. I usually end up making a wisecrack remark because I'm so sick of his crap.

THERAPIST: It's understandable that you're upset with him. Can you give me an example of what you say?

CSO: Sure. The last time he was late . . . and drunk . . . I told him to find his own dinner. He came over and grabbed me by the shoulder and pulled me over to the fridge. He made me stand there staring into it until I pulled out some leftovers for him. Then he steered me over to the microwave to heat it up. The whole time he was digging his fingers into my shoulders. It scared me.

THERAPIST: I bet it did. And there's no reason for him to be rough like that . . . ever. Was this an unusual response for him? Have you ever told him to find his own dinner, and in response, he's gone ahead and done so . . . without touching you or otherwise threatening you?

CSO: I don't know. It's easier to remember the times he *did* threaten me, like the time I stuffed his dinner down the garbage disposal because he was late. When I pointed to where his dinner was, he backed me up against the wall and screamed at me. He had me worried. (*Pause.*) What was your question?

THERAPIST: Julia, I'm trying to see if there's something different about these two times: when Justin comes home late and drunk and ends up physically threatening you, and when he comes home late and drunk and *doesn't* physically threaten you. What do you think?

CSO: Well, if I stay away from him, he doesn't bother me. It's just hard to do that sometimes. I have things I need to do around the house with the kids. But that can't be the only thing, because sometimes I'm around him, and he doesn't touch me.

THERAPIST: Well, this sounds like a good time to look at this chart I've been jotting stuff down on, because I think it can help us sort this out. (*Shows client the chart.*) As I explained a little while ago, this is very similar to the chart we used to outline Justin's drinking problem. You can see that I've already filled in some information, based on what you've just told me.

Note: The therapist decides to introduce the functional analysis chart (Figure 4.1) and thus more formally complete the exercise, in part, because the client is having trouble pinpointing the triggers for the violence. (Figure 4.2, end of chapter, provides a sample functional analysis for this case.) Importantly, the therapist already senses that one of the triggers appears to be the CSO's angry comments or actions toward the IP during the high-risk period. If additional information supports this notion, the therapist will gently guide the CSO to discover this connection herself. Finally, notice that the therapist also took advantage of the opportunity to remind the CSO that there was no justification for the IP's aggressive behavior.

THERAPIST: Let's start with the external triggers in column 1. I filled in item 3, since you said the trouble usually happens when your husband is late for dinner and has been drinking. As far as the other external factors, does it usually happen in the same place? And is anyone, besides you, there to witness it?

CSO: He doesn't get rough with me if the kids are watching, if that's what you mean. They're at least in another room. As far as *where* it happens . . . I'd have to say, the kitchen. If I'm already busy with the kids in the bathroom or bedroom, he doesn't come near me. If I'm in the living room watching TV, he might yell at me, but he doesn't get close enough to touch me. That's pretty interesting. I hadn't thought of that before. What is it about the kitchen? Do you think maybe he was beaten up in the kitchen when he was growing up?

THERAPIST: That's certainly possible. But I would guess that either it has more to do with him being close enough to grab you, or with the type of interaction that tends to take place between the two of you in the kitchen.

CSO: What do you mean?

THERAPIST: Let's see if you can answer that question yourself after finishing the first and second columns of this chart here. It doesn't matter what order you do them in. What would you say in response to this question about your own behavior: "What is the last thing you say or do right before he gets aggressive?" And column 2, "Internal Triggers," asks about Justin's thoughts and feelings right before he gets violent. What do you think?

CSO: Oh, I get it. So what's going on between the two of us? Well, he's usually pissed at me about the dinner. At least, that's what he's yelling about.

THERAPIST: Does he *always* yell at you about the dinner when he's late?

Note: The therapist continues to help the client discover the connection between her own behavior and the violence. In exploring the husband's behavior prior to the violence, the therapist would have asked directly about any substance use if the CSO had not mentioned it (refer to the last two questions in column 1).

CSO: Well, he has nothing to yell about if I've waited on dinner until he gets home, or if I offer to fix it for him. I just get sick and tired of doing that, though, and so sometimes, when I can't stand it anymore, I let him know it. Oh . . . wait . . . maybe it has more to do with how *I* handle him being late. Come to think of it, I guess I *have* been able to tell him to get his own dinner without him getting upset. Maybe it depends on *how* I say it . . . like how pissed off I sound at the time.

THERAPIST: Sounds like a critical piece of this is how you handle your own anger toward him when he's late—anger that is very justifiable, by the way. Unfortunately, though, it might be putting you in harm's way.

CSO: I guess, in some way, I knew that. So what am I supposed to do? I can't just let him keep being late and drunk all the time. And what about *my* feelings?

THERAPIST: You're raising excellent issues. But remember, our first priority is to keep you safe, so we'll need to come up with safer ways for you to express your anger and frustration. Then I'll help you come up with ways to influence Justin's drinking.

CSO: I definitely need help with my frustration. I've had it!

THERAPIST: OK. First, let's go ahead and fill in the last few questions about triggers in the first column. You said that his aggressive outbursts might depend somewhat on what you say to him about his dinner, right?

CSO: Yes. Let me think a minute. (*Pause.*) OK. The last time he got rough was after I said something like, "That's OK. I'll make a second dinner tonight. I'm just your personal maid anyway." And the time before that was the garbage disposal incident. He asked me if I'd already put his dinner away, and I said, "Yes, I sure did put it away for you" and pointed to the disposal. At least I didn't yell at him either time. That only gets him fired up even worse.

THERAPIST: It's good that you recognize the danger in yelling at him. As far as these two recent situations go, what would you guess Justin was thinking when you made those comments or gestures? (*Points to the first question in column 2 on the chart.*)

CSO: He was probably thinking, "How dare she! I work hard all day. The least she can do is get my #*! dinner for me without showing any attitude."

THERAPIST: I think you've touched on something important. Do you know what he'd be referring to by "showing attitude"? *That* might be a critical piece, because you said a few minutes ago that sometimes you *can* get away with not fixing his dinner when he's late without him getting physical.

CSO: That's true. Yes, "showing attitude" would be saying something kind of, oh, sarcastic, I guess.

THERAPIST: So when you say something sarcastic about his dinner, I would guess that he's feeling your anger and frustration, even though you're not yelling at him, right?

CSO: I never really thought of it that way. You might be right.

THERAPIST: If that's the case, should we modify your answer to this second question? I've written that he's pissed at you about dinner at those times he gets violent. Can you be more specific?

Note: The therapist is trying to be as precise as possible about the CSO-related triggers, so that the client can recognize the sometimes subtle distinction between the kind of behavior she exhibits that contributes to violent outbursts and the kind of behavior that does not have that effect. Notice that the therapist is allowing the CSO to discover the role of her sarcastic remarks on her own, and without any judgment of them.

CSO: Let's change this answer to Justin being pissed at me for making a sarcastic comment about getting his dinner. You know, I'd be better off if I didn't say anything. The more we talk about this, the more I realize that he usually goes ahead and gets his own dinner without a word, if I'm busy in the other room with the kids. But if I'm there in the kitchen still cleaning up, we fight. Oh—that's the kitchen connection, I guess. It's just so hard to bite my tongue sometimes.

THERAPIST: That's totally understandable, Julia. And my job isn't to take away your voice but to help you find a safer way to express yourself until we get a better long-term solution. This next question is a little different. We've been talking about triggers for violence; things that in some way might contribute to your husband getting abusive. I'm interested now in other things that you notice going on right before Justin gets violent—things that might not actually be a trigger for it. In other words, are there other "red flags" that signal he's about to get aggressive? Do you see the distinction? These red flags are important to identify, if we haven't already, because if you can reliably recognize them and respond, you should be better able to avoid getting hurt. So can you think of any other signals for violence that might not actually be *triggering* the outbursts? For example, what does he say or do that let's you know he's about to get violent?

CSO: Well, I can picture him wildly waving his finger at me and yelling for a minute or so . . . right before he grabs me. Sometimes he paces and sort of mumbles to himself. I think he's trying to settle himself down. I know I should back off when he does either of those things, but sometimes I'm just too stubborn.

THERAPIST: In a minute we can talk about a safer way to respond when you notice these signals . . . and feel stubborn. Good job, though, at coming up with these. They're exactly the kind of red flags I'm talking about; things he says or does that aren't technically triggers but *are* signs of danger. I'll add them to the chart at the bottom of the second column.

Note: In addition to outlining triggers for domestic violence, this particular functional analysis interview is recognized as an opportunity to inquire about other red flags for IP aggression. The objective is to identify the full chain of events that signals the impending violent episode, regardless of whether each identified behavior plays a role in initiating it. Equipped with this information, the CSO is better able to develop a plan to avert the abuse.

THERAPIST: As far as outlining the violence itself, we've already discussed Justin's actual behavior in two situations. In the third column I've written that he grabbed you by the shoulders and steered you across the room, first to the fridge and then to the microwave, while digging his fingers into your shoulders. For the second situation I wrote that he backed you up against the wall and screamed at you. Are there other examples of his violence toward you in the kitchen when he's late and drunk and you've said something sarcastic?

CSO: Oh, I'm sure there are other examples. Mostly it's shoving, slapping, and if you count nasty comments, then he's in my face and yelling at me a lot.

THERAPIST: Then I'm adding these to the chart as well.

Probably the biggest discovery for clients at this point in the functional analysis is that the violent behavior is fairly predictable. With this realization comes the belief that the IP's aggressive behavior should be avoidable on most occasions. As CSOs arrive at these conclusions, remind them that although some of their behavior might have acted as a partial trigger for the violence, the violence is never justifiable or acceptable. A common discovery for therapists during this first half of the functional analysis is that there are often multiple examples of abusive IP behavior in response to similar triggers. It is advisable to note these as well, in order to monitor the reduction of all violence. Importantly, ideas for responding differently begin to surface at this early stage of the functional analysis, but the consequences of the aggression should be explored before any final decisions are made regarding how to proceed with a prevention plan.

A FUNCTIONAL ANALYSIS OF VIOLENT IP BEHAVIOR: OUTLINING THE CONSEQUENCES

As mentioned in Chapter 3, many CSOs have trouble accepting the fact that their IPs experience a host of positive consequences from abusing substances. The concept is even more elusive when applied to their IPs' violent behavior. But clients *do* understand that *something* is keeping the aggressive behavior going; they simply have never thought of it in terms of "positive consequences." They have less difficulty acknowledging that negative consequences are associated as well; you simply need to be sure that the consequences they identify are the *IPs'* and not just their own. The dialogue between the therapist and Julia (CSO) continues, first by exploring the husband's perceived benefits in behaving aggressively, and then by moving on to the longer-lasting complications that ensue:

THERAPIST: You can see here, Julia, that the next part of the functional analysis involves outlining what Justin might see as the short-term positive consequences of his violent behavior. Does that sound strange to you? Does it seem odd to think that Justin gets something positive out of being violent?

CSO: Well, he must get *something* out of it, because he sure does it enough!

THERAPIST: My thoughts exactly. And do you remember doing this part of the chart for his drinking? Do you remember *why* we looked at the positive things Justin got out of such problematic behaviors?

CSO: It had something to do with keeping the behavior going. He was going to keep doing that stuff unless we found out why. No . . . that doesn't sound right.

THERAPIST: Actually, you're very close. It *does* have to do with the behavior continuing and needing to figure out why, but there's an important step that involves helping him find another, healthier way to get those same, or similar, positive outcomes. So what in the world would Justin find positive or rewarding about hurting or threatening you?

CSO: I've been thinking for some time now that it makes him feel like a big man; powerful. Is that what you mean?

THERAPIST: If you think feeling powerful is experienced as rewarding by your husband, then yes. And it makes sense, because when does he often get violent? When you're standing up to him in some way, such as by being sarcastic.

CSO: He has to show me who's boss, I guess. But that's stupid. Everybody knows he's the boss.

THERAPIST: But he must feel threatened for some reason when you're sarcastic. Physically overpowering you might make him feel tough again. What else does he get out of being physically aggressive toward you?

CSO: I guess the obvious thing is that I make him his dinner—so he gets what he wants there. But how do we fix that? If I *don't* get his dinner for him in those situations, he'll be even worse! Geez . . . if he just asked me nicely, I'd probably fix his stupid dinner anyway!

THERAPIST: Well, we definitely don't want to make things worse. But let's wait a few minutes before we figure out how to fix the problem, OK? I don't want you to assume that we're going to have you stop everything you've been doing. What I'm hoping is that we can find a way to make some early changes so that the situation doesn't even get close to being violent. OK. So he gets you to do something for him, like make his dinner. What else does he get out of it?

CSO: I bet it makes him feel like he's a priority, because I drop everything and wait on him when he threatens me. That's one of his regular complaints about me these days: that I never make him a priority anymore.

THERAPIST: Julia, you're doing a terrific job coming up with these "rewards." Some people have trouble with this part. Just to make sure we haven't missed any other positive things he might experience, let me ask these other two questions in the fourth column. First, about his thoughts: What do you think he's saying to himself right *after* he's aggressive with you in the kitchen?

Note: The therapist begins this segment by quizzing the client about the purpose of recognizing the benefits her husband might experience from being abusive. She then praises the client's good work in outlining the IP's positive consequences. A fair number of CSOs cannot transcend their own negative experience of the violence to envision what might be perceived by the IP as an advantage of it. The therapist then moves to the formal questions, as the added structure is often helpful in eliciting more ideas in this section.

CSO: What's he saying to himself? I don't know. I never thought about it. Let's see. He's probably saying, "That should put her in her place," or "I shouldn't have to fight for what I deserve."

THERAPIST: I'll jot those down. And when he's thinking these things, how do you suppose he's feeling?

CSO: Superior. Pleased with himself. But I know it doesn't last long.

THERAPIST: No, I don't imagine it would. But in the meantime, you've suffered terribly. OK. So these feelings answer item 3 here. These thoughts and feelings seem right in line with what you're guessing he gets out of the violent acts; namely, feeling powerful. But you added the idea that he "deserves" supper. Good. That will help us later as we come up with a plan. Let's move on to the last column, where we list the negative side to the violence for him. Just like when we did this for his drinking, I'll list all the negative consequences you know of, and then I'll put an asterisk next to those you think Justin would agree with. What do you think?

CSO: That's easy. I lose respect for him when he hurts me.

THERAPIST: I'll put that down under Interpersonal consequences. Now, do you think he'd agree it's a negative outcome? Is he even aware of it?

CSO: I haven't exactly talked to him about it, so I don't know. Does that mean we shouldn't mark it down?

THERAPIST: I'm putting them all down anyway. It's a good one to remember; we just need to make sure *he* knows about it eventually, otherwise it won't influence his behavior that much. OK. Back to the question of whether he'd agree this is a negative consequence. Assuming he knows you lose respect for him, does he care?

CSO: I'm not sure.

THERAPIST: Then for now I won't put an asterisk next to it. Again, if it feels to him like a downside of his battering, there's more of a reason for him to stop the violence. How about some other negative consequences of his abuse that directly involve your relationship with him?

Note: CSOs often readily list negative consequences, but ones that are experienced by the *CSO*, not the IP. Although the distinction should be made by placing an asterisk next to the ones the IP would agree are negative, it is best to note all of them, as the information may be useful later.

CSO: I carry a grudge for a while afterward. Does that count?

THERAPIST: Sure. Do you think it bothers him, and does he see it as connected to his aggressive acts?

CSO: Yes, I think it bothers him when he notices that I'm not talking to him. Of course, he has to be sober to notice. He tries to get me in a good mood by doing something nice for me.

THERAPIST: And does it work?

CSO: What do you mean?

THERAPIST: For starters, does he get you in a good mood?

CSO: Usually. Why?

THERAPIST: I'm trying to see the extent of the negative consequences he experiences for his violence. Based on what you've said, he has to deal with you not talking to him for a short time afterward. But my guess is that he thinks all is forgiven once you're in a good mood again.

CSO: Well, I wouldn't say *all* is forgiven. Oh . . . but *he* might see it that way. I get it.

Note: The therapist pointedly inquires about the CSO's reaction to the IP's efforts to be forgiven in the aftermath of a violent episode, because this might be a potential area for intervention later in treatment. If the IP's negative consequences are not particularly potent, he is less likely to alter his behavior.

THERAPIST: Julia, the fact that he *does* care whether or not you're talking to him is a good sign. It gives us more to work with, because it shows that he values his relationship with you. But for now, let's continue with listing the negative consequences of his violent acts in these other areas so that we can get a complete picture. Since emotional consequences are often related to the interpersonal consequences area we just covered, let me ask next if he experiences any negative *emotional* repercussions of his aggression?

CSO: Like I just said, he seems upset because he sees me upset.

THERAPIST: Could you say a little more about the emotion you think he's feeling when you say he gets "upset"?

CSO: He seems worried. *You* know . . . "upset."

THERAPIST: Worried. Thank you. That helps. And are they any *physical* consequences of his aggression for him?

CSO: Well, I don't shove him back, if that's what you mean. No, I can't think of any way he suffers physically. But I see down the list here it asks about his job. I know that at least one of his coworkers suspects something, because Justin has accused me of telling "stories," as he calls them, about our personal time at home. I haven't told his coworkers a thing, so I don't know who they heard it from. But he seems concerned about people at work knowing about the way he treats me.

THERAPIST: Good. That gives us even more to work with. What about these other areas?

CSO: Legal? I don't know. He knows I'll never call the cops on him, but I think he's a little worried that I'll get sick of it, once and for all, and divorce him someday. Is that a legal consequence?

THERAPIST: Worrying about a possible divorce could fit either the legal or interpersonal category. No need to put it in both places, though. Would it feel like more of an interpersonal or a legal consequence to him?

CSO: I *hope* it feels more like an interpersonal and not just a legal consequence!

THERAPIST: Then let's add it to the interpersonal item. Any financial consequences, or other consequences that aren't listed here?

CSO: There'd be financial consequences if we got divorced, but there really aren't any now. There'd be more consequences if people knew about the violence.

THERAPIST: We can talk later about whether it would be a good idea to confide in more people. For now, let's step back and see what we've learned about the setting in which the domestic violence often occurs, including what Justin seems to get out of it. From there, we'll go ahead with a plan.

A FUNCTIONAL ANALYSIS OF VIOLENT IP BEHAVIOR: USING THE INFORMATION TO FORMULATE A PLAN

As with all functional analyses, the final phase entails stepping back to review the overall picture of the context for the behavior of interest, and then discussing how this information can be used to formulate a change strategy. To assess clients' degree of understanding, have *them* summarize what they just learned about the triggers, the additional red flags, and the consequences of the problem behavior. In Julia's case, you would want her to mention the following points when referring to the violent episode:

TRIGGERS

External Triggers

The violent behavior occurs on evenings when Justin comes home drunk and late for dinner; it takes place in the kitchen when the children are in the other room; it is often sparked by a sarcastic comment from Julia in response to his demand for dinner.

Internal Triggers

The intoxicated IP strikes out in anger when he thinks his wife is showing "an attitude" about doing something for him (i.e., preparing his dinner) that he feels he deserves.

Potential Interventions

Based on these triggers, partial intervention strategies that might be considered are listed below (the sections of this book that deal with the relevant procedures are noted in brackets):

  • Suggesting that Julia regularly leave the kitchen and go to another room with the children when she hears her husband arriving home late; leaving his dinner accessible and easy for him to heat up [instruction in how to withdraw rewards at times of problematic behaviors (Chapter 7) and problem-solving training (Chapter 7)].
  • Teaching Julia safer methods and times for expressing anger toward her husband; demonstrating a strategy for resolving her frustra-

tion with him in the meantime [communication training (Chapter 5); problem-solving (Chapter 7)].

Interventions deemed appropriate for the case would be taught to the CSO as part of CRAFT.

RED FLAGS

Justin's waving his finger at Julia and yelling, or pacing and mumbling, constitute the red flags for impending violence in this case. The crucial first response to most red flags involves putting physical distance between self and the IP as quickly as possible. Thus, Julia would be advised to put aside her "stubborn" feelings and step back at the appearance of any red flags. The next move would depend on the established protection plan, as described later in this chapter.

CONSEQUENCES

Positive Consequences

Julia should mention that treating her aggressively makes Justin feel powerful and superior at a time when he believes his power has been threatened by her; it also makes him feel that he is a priority in her life; and it gets him his dinner in a hurry.

Negative Consequences

Once sober, Justin gets upset when he sees that Julia is upset and is not talking to him; he worries about a possible divorce; he also is upset that coworkers might know about the abuse.

Potential Interventions

Although the choice would obviously depend on many unmentioned individual case factors, potential intervention strategies that are outgrowths of these consequences are listed below, with the relevant CRAFT procedures noted in brackets:

- Teaching Julia to refrain from behaving in a way that the IP would perceive as challenging his authority (e.g., being sarcastic) during a high-risk time, thereby eliminating his perceived need to prove his power [communication training (Chapter 5); problem-solving instruction (Chapter 7)].
- Suggesting that Julia devise a plan for helping her husband feel like a priority more often; and teaching her *how* and *when* to reward appropri-

ate behavior [problem solving training (Chapter 7); instruction in how to reward appropriate behavior (Chapter 6)].

• Showing Julia how to explore the divorce issue openly with Justin [communication training (Chapter 5)].

• Teaching Julia how to change her pattern of giving in later to his attempts to reconcile, but without any discussion of how to avoid the problem in the future [communication training (Chapter 5); instruction in how to withdraw rewards (Chapter 7)].

• Teaching Julia how to work *with* Justin to address the problem of his dinner not being ready [communication training (Chapter 5); problem-solving instruction (Chapter 7)].

• Practicing with Julia various ways to discuss the issue of Justin's coworkers knowing about the abuse, and then deciding how to proceed from there [communication training (Chapter 5); problem-solving instruction (Chapter 7)].

Notice that the basic procedures recommended for approaching the violence problem from the perspective of the *triggers* (e.g., communication training) are mostly the same ones outlined for generating a solution while considering the *consequences*. The fact that the requisite behavioral skills are relevant for a number of different CRAFT procedures should be pointed out to CSOs, since it may help them feel less overwhelmed at the prospect of learning so many techniques. Regardless, the elements needed in order to ensure the CSO's safety must be addressed first. Despite the fact that conceivably, domestic violence would decrease in conjunction with the reduced use of alcohol or drugs (Leonard, 2000; O'Farrell & Fals-Stewart, 2003; O'Farrell & Murphy, 1995), it would be a mistake—and possibly dangerous—to rely on that kind of a sequence of events. Even if a decrease occurred, "less" violence is still too much when it is happening at all.

As mentioned in the previous chapter, CSOs sometimes feel responsible for their IPs' problem behavior when they see how their own words or behavior have functioned as a "trigger." This reaction is of particular concern when domestic violence is involved, because many victims have been told repeatedly by their aggressors that *they* provoked the violent act themselves. Consequently, it is critical to remind CSOs that there is *never* an excuse for violence, and that most loved ones would never respond to the CSOs' behavior—*regardless* of what it is—with aggression. In addition, be sure that CSOs understand that their "triggering behavior" is only one segment of the complicated path that leads to violent IP outbursts, and that they *should not underestimate the contributing role of the alcohol or drugs*. One final point to raise with CSOs before closing the functional analysis discussion is whether additional antecedents to violence should be explored. In essence, you are asking if the information gleaned about the episode selected for the functional analysis is representative of other episodes. If you are concerned that it might not be, then novel triggers (and a relevant safety plan) usually can be identified without conducting another entire functional analysis.

PREVENTION OF DOMESTIC VIOLENCE

DEVELOPING SAFER CSO RESPONSES

It is advisable to have at least a brief discussion about the prevention of violence with all clients, regardless of their history. For those clients with neither past violent episodes nor serious threats, you can ask them to imagine the most dangerous situations that might arise as they change their behavior toward the IP. Depending on the likelihood of IP aggression, you might simply assist these CSOs in tracing the chain of events that could lead to problems, without conducting a formal functional analysis. If there is a history of physical abuse with the IP, you will already have completed a functional analysis of the violence.

Regardless of how the triggers to (potential) IP aggression are identified, the objective is to use this information to develop a method for preventing future abuse. At the heart of the plan is the belief that IP violence is usually predictable and, consequently, often avoidable. Successful avoidance requires that CSOs learn to respond to the earliest warning signs in a way that either takes them out of harm's way or minimizes the chance of an aggressive outburst in the first place. In the illustration just presented, which utilized the functional analysis to outline the IP's violent episodes, it became clear that the safest course of action for the wife was to stay out of the high-risk area (the kitchen) at the high-risk time (when the husband came home late and was drunk), and to leave his prepared dinner easily accessible. Furthermore, it would be important to avoid expressing her anger to him through sarcastic remarks. The sequence of events that preceded the violence was scrutinized to identify any red flags (e.g., waving finger, yelling, pacing, mumbling) that were *not* also triggers, with the goal of providing the CSO with the best possible chance to avoid or escape a risky situation as early as possible.

Several additional examples of common IP triggers and the resultant violence are supplied, along with recommended safer CSO responses, in the following material.

Trigger

An IP cannot find his liquor bottles in their usual hiding place, which means that his wife (CSO) has disposed of them. He screams at her and proceeds to shove her around the room, until she admits that she has taken them. He then makes a trip to the liquor store to buy more.

New CSO Response

First, the wife would be advised *not* to discard the husband's bottles. Not only does the act infuriate him and trigger verbal and physical violence, but it is ineffective in stopping the drinking. Instead, the drinking would be dealt with over time, by teaching the CSO other CRAFT procedures, such as how to reward sober behavior and to withdraw rewards during drinking periods.

Trigger

An inebriated mother (IP) starts slapping her 18-year-old daughter (CSO) when the daughter refuses to make dinner for the family a fourth night in a row. At that point the sobbing daughter gives in and cooks.

New CSO Response

In the interest of safety, the daughter would be asked to resist defying her mother over the dinner issue, for now, particularly if she is drunk. In addition to helping the CSO find a better method for dealing with the mother's alcohol use, the daughter would be offered communication skills training to develop safer ways to express her anger as well as to talk with her mother about dinner preparation issues.

Trigger

A 21-year-old father (IP) with only part-time work hates to have his afternoon nap disturbed when he has been smoking marijuana. If his 6-month-old son's crying wakes him up and his young wife (CSO) does not attend to the baby immediately, the IP angrily accuses her of intentionally waking him and proceeds to push her around the house roughly.

New CSO Response

According to the CSO, the safest response is to take her son out for a walk as soon as he wakes up and begins crying, so she would be advised to do this until a better long-term solution could be adopted in terms of her husband's drug use and employment problem. Any passive–aggressive behavior on her part would be addressed through problem-solving methods and communication training.

Trigger

A 24-year-old brother (CSO) has been beaten up rather severely by his older brother (IP), during several past attempts to get the IP away from an illicit drug party scene.

New CSO Response

A variety of options would be generated through problem-solving, such as having the CSO avoid these drug parties, for now, or notifying the police if he is truly concerned about his brother's safety in the situation. Again, the drug use itself would be the focus of other CRAFT procedures.

REPERCUSSIONS OF NEW CSO RESPONSE

Perhaps an obvious issue to consider at this point is whether a new type of CSO response may minimize domestic violence while, at the same time, actually making it easier for the IP to continue drinking or using drugs. In fact, this outcome may occur—temporarily. Nonetheless, the long-term outcome should be quite different, once the CSO is proficient in the various skills taught within the CRAFT program. Consider one example in the case of Julia and Justin. If the company of his wife and the children during dinner was at all reinforcing to Justin, then hopefully his decision to arrive home late (and drunk) would eventually be influenced by the fact that he is no longer spending time with his family. In order to arrive home earlier, he would have to forfeit some of his drinking time. (The relevant "time-out" from positive reinforcement procedure is outlined fully in Chapter 7). Additionally, other CRAFT procedures would be introduced to address the substance abuse directly.

Interestingly, you will soon notice that the safety plan for one client is built around a CSO behavior (e.g., having dinner readily available for a late, drunk IP) that will be discouraged for another CSO, in an effort to allow the natural consequences of the IP's substance use to be experienced. The critical distinction is whether or not a CSO is likely to be the victim of domestic violence as a result of her or his actions.

DEVELOPING SAFER RESPONSES WITHOUT KNOWING THE TRUE TRIGGERS

The previous section focused on changing certain CSO behaviors that had been triggers for violence. Periodically, CSOs report that they are not even physically present when the chain of events begins and therefore cannot be viewed as a trigger. These CSOs anxiously state that their IPs' outbursts seem unpredictable, since what are harmless remarks or behavior on most occasions are responded to with IP attacks on other occasions. Upon questioning, however, many of these CSOs are able to identify characteristic IP behaviors which signal that violence is imminent. So although the clients are unaware of the actual trigger, they typically can predict the occurrence of violence after all. Consequently, they can learn to avoid it by implementing procedures similar to those just outlined when triggers are known. In the functional analysis section, these precursors were called *red flags* to distinguish them from triggers. Some common examples of recognizable precursors with unknown early triggers follow. Assume that the IPs' substance abuse occurs regularly in the scenarios below and therefore that substance abuse alone is not the trigger:

• A wife (CSO) states that when she hears her husband (IP) screech to a halt in the driveway, kick the front door closed, and slam his keys down on the table, she knows there is a good chance he will be aggressive if *anything* upsets him within the next hour.

• A husband (CSO) says that if arrives home from work to find his wife (IP) lying on the couch and neglecting their crying daughter, while obviously high on her prescription pills, he is quite certain that she will throw household items at him the moment he opens his mouth (regardless of the nature of the comment).

• A sister (CSO) reports that her brother (IP) periodically pushes her around roughly for no apparent reason if he is intoxicated and is "showing off" for his friends.

Situations such as these tend to be extremely uncomfortable ones for CSOs, because apparently they can secure their own safety only by staying away from the IP and saying nothing. In truth, it is as if the IP were waiting for an excuse to enact aggression toward someone, and the CSO is a convenient target. Again, a safe course of action in response to these identified precursors would be developed first, and a long-term plan that added CRAFT procedures geared at influencing the IP's substance use directly would follow.

DEVELOPMENT OF PROTECTION PLANS FOR SERIOUS ONGOING VIOLENCE

EXITING QUICKLY

It is critical for CSOs to understand from the start that they should flee the situation immediately, if they believe they are in grave danger. Grave danger typically is defined as the threat or experience of injuries requiring hospitalization or emergency medical care. However, encourage CSOs to "go with their gut" and adhere to their own interpretation of grave danger.

In preparation for the possibility that CSOs may need to leave their homes in a hurry, mentally walk them through the event. Be sure to stress the following points:

- Be cognizant of the closest and safest exit routes.
- Guard against being backed into a corner or steered into remote sections of the house (e.g., basement, laundry room).
- Keep a bag of essential items packed (e.g., important documents, money or checkbook/credit card, small medication supply, change of clothing) and stored secretly in an accessible location in the home, the car, or at a friend's.
- Have a specific destination planned and transportation available (as described below).

Temporary Refuge

An effective protection plan includes knowledge of a specific destination, should CSOs need to escape in a hurry. One reasonable option is a safe house, such as a domestic violence shelter. The names of these types of shelters vary by community, so you should have a local listing available, complete with addresses and phone numbers. These listings often include women's cooperatives, victims' advocacy services, and rape crisis centers (see domestic violence listings in Levin & Greene, 2000, p. 13). Since you do not want to take the risk that violent IPs will inadvertently find in their own homes such a listing of all the local safe houses, direct CSOs to select one from the list and memorize its address and/or phone number. Arrangements for transportation to the safe house should be discussed in advance, with the realization that many shelters offer this service. As an alternative to a community-sponsored shelter, CSOs may instead choose to take refuge at the home of a family member or friend. As explained previously, if CSOs choose this option, you should determine whether these individuals are aware of the domestic violence situation, or whether a conversation explaining the problem should be rehearsed. Lastly, transportation details would need to be considered.

Legal Interventions

Regardless of the protection plan decided upon, remind all CSOs that calling 911 is always an option if they feel threatened. Sadly, the police receive many requests to respond to domestic violence situations. In some

counties the authorities offer the victims transportation to domestic violence shelters or to hospitals at the time they respond to the call.

Another legal option for victims of domestic violence is to petition
the district court for a temporary restraining order against the offender.
An order of protection can be issued in many states if a serious threat of
violence exists, even if the violence has not yet occurred. Although the
exact procedure involved in applying for a restraining order varies by
state, clients can typically obtain the necessary forms from the police or
clerk's office in the local courthouse. A petition describing the nature of
the complaint is completed while under oath. Ordinarily, clients do not
need an attorney to file it. In most states a hearing is scheduled within 10
days to determine whether a 90-day restraining order is needed. Both parties are expected to be present. The specifics of a protective order, if one
is issued, may vary widely, depending on the situation. For instance, the
court may order the offender to maintain a minimum distance from the
victim, to provide temporary child and/or spousal support, or to arrange
for the maintenance of the property during the 90 days. Decisions also are
made at the hearing about constraints on communication, a child visitation schedule, and the consequences of violating the order. Counseling is
often recommended as well, because the restraining order is viewed as
only a temporary solution to a serious relationship problem. A request
may be made by either party during the 90-day protective order to review
the hearing, with the objective of amending the order. Likewise, the
restraining order may be extended at the end of the 90 days, upon the
petitioner's request, if the court sees it justified (Meyers et al., 1996).

HELPING VICTIMIZED CSOs
DEAL WITH THEIR GUILT AND ANGER

Once CSOs have a prevention plan and, if necessary, a protection plan in
place, you should address their feelings about the domestic violence.
Often therapists are surprised to discover that many victims feel guilty
over what they perceive as the role they have played in provoking the violence, or for involving the IP in the legal system by filing a report.
Although it is sometimes useful to normalize this guilt reaction, it is
always important to remind clients that violence by *anyone* under *any* circumstances is never a normal or acceptable reaction. Follow up this point
by asking CSOs to enumerate the ways in which their own and their IP's
lives would improve if the violence stopped. Additionally, discuss the evidence for an association between decreased violence and decreased substance use. Finally, highlight the fact that less violence in the household
implies more opportunities to invite the IP to enter treatment.

Some CSOs are not able to get in touch with their anger about being victimized until they have set aside the guilt, whereas others are cognizant of their anger, at some level, from the start. Regardless, CSOs need to proceed cautiously when it comes to expressing their anger toward the IP, since it could partially trigger a violent episode. As noted previously, it is important for CSOs to cease their displays of anger altogether, if those displays are instrumental in leading to abuse. However, it is also crucial for clients to have the opportunity to safely discuss their resentment and frustration. Since it may take a considerable amount of time and treatment before it is reasonable to have such a conversation with the IP, encourage CSOs to discuss these strong feelings during therapy sessions in the meantime. As was explained in Chapter 2, the use of therapy time to express anger toward the IP needs to be constrained, however, as some CSOs would otherwise spend the bulk of each session on the topic. Instead, you show them how to move forward, rather quickly, in order to promote positive changes, as opposed to remaining stuck with their anger.

SUMMARY

The first objective of this chapter is to underscore the fact that clinicians are likely to have to deal with violence issues if they deal with relationships in which there is substance abuse. The second purpose is to stress the need for caution: Given that CRAFT involves asking clients to modify the way they interact with a substance-abusing loved one such that it discourages use, the likelihood of facing a disgruntled IP is high. This chapter provides fundamental information for assessing risk and for developing a safety plan. In the process, it supplies a second example of a functional analysis of a problem behavior.

FIGURE 4.1.   CRAFT FUNCTIONAL ANALYSIS OF A LOVED ONE'S VIOLENT BEHAVIOR

External Triggers	Internal Triggers	Violent Behavior	Short-Term Positive Consequences	Long-Term Negative Consequences
1. *Who* else is present besides you when your loved one gets violent?	1. What do you think your loved one is *thinking* about right before getting violent?	1. *What* does your loved one's violent behavior usually consist of?	1. What do you think your loved one *likes* about getting violent?	1. What do you think are the negative results of your loved one's violence in each of these areas (* the ones he/she would agree with): a. Interpersonal:
2. *Where* does the violence usually occur?	2. What you think he/she is *feeling* right before getting violent?		2. What pleasant *thoughts* do you think he/she has during or right after the violence?	b. Physical: c. Emotional: d. Legal:
3. *When* does the violence usually occur? [Alcohol/drugs involved?]	**Other "Red Flags":** What is the last thing your *loved one says/does* before getting violent?		3. What pleasant *feelings* do you think he/she has during or right after the violence?	e. Job: f. Financial: g. Other:
4. What is the last thing *you say/do* right before your loved one gets violent?				

From *Motivating Substance Abusers to Enter Treatment* by Jane Ellen Smith and Robert J. Meyers. Copyright 2004 by The Guilford Press. Permission to photocopy this figure is granted to purchasers of this book for personal use only (see copyright page for details).

External Triggers	Internal Triggers	Violent Behavior	Short-Term Positive Consequences	Long-Term Negative Consequences
1. *Who* else is present besides you when your loved one gets violent? Nobody. 2. *Where* does the violence usually occur? In the kitchen. 3. *When* does the violence usually occur? [Alcohol/drugs involved?] When he's late for dinner and is drunk. 4. What is the last thing *you say/do* right before your loved one gets violent? "I'm just your personal maid." [a sarcastic remark]	1. What do you think your loved one is *thinking* about right before getting violent? How dare she! I work hard all day. The least she can do is get my #*! dinner without showing any attitude. 2. What you think he/she is *feeling* right before getting violent? Pissed at me for making a sarcastic comment about getting his dinner. **Other "Red Flags":** What is the last thing your *loved one says/does* before getting violent? Waves finger at me & yells; paces & mumbles.	1. *What* does your loved one's violent behavior usually consist of? Grabs me by shoulders and steers across room (to fridge or microwave); digs in fingers. Backs me up against wall and screams. Shoves, slaps, yells.	1. What do you think your loved one *likes* about getting violent? Makes him feel like a big man; powerful. His dinner gets fixed. Makes him feel like a priority. 2. What pleasant *thoughts* do you think he/she has during or right after the violence? That should put her in her place. I shouldn't have to fight for what I deserve. 3. What pleasant *feelings* do you think he/she has during or right after the violence? Feels superior; pleased with himself.	1. What do you think are the negative results of your loved one's violence in each of these areas (* the ones he/she would agree with): a. Interpersonal: He loses my respect. I won't talk to him for awhile.* He's worried about a possible divorce.* b. Physical: c. Emotional: He gets upset (worried because I'm upset.* d. Legal: e. Job: He's concerned that coworkers know.* f. Financial: g. Other:

CHAPTER 5

IMPROVING COMMUNICATION SKILLS OF CONCERNED SIGNIFICANT OTHERS

Teaching communication skills to CSOs is an important component of the CRAFT program, and yet the reason for this is not immediately obvious to many CSOs *or* therapists. The explanation begins with a fact: Communication problems are routinely found in relationships involving individuals who abuse substances (Epstein & McCrady, 1998; O'Farrell & Fals-Stewart, 1999, 2003). More importantly, behavioral marital or family therapy for individuals with alcohol or drug problems regularly includes communication training, and generally the therapy has produced favorable outcomes in terms of reduced use (Bowers & Al-Rehda, 1990; Epstein & McCrady, 1998; Fals-Stewart et al., 2001; O'Farrell, Cutter, & Floyd, 1985). So in some ways CRAFT's communication training with CSOs is similar to a segment of behavioral couples therapy but with only half of the couple (i.e., the willing participant) present. As with other components of the CRAFT program, CSOs benefit from the communication skills training, regardless of whether the IP ever participates in couples or any other type of therapy. These additional advantages are enumerated below.

RATIONALE FOR TEACHING COMMUNICATION SKILLS

There are numerous reasons for spending time on teaching communication skills to CSOs, but it is only necessary to review those that are relevant to, and thus will be meaningful for, your CRAFT clients. Generally speaking, most individuals can benefit from taking a look at their current communication style. It is easy for people to fall into the habit of only vaguely expressing what they want, blaming others for their problems, allowing resentment to build up, and delivering messages in a negative manner when they could almost as readily be stated in a positive way. These types of communication problems, and others, are particularly salient in relationships where substance abuse is an issue (Epstein & McCrady, 1998; Monti, Kadden, Rohsenow, Cooney, & Abrams, 2002; Murphy & O'Farrell, 1997; O'Farrell & Birchler, 1987; O'Farrell & Fals-Stewart, 1999, 2000, 2003). At times, these problematic interactions may even trigger episodes of alcohol or drug use (Maisto, McKay, & O'Farrell, 1995; Maisto, O'Farrell, Connors, McKay, & Pelcovits, 1988; McCrady, 1989). Not surprisingly, then, communication training is an essential component of couples work within the addictions field. Individuals must learn to change their dysfunctional interactional patterns if an atmosphere supportive of sobriety is going to be realized (O'Farrell, 1995; Project MATCH Research Group, 1992). Research supports the inclusion of communication skills training in relationship counseling, because reduced substance use is often found for participants in these comprehensive substance abuse programs (Bowers & Al-Rehda, 1990; Epstein & McCrady, 1998; Fals-Stewart et al., 2000, 2001; Monti et al., 1990; Stanton & Shadish, 1997). Many of the programs detect improved marital adjustment as well (Fals-Stewart et al., 2001; McCrady, Stout, Noel, Abrams, & Nelson, 1991; O'Farrell et al., 1985; O'Farrell & Fals-Stewart, 2000).

Additional reasons why CSOs can benefit from attention to communication skills, even though their IP may not currently (and may never) be in treatment, is that, for one thing, positive communication is contagious! It is natural for others to follow suit and utilize positive communication when the person with whom they are interacting is doing so. It is also the case that positive communication can enhance happiness in certain other life areas, such as when an individual starts acting assertively or becomes more sociable. In turn, this improved communication increases access to support systems (Monti et al., 2002), which is an added advantage for many CSOs who have become socially isolated.

Although positive communication often requires more thought and effort than negative communication, the payoff is usually better, because the communicators are more likely to get what they want. As noted, the old adage "You catch more flies with honey than with vinegar" holds true. Individuals are better able to listen and more willing to respond appropriately when they do not feel as if they are being verbally assaulted. Positive communication can also be a powerful and inexpensive reinforcer when used to compliment someone or to share heartfelt feelings.

Another reason why it is imperative for CSOs to develop a positive communication style is because the skills that comprise such a style form the foundation for other CRAFT procedures that are introduced later in treatment. For instance, clients are taught to present verbal explanations for some of the changes in their behavior toward the IP, such as why they are suddenly offering small rewards when the IP is clean and sober, and why they are starting to withdraw reinforcers (e.g., leave the room) when the IP is using substances. Furthermore, throughout the CRAFT program, CSOs are prepared to invite the IP to sample treatment when appropriate occasions arise. It is paramount to the success of these procedures that good communication skills are already in place.

As noted, you only need to present the rationales that are relevant to CSOs. Table 5.1 outlines the various reasons just mentioned for teaching CSOs communication skills.

DESCRIPTION OF THE GUIDELINES
FOR POSITIVE COMMUNICATION SKILLS

There are many valid ways to teach good communication skills (e.g., Christensen & Jacobson, 2000; Monti et al., 2002). One common component stressed is the selection of a suitable time (as well as a backup time) to have any significant conversation. "Good timing" ideally entails a CSO initiating the communication when the IP is clean/sober and not hungover, and on an occasion when both the CSO and IP are in reasonably good moods. Guidelines for an approach to determine the *content* of the conversation, built upon procedures introduced in the Community Reinforcement Approach (Hunt & Azrin, 1973; Meyers & Smith, 1995), are listed below. Suggestions regarding how you might actually work with CSOs to incorporate them follow. In terms of presenting the guidelines to the clients, provide a brief overview of each point and its purpose, along with illustrative examples that contrast "problematic" and "improved" versions of the communication. Samples are provided, but you may want to use your own examples if they are more applicable to your client. You might also give your clients index cards containing the outlined points, so that they can be taken home and easily accessed (see Figure 5.1, end of chapter). Inform CSOs that they are not expected to memorize the seven guidelines, nor do they have to worry about trying to add all of them to their conversations with the IP. Instead, invite CSOs to practice incorporating just a few of the suggestions into their communication style. Proceeding in this gradual fashion will facilitate a smoother transition to a positive (albeit initially awkward) mode of communicating. Remind CSOs that the objective is to use enough of the guidelines to improve their verbal interactions with the IP, such that they are heard and understood and their IP is open to discussion. Encourage them to practice these skills with

TABLE 5.1. RATIONALE FOR COMMUNICATION SKILLS TRAINING

1. Most relationships involving an individual who abuses substances have *a communication problem* that *interferes* with achieving or maintaining a clean and sober lifestyle.

2. *Effective couples therapy* in the alcohol and drug field typically includes communication skills training.

3. Positive communication is *"contagious"*; it is often adopted by others who hear it.

4. CSOs can *increase satisfaction in multiple areas* of their lives by using positive communication skills (e.g., assertiveness) when dealing with individuals aside from just the IP.

5. Improved communication opens the door to *larger social support networks.*

6. *CSOs are more likely to get what they want* through positive as opposed to negative communication, because the listener is less likely to act defensively ("You catch more flies with honey . . . ").

7. Positive communication (e.g., a compliment) can serve as *a powerful reinforcer* for a loved one.

8. Good communication is *the foundation* for other CRAFT procedures (e.g., verbally linking reinforcers with specific IP behavior, inviting the IP to sample treatment).

---

family members or friends other than the IP at first, so that unanticipated real-life issues that arise can be addressed.

Note that the guidelines and examples below are worded to reflect a CSO delivering a message/communication to an IP. As mentioned, skills learned through communication training are not intended to be limited to CSO–IP interactions. Ideally, the CSO would use newly acquired communication skills in conversations with others as well, both at home and in the community.

GUIDELINES FOR POSITIVE COMMUNICATION SKILLS

1. Be Brief

Explain that lengthy communications tend to be a "turnoff" to many would-be listeners, which is the last reaction anyone wants to elicit when they are trying to be heard. Long communications tend to include irrelevant information that diverts attention from the main point. To make matters worse, much of this irrelevant information is emotionally-charged "old stuff" that upsets the listener and arouses his or her defenses. Those

IPs (or whomever else the message is directed toward) who manage to stay tuned in and calm for the duration will likely miss the point or will only hear a version of it that is prejudiced by their own strong reactions.

EXAMPLES

- *Problematic.* "I don't know what to do about you always coming home late. I worry and worry. I don't remember being late all the time when I was young and still living in my parents' home. We had rules. And I wasn't out drinking half the night every other day. Ya know, at the very least, it wouldn't kill you to call."
- *Improved.* "Could you agree to call me tonight if you're going to be out past midnight? That way, I won't have to worry about whether you're safe."
- *Problematic.* "I can't believe you didn't make those phone calls! What have you been doing all day? I don't ask you to help much with my business. Don't you want me to be successful? You're just like my mom. You agree to help, but then you somehow always end up being too busy, or you have to take your pills and lie down. I dealt with that *all* the time growing up. No thanks. I'll do it myself."
- *Improved.* "You didn't get a chance to make those calls? Do you have time to sit down now and get them started?"

2. Be Positive

Positive refers to the type of wording CSOs should use in a communication, whenever appropriate and feasible. It means *avoiding* blaming, name calling, and overgeneralizing at all costs. Communications delivered in accusatory tones are invariably met with defensiveness and arguments. Such defensiveness is much less likely to happen when CSOs rely on upbeat, positive wording. Using positive language also means stating things in a way that indicates what is *wanted* as opposed to what is *not wanted*. This emphasis appears to be particularly relevant for situations in which an individual is making a request or discussing a problem. Unfortunately, saying what is *not* wanted is a type of communication that is fairly typical for a person who is upset, frustrated, or angry. A negative interaction is almost guaranteed at such times, with the end result again being a defensive IP. The other distinct advantage to phrasing a request in terms of what is *wanted* is that IPs have a much better idea of what new behavior is expected to replace their old behavior. If CSOs only instruct their IPs to *stop* doing something, it is not always clear what should be done instead.

EXAMPLES

- *Problematic.* "I hate it when you get drunk and make an ass of yourself when we're out with friends."

- *Improved.* "It's nice socializing with you when you're sober, because your great sense of humor comes through."
- *Problematic.* "If I hear you whine like a spoiled brat one more time about wanting your own TV, I'm going to get rid of the one we have."
- *Improved.* "Let's sit down tonight and discuss some of the creative ideas you've come up with for earning money to get your own TV."

3. Refer to Specific Behaviors

State that vague requests often go unanswered. Explain how most IPs are, at best, ambivalent about (if not outright opposed to) giving CSOs what they want when it is even distantly associated with the substance use domain. Therefore it would not take much of an obstacle for an IP to passively "decide" not to bother doing anything. It is somewhat more difficult to make such a decision if an IP knows exactly what is being requested. Importantly, teach CSOs to refer to *behaviors* instead of thoughts or feelings, because an *observable* change is easier to detect, measure, and reinforce.

EXAMPLES

- *Problematic.* "You never lift a finger around the house. Can't you help out once in a while?"
- *Improved.* "I'd really appreciate it if you'd stack the dirty dishes in the sink every night after dinner."
- *Problematic.* "You said over a month ago that you'd get some help for your problem, but you haven't done a thing. You *need* help."
- *Improved.* "There's an AA meeting every night at 7 P.M. at the fire station down the street. Would you be willing to go with Bubba tomorrow night if he picks you up?"

4. Label Your Feelings

Invite CSOs to briefly describe their feelings to the IP when they are in reaction to the problem behavior being discussed. If feelings are stated in a calm, nonjudgmental, nonaccusatory way, IPs are more apt to hear them and empathize.

EXAMPLES

- *Problematic.* "Your inconsiderate behavior is driving me nuts. I'll be lucky if I don't have a nervous breakdown from the stress."
- *Improved.* "I get nervous and preoccupied when I see that the bills haven't been paid on time. I wonder if you could help me with them?"

- *Problematic.* "I have never been so humiliated in my entire life. How could you get high before meeting my parents?"
- *Improved.* "I was really embarrassed for both of us when you started laughing and talking really loudly to my parents at dinner."

5. Offer an Understanding Statement

Encourage CSOs to verbalize some understanding of the issue under discussion from their IP's perspective, even though it might be difficult to do so. The reason is simple: IPs are less likely to get defensive and more likely to listen if their CSO expresses empathy.

EXAMPLES

- *Problematic.* "I don't get it. I could think of a million fun things to do if I suddenly had more free time."
- *Improved.* "I bet at first it's going to be hard finding people who don't get high and who you actually enjoy spending time with."
- *Problematic.* "Well, what did you expect? Did you think I was going to keep letting the kids have dinner with you when you show up drunk every night?"
- *Improved.* "It must feel strange to not have the kids eat dinner with us, but I felt like I needed to do that for now while you're struggling."

6. Accept Partial Responsibility

Ask CSOs to take a close look at a problem situation to see if there is a small piece of it for which they can accept some of the responsibility. The purpose is to show IPs that their CSO is not simply interested in blaming them for problems, but instead is willing to consider their own role. This type of message is disarming to IPs and often helps them be less defensive and more open to discussion of the problem at hand. But be prepared: Some CSOs are likely to become angry or confused when you explain this component of a good communication. They may be unable to see beyond the many "disasters" resulting directly from the IP's substance use and consequently oppose any notion of taking responsibility for anything remotely associated with the IP. Explain that you ask CSOs to verbalize their partial responsibility because they are more likely to get what they want in the long run. In other words, their IP is more apt to be willing to communicate and work on problems. For those CSOs who remain unswayed, it might be a good time to remind them that it is not necessary to utilize all seven recommendations to create a positive conversation. They can certainly improve their current communication style by adding a few of the other components with which they feel more comfortable.

EXAMPLES

- *Problematic.* "How could you forget to call the repairman? We just talked about it last night!"
- *Improved.* "You didn't call the repairman? You know, when I got to work I was thinking that I should have left my checkbook out on the table at home as a reminder for you to call."
- *Problematic.* "I *knew* you weren't going to show up for our session. Why should you remember something as insignificant as that?"
- *Improved.* "I don't know why I didn't remind you about our session today; it's not like I didn't talk to you."

7. Offer to Help

Finally, encourage CSOs to make an offer to help their IP in some way with the problem under discussion. Although often it is worthwhile for CSOs to offer specific types of help, of their own choosing, it is also useful for CSOs to inquire generally, "How can I help?" IPs tend to experience offers of assistance as nonblaming, supportive acts, and so they are more inclined to respond positively.

EXAMPLES

- *Problematic.* "So I see that, once again, you have no will power; you drank the chilled bottle of wine I was saving for Saturday's party."
- *Improved.* "When I replace that bottle of wine I'd been saving for the party, maybe I should keep it at work until I'm ready to use it so it's not right out there tempting you."
- *Problematic.* "So you're stressed. Don't tell me you're going to use that as an excuse to get crazy and high."
- *Improved.* "How can I help?"

WHEN TO INTRODUCE COMMUNICATION SKILLS TRAINING

When employing a behavioral approach to treatment, not only do you need to know *how* to teach the requisite skills but *when* to introduce them. You must watch for a time when the client will benefit maximally from the training; a time when the CSO recognizes (at some level) a need for the skill because of a resultant problem she or he is currently facing. Sometimes you can directly observe communication deficits when CSOs participate in role plays in session. On other occasions clients essentially identify their own communication problem by reporting that they do not know how to ask for something, or are uncertain how to discuss a topic. And with others, the need for communication training becomes clear when reviewing the reasons for incomplete or unsuccessful homework assignments. In each of these circumstances you should immediately label and comment on the noted communication problem. If at all possible, proceed directly to communication skills training, using the real-life problem the CSO has presented as your illustrative example.

ILLUSTRATIVE CASE USING THE GUIDELINES FOR POSITIVE COMMUNICATION: ASSERTIVENESS PROBLEM

Two sample cases follow in which positive communication skills training is used. You will note an extensive reliance on role playing. If you do not routinely use role plays in your work, please refer to the section on "The Use of Role Plays" after the first sample case. In the cases themselves, note also the timing of when the communication training procedure is introduced, and the aspects of the guidelines chosen by the therapists to emphasize, given their particular clients' situation and needs. The first case example involves a wife (Tassie) as the CSO. Her husband, the IP, has a long history of polysubstance abuse. Although the CSO used to occasionally join in, she stopped using all drugs almost 2 years ago. Assume the CSO has attended three CRAFT sessions thus far. The conversation begins at the start of the fourth CSO session, with the wife reporting on her progress on an assignment to generate a list of small positive rewards that she can use to reinforce her husband when he is clean and sober (Chapter 6 describes this procedure):

THERAPIST: Tassie, how did the assignment go this week?

CSO: OK, I guess. I came up with a few things to use as rewards. But it was sort of upsetting because Marcello found my list and started making fun of me and my therapy. I didn't know what to say.

THERAPIST: I imagine it *would* be upsetting to have him put down the things you've been working so hard at. What *did* you say?

CSO: Nothing. I just left the room. But then I got annoyed with myself. Why don't I stick up for myself? It happens a lot. And I didn't feel like working on the list anymore after that.

THERAPIST: Sounds like this would be a good time to work on communi-cation skills—ways to help you say what you'd like to say, *and* in a way that Marcello can listen.

Note: The therapist sees this exchange as an ideal time to introduce positive communication skills training. Not only has the CSO identified a need, but it is clear that the CSO's unassertive behavior is interfering with her ability to complete her assignments. Given the problem identified, the therapist will emphasize assertiveness aspects of communication skills.

CSO: If you think it'll help. There are lots of times when I don't know what to say to him.

THERAPIST: How about if we start with the situation you just described? Let's redo your part of the experience using some positive communi-cation skills. Here's a list of seven points or guidelines for improving conversations. (*Hands CSO an index card resembling Figure 5.1.*) Let's just go over the list first, and then maybe you can tell me the ones you think you need help with. [Assume the therapist explains the "Guide-lines for Positive Communication Skills" and provides examples.] As you think back over some of the problems you've had talking to Marcello, do you see a good place to start?

CSO: Well, I know what I *don't* have trouble with: being brief! I hardly say anything at all when I'm upset with him. And I *do* tell him my feel-ings. But I'm not sure I talk about specific behaviors, like #3 suggests. I think I just sort of complain about things he does, in general.

THERAPIST: Then that's a good place to start. And I think it's great that you're already using some of the parts of a good conversation; you're being brief and you're labeling your feelings. Good for you!

Note: The therapist assesses the CSO's ability to identify her communica-tion strengths and weaknesses, and then takes the opportunity to rein-force her. He will decide for himself once he has observed her in a role play whether she needs assistance with some of these guidelines that she considers areas of strength. For instance, being brief (guideline 1) does not imply that the CSO should walk away and say nothing, which appar-ently she does on some occasions. Next he provides a brief description of the purpose and format of a role play, and then begins it himself.

THERAPIST: Now let's reenact the situation that happened this week when Marcello found your list of rewards. We'll do a role play, with me pre-tending to be Marcello. Pretend the conversation with him is actually happening again . . . *right now*, but this time, try responding to him differently. Feel free to refer to the guidelines on that card I gave you, as you try to add a few of the seven skills we just reviewed. Oh . . . and don't worry if I don't say exactly what your husband said—or would say. It will come across good enough to serve our purpose here, which is to allow you the chance to practice in a safe setting and to get specific feedback. I'll start it off. (*as Marcello*) What's this list? Don't tell me . . . are these ways for you to manipulate me? What has that therapist got you doing now? (*Laughs critically.*)

CSO: (*In role play*) I don't like it when you laugh at me. Maybe this seems funny to you, but it's important to me. (*To therapist*) I don't know what else to say.

THERAPIST: Fine. Let's stop the role play for a minute and see what we've got. Can you tell me the things you liked about your conversation? And then we can talk about what you might want to try differently next time.

Note: The therapist invites the client to highlight the positive aspects of the conversation first. He will then ask her to describe what area she needs to work on, before adding his own suggestions. Note that he will not identify all the weak points of the communication at once; instead, he will gradually add other suggestions if they do not occur naturally in the repeated role plays of the same conversation.

CSO: Like I said before, I'm usually brief and can say my feelings. But I tried adding #5 on the list: an understanding statement. It didn't feel very different, though. Maybe I'm not doing it right.

THERAPIST: Well, let's see what I come up with. You were definitely brief. I'm not sure you really expressed your feelings, though. You said that you didn't like it when he made fun of you, but you didn't really say *how* that felt. You made a really good effort overall, though.

Note: The therapist uses the "sandwich" technique for giving feedback: sandwiching constructive criticism in-between two positive comments.

CSO: I didn't tell him my feelings? Oh . . . you're right. I should have told him that it hurts my feelings or makes me feel put down when he laughs at me.

THERAPIST: Good. That's a feeling. For your understanding statement, you said, "I can see why this might seem funny to you." I bet you could come up with something that has a little more empathy in it; something that shows you're really trying to see things from his perspective. Your comment almost sounds sarcastic, doesn't it?

CSO: I hadn't thought of it that way, but I guess you're right. How about, "I know it must seem odd to have me doing things differently all of a sudden." Is that an understanding statement?

THERAPIST: That's a real good one. It sounds sincere. Can you put these all together now and give it another try?

Note: The therapist does not mention that the CSO never really answered the IP's question. He will see if this point is corrected naturally during the next role play.

THERAPIST: (*As Marcello*) Tassie, what in the world are you up to now? Don't tell me it's more "homework" from your therapist. (*Laughs sarcastically.*)

CSO: (*In role play*) Marcello, I guess this must seem strange to have me doing different things all of a sudden, but it hurts my feelings when you laugh at me.

THERAPIST: Tassie, that was good. Can you tell me what you liked about your conversation this time?

CSO: I talked about my feelings this time, and I tried not to sound sarcastic when I gave my understanding statement.

THERAPIST: You didn't. It was good. Are there things about it you'd like to change still?

CSO: I'm not sure. What do *you* think?

THERAPIST: I think it sounded much better. But I wonder if you're really answering his question about what you're doing. You said you were doing things differently, but you didn't say what it was. I'm not sure he really wanted to know, though. Was he just looking for a way to harass you, or do you think he was curious?

Note: The therapist does not want the CSO to miss a potential opportunity to explain CRAFT to her husband.

CSO: I'm not sure. I don't mind telling him what I'm doing. Actually, I got so upset at the time it really happened that I didn't see it as a chance to tell him about my assignment.

THERAPIST: Like I said, I'm not sure he wanted to know. It's something to think about if it happens again, though.

CSO: But what if I try to explain things to him and he just keeps laughing at me?

THERAPIST: That's a good question. He might. What would that be like for you if he did?

CSO: I guess, not any worse than it already is. I think it's worth trying.

Note: This is an important point, because although the chances of an appropriate response from the IP increase when the CSO's message is delivered in a positive manner, ultimately, the CSO cannot control the IP's reaction.

THERAPIST: OK, then. Let's try it again. Don't worry about adding anything new, unless maybe you want to explain more about your assignment. Let's just practice what you've been saying already.

Note: The therapist does not want to overwhelm the client by having her add too many new components to her conversation. At this point he simply is interested in having her practice a basic, good conversation within the session so that she is more likely to deliver it at home. He also uses each role play as an opportunity to slightly alter his portrayal of the husband's comments, so that the CSO can get practice in responding to a variety of statements.

THERAPIST: (*As Marcello*) What's this nonsense? Don't tell me this is part of your therapy again!

CSO: (*In role play*) As a matter of fact, it is. And it hurts my feelings when you call it "nonsense." I guess maybe it would seem a little silly to me, too, if I didn't see what went on during the therapy sessions. Hey, maybe it would help if I told you about it. Want to hear?

THERAPIST: Very nice job! Tassie, I can see that I'm working with a pro here. You just needed a little guidance. So what did you like about your conversation this time?

CSO: I think I gave a pretty good understanding statement. I'm not sure if I really gave my feelings, though. Maybe. I said he hurt them. And I was brief, sort of. I also tried to see if he really wanted to hear about my assignment. I didn't come right out and tell him, though. Was that OK?

THERAPIST: It was great! Like I said before, don't worry about saying things a specific way. Just try to add some of the suggested pieces from the guidelines to your conversation, but say them in a way that you're comfortable. Actually, by asking him if he wanted to hear about your assignment, you were offering to help—which is guideline 7—so you get bonus points. (*Laughs.*)

CSO: Well, I need them! I don't think I could add much more without it sounding too rehearsed.

THERAPIST: There's no need to add anything. And as far as whether you made your feelings clear enough when you said you felt "hurt," I think Marcello would get the message.

Note: Although the communication is not perfect, it is much improved over the original attempt and probably will result in a more positive reaction from the IP. The therapist does not encourage the CSO to add any more of the seven conversation components, because she appears to be incorporating as many as she can reasonably handle at the moment.

THERAPIST: Now, we just need to discuss what you think Marcello's reaction will be to this new type of communication. Hey, a good way to sort this out is to have you play Marcello and for me to play you in what we call a "reverse" role play. In playing you, I'll communicate in the way you just did so that you can imagine how Marcello would respond. If it's not the type of response you want, we may need to take another shot at the conversation. Then we'll finish up with an assignment for the week that's related to being assertive with your husband.

The therapist made a number of clinical decisions involving the communication training procedure illustrated in the dialogue, including (1) the determination of when to introduce it so that it would be most meaningful, (2) how many role plays to conduct, and (3) what level of competence to expect. The issue of selecting a suitable time to approach the IP was not emphasized, because the rehearsed conversation was intended to be in response to an IP remark.

THE USE OF ROLE PLAYS

As mentioned previously, in line with most behavioral or cognitive-behavioral treatments, CRAFT relies heavily on the use of role plays to teach communication skills (Monti et al., 2002; O'Farrell & Fals-Stewart, 2003; Smith, Meyers, & Milford, 2003; Spiegler & Guevremont, 2003). The notion of rehearsing conversations during sessions while playing the role of a client's spouse, parent, child, friend, or whomever, may seem antithetical to the basic clinical training of some therapists. Nevertheless, this format for communication skills acquisition is considered a critical component of CRAFT, and counselors are strongly encouraged to "sample" and then adopt role playing as part of their therapeutic style. Role plays provide a unique opportunity for you to observe and assess, firsthand, the CSOs' degree of communication abilities. Role plays also enable CSOs to practice difficult conversations in a safe environment and in a manner that allows for realistic feedback from the other person being role-played (by you). Finally, role plays present many opportunities for positive reinforcement, since clients improve with each repetition.

Advocates of behavioral rehearsal in the form of role plays usually adhere to a relatively common format. As the therapist, you:

- Have *CSOs describe* the problem situation and the anticipated IP reaction in some detail, so that your portrayal of the IP is experienced as believable.
- Ask CSOs to imagine that the situation is *actually happening* to increase the chance that they will converse in a natural fashion, and will feel the emotions that typically are associated with the scenario.
- *Model* the desired behavior by starting the role play conversation yourself, thereby making it easy for the CSOs to simply join in.
- Continue the role play for only a *brief* period of time, so that very specific feedback can be offered shortly after the CSOs' words are spoken.
- Invite *CSOs* to *comment first* on their performance, starting with what they liked about it, and finishing with what they think needs improvement.
- Have clients be as *specific* as possible with their own *observations*, thus enabling you to evaluate their understanding of their strengths and weaknesses.
- Provide your own *specific feedback*, at times using the *sandwich technique*: providing a positive remark, followed by constructive criticism, followed by another positive comment.
- *Repeat* the role play so that the client can practice incorporating the feedback, and you can present various possible IP reactions.
- Repeat the specific *feedback* component, again starting with the client.
- If necessary, *repeat the entire process again* until sufficient improvement is demonstrated.
- Assign *homework* related to the role-played communication and discuss the possibility that the IP might not respond as desired.

- ***Common Therapist Errors:*** Allowing the role-played conversation to run too long, providing only vague feedback, overwhelming the client with too much feedback, and failing to repeat the role play.

In most circumstances the individual who is most reluctant to participate in a role play is not the client but the therapist! This resistance stems from a variety of factors: lack of conviction about the value of role plays, low confidence in one's ability to "act" the part properly, or sheer embarrassment. You can test the value of role plays by trying a few with clients and seeing if their communication improves. The concerns about not being a good "actor" and the related self-consciousness tend to disappear with practice, as you learn that your acting skill is really inconsequential. Yet, therapists are not *always* alone in their resistance to engage in role plays, as some clients initially are wary about participating as well. For the most part, this wariness can readily be addressed by reviewing the purpose of the role play and then by simply starting in. Clients always respond; albeit, at times they need to be encouraged to converse as if the situation were actually happening at that very moment, instead of talking *about* the situation and how they *would* react. In other words, remind the client to stay in the role.

REVERSE ROLE PLAYS

The dialogue between Tassie and her therapist ended with the therapist preparing to start a reverse role play. In CRAFT a reverse role play means the therapist plays the part of the CSO, and the CSO plays the IP. What purpose does a reverse role play serve? When CSOs put themselves in their IP's role in a situation, they gain a sense of how their own real-life communication would be experienced by the IP and the types of problematic reactions that might arise. These anticipated difficulties can then be addressed: The CSOs might slightly alter the wording of their comments, perhaps to emphasize a point better or to decrease the chances of inciting an argument. In the opposite direction, the decision that a particular area of conflict is unsafe to tackle due to a predictably violent reaction by the IP, might emerge from a reverse role play.

As an example of a moderate reaction, assume in the sample case that Tassie discovered, in the course of playing Marcello's part, that the critical feature regarding how he received her assertive comments was his mood at the time. If Marcello often were in an irritable mood when he directed his demeaning remarks to her (irritable mood defined by the CSO as making negative comments about a variety of topics, frowning continually, not joking around), a reverse role play might have helped Tassie realize it would be best to postpone the bulk of the conversation at such a time. So she might simply tell him her feelings were hurt by his comment and that she would discuss it with him later. When he later appeared to be in a better mood, she could refer back to his negative comment and offer her rehearsed assertive response. Although Tassie may have understood the importance of selecting an opportune time for approaching her husband by discussing it with her therapist, the impact tends to be more pronounced if a client experiences the value of timing during a role play. Another important benefit of reverse role plays, in general, is that CSOs tend to experience empathy for the IP during the exercise, as they gain a more vivid appreciation of the IP's own perspective in their struggle. This empathy is particularly helpful for CSOs who are extremely angry with their IPs.

ILLUSTRATIVE CASE USING THE GUIDELINES
FOR POSITIVE COMMUNICATION: MAKING A REQUEST

This second case involves a 45-year-old son (CSO) who is learning how to make a request of his 70-year-old widowed father (IP). The son (John) visits his father about three times a week. The father has a longstanding alcohol problem that is substantially contributing to an overall decline in health. He has never been amenable to treatment. Assume this is the middle of the second CSO session. The therapist just asked John to identify some nondrinking, pleasurable activities that his father was already participating in, to some degree, or which he used to enjoy. She told John that his task was to encourage and support his father's selection of these activities over drinking, such as by suggesting the activities or by accompanying him to the event. The dialogue begins with John's reaction to the request for a list of pleasurable activities:

CSO: As far as fun activities he does now that don't involve alcohol . . . hmmmm . . . I can't think of any. There are a lot of things my dad *used* to enjoy doing, but he stopped most of them when my mom died. He really used to like golfing and fishing. He hasn't done either of them in years, though. I wouldn't even know how to suggest them. When I've made suggestions in the past, he's told me to stop trying to control his life.

THERAPIST: Well, we've got two issues here: whether these activities are good ones to try to get him to sample again, and if so, when and how to present the suggestion to him. So you say he always really enjoyed fishing and golfing?

Note: First the therapist tries to determine how reinforcing these activities are for the IP, which is a critical factor if they are going to compete with drinking. If they are promising reinforcers, she will opt to focus on them, despite the fact that they are not ongoing activities. Typically ongoing activities are preferable, since it is often easier to increase their frequency than to introduce a new one (Chapter 6 provides a detailed explanation of this procedure).

CSO: Yup. He'd golf and fish every week. I think it relaxed him. Part of it was the good friends who went along. But they've either moved out of town or are too sick to get out now. I wouldn't mind going with him, but like I said, he tells me to butt out when I try to get involved.

THERAPIST: As we discussed before, part of his lack of interest in things might have to do with him being depressed. Still, we might be able to influence his reaction to you if we work on the way you make your request. How about if we talk about ways to invite your dad to go fishing or golfing?

Note: The therapist decides to focus on these particular pleasurable activities because they apparently have a history of being reinforcing for the father. She also plans to use this opportunity to teach positive communication skills, if the CSO's self-reported need for assistance proves to be valid when observed in a role play.

CSO: It wouldn't hurt to talk about it. I seem to have a knack for upsetting him these days.

THERAPIST: I can't promise that your dad won't get upset once you've learned a new way to talk to him, but we can at least decrease the chances that he will. So pick the activity: golf or fishing? It's good to pick one that's fun for you too.

CSO: Fishing. I have fond memories of him taking me fishing as a kid.

THERAPIST: Fine. Go ahead and pretend that I'm your dad. Ask me to go fishing with you, like you normally would. That way I can get an idea of what your dad might be reacting to, and what we should work on. Make believe you've just come over to my house, and it's a good time to talk. Pretend you're really having this conversation with your dad right now. I'll start it off. And don't worry if I don't say things exactly like your father would. Just try to stay in the role. (*As father*): Hey, John. How ya doin'?

CSO: (*In role play*) Great, Dad. How about you?

THERAPIST: (*As father*) Not too bad, all things considered.

CSO: (*In role play*) Ya mean, like considering the booze? Ummm. Nope, I'm not going to mention that anymore. OK. So, Dad, I know you've heard me say this a million times before, but I think you need to get out more. How about we do a little fishing?

THERAPIST: (*As father*) What? What are you talking about? What does fishing have to do with my drinking?

CSO: (*To therapist*) I think I need help already. I can hear him asking something like that.

THERAPIST: OK. This is a good place to stop anyway. John, in looking back at your conversation, what do you like about what you said?

CSO: I came right out and said what was on my mind. And I know he listened, because he answered me back about it.

THERAPIST: Yes, he did hear you. But I wonder if he would have agreed to go fishing. That's the outcome you're really looking for, right?

CSO: Yes. Hmmmm. I don't know if he'd agree to go. It didn't sound too promising. As a matter of fact, it sounded a lot like our conversations always do.

THERAPIST: Can you take a look at what you said and figure out what needs some polishing yet?

Note: Being uncertain of John's communication skills, the therapist decided to obtain a sample by having him do a role play without first explaining the Guidelines for Positive Communication Skills. She invited John to evaluate his own performance before offering feedback herself. She made sure he first commented on the positive aspects of his conversation before moving to the parts requiring improvement.

CSO: Maybe I shouldn't have brought up the booze at all. It was habit. I know he doesn't like it when I mention it.

THERAPIST: You're probably right. And in playing your dad, I can say that it automatically got me defensive, and even annoyed, when you started off with a negative comment.

CSO: It did? Yeh, I guess I can see that. What did the rest of it feel like?

THERAPIST: To tell you the truth, as soon as you made the comment about the booze, I only half-listened to the rest because I was annoyed. And being annoyed, I didn't feel like agreeing to do *any-thing* with you. But I *did* get the feeling you cared about me, because why else would you want to take me fishing?

Note: The therapist tries to balance the constructive criticism with some positive remarks.

CSO: So I made you mad? And as soon as you were mad, the rest didn't really matter?

THERAPIST: Not as far as getting me to go fishing.

Note: One advantage of role plays is that you can describe your reactions to the CSO's comments that might be experienced by the real IP. These are then factored in when determining how to improve the conversation. The valuable message for this CSO is that starting a conversation with negative remarks (especially general ones that are irrelevant to the topic at hand) sets the listener up to respond defensively. The battle has already been lost at this point.

THERAPIST: So based on this feedback, what do you think you'd do differently next time?

CSO: For starters, I'd skip the booze comment. I know it doesn't help. I just get frustrated, I guess.

THERAPIST: That's totally understandable. But keep in mind what you're trying to accomplish; namely, to get your dad to do fun, healthy things with you. You're more likely to accomplish this if you hold off expressing those frustrated feelings to him. It doesn't mean you have no right to feel frustrated, just that there will be better times and ways to talk with him about it.

Note: The therapist validates the CSO's feelings while, at the same time, pointing out that he has much to gain by waiting for a more suitable time and developing a more agreeable manner to express them.

CSO: You're right. I just have to remind myself before I go to see him.

THERAPIST: John, before we redo the role play, I'd like to go over some guidelines for conversations that I think you'll find helpful. (*Explains the Guidelines for Positive Communication Skills, provides examples, and hands him the card resembling Figure 5.1.*) Which of these things would you like to try doing in your conversation with your dad?

CSO: Like #3 says, I could be more specific about what I'm asking him to do. Maybe he'd be tempted to go if I said exactly when and where I wanted to take him fishing.

THERAPIST: Now you're talking! Yes, I bet he'd be tempted. Not only does the *where* bring an enticing picture to mind, but the *when* makes the invitation much more real. It's not a vague, general offer anymore. Good. Shall we try that, or would you like to add something else?

CSO: Let's see. We talked about #2 already. I'm *not* going to start off saying anything negative about his drinking. And I'm going to give him more details about the fishing. I could add one small thing still. What's this "partial responsibility" thing again?

THERAPIST: Accepting partial responsibility means taking a little bit of the responsibility for the problem you're discussing. It *doesn't* mean you're taking responsibility for your dad's drinking problem. In this situation, maybe you could take partial responsibility for him being reluctant to go.

Note: It is common for CSOs to question or react to the statement about partial responsibility (guideline 6), because they immediately assume it means taking responsibility for the IP's substance abuse problem. As mentioned, that is not the intended use of this suggested conversation enhancer. Instead, the CSO should accept responsibility for a small piece of a different problem currently being addressed.

CSO: Partial responsibility for dad being reluctant to go . . . Hmmmm. I could say that I don't blame him for thinking twice about agreeing to go, since I usually spoil it by bringing up his drinking when we're together for any length of time. Of course, then I'd have to promise I wouldn't do that, or he'd never go.

THERAPIST: Keeping that promise would be important because, remember, the activity is supposed to be fun for him so that it competes with his drinking. If he doesn't have fun, he won't want to do it again.

CSO: That makes sense. Sure, I could try hard not to mention alcohol.

THERAPIST: You know, John, you've hit the jackpot with your idea about accepting partial responsibility. If you say what you've just told me, you're actually doing a lot more than just accepting partial responsibility. Look at these last three guidelines and tell me what else you're doing. You said you wouldn't blame him for not wanting to go, since you often end up talking about his drinking. And then you said you'd tell him you wouldn't bring up the topic this time. What does it sound like you did *besides* take partial responsibility for the problem?

CSO: According to this list (*Refers to index card*), it looks like I made an understanding statement. Is that what you mean?

THERAPIST: Yes, that's a big part of it. And when you said you wouldn't bring up the topic during the fishing trip, what did that sound like?

CSO: An offer to help?

THERAPIST: Definitely! You're much better at this than you realized.

Note: The therapist would never have urged the CSO to add this many changes (guidelines 5–7) to his original conversation, but he happened upon them naturally. The therapist knew that John did not realize he had incorporated so many of the guidelines, so she helped him discover this rather than just pointing it out. Next she will ask him to synthesize and practice delivering as many of these points as comfortably possible for him, and then she will offer feedback.

THERAPIST: OK. Now it's time to put these ideas together and practice saying them in round 2 of our role play. Don't worry if you can't incorporate all of them. Remember, adding any of them will help. So here I go as your dad again. (*As father*) Hey, John, it's good to see you. What's up?

CSO: (*In role play*) Dad, I was wondering if you'd like to go fishing with me this Saturday morning. We could go to that spot you really like upstream—Fawn's Leap. I promise I won't even say anything about how you drink too much.

THERAPIST: (*As father*) You and that darn drinking talk. Well, I'm not sure. (*Pauses.*) I haven't been fishing in a long time. I don't even know where my equipment is. It sounds like too much of a hassle.

CSO: (*In role play*) Aw . . . come on, Dad. It'll be fun. If you don't want to bother looking for your stuff, I can loan you some of mine. Or I'll help you look for yours, and we can see what kind of shape it's in.

THERAPIST: (*As father*) I don't know. Give me a day to think about it.

CSO: (*In role play*) All right.

THERAPIST: Phew! You were working hard, John. Good job. Tell me what you liked about your conversation this time.

CSO: Well, I know what I *didn't* like! I couldn't even get *you* to agree to go. How am I ever going to get my dad to say "yes"?

THERAPIST: I was trying not to make it too easy. I was trying to act like I thought he might. But the important thing for now is to look at what *did* seem to work well and what might still need our attention.

CSO: I know. It's just that you sounded so much like my dad, it made me wonder if I'll ever be successful.

THERAPIST: Well, I can't guarantee that he'll ever say "yes" to fishing, but I *can* guarantee that your conversations with him will improve. You've already gotten a lot better. And even if the fishing never happens, maybe you'll be able to get him to do some other nondrinking activity with you. That's what's really important anyway.

Note: The therapist encourages John to focus on the positive aspects of his improved conversation first. She then praises his efforts, acknowledges his feelings, and reminds him of the main purpose of the exercise.

CSO: Well, I thought I added a few good things to my opening line; things that we talked about. Let's see. I was specific about the fishing. I said we'd go Saturday morning, and I picked one of his favorite fishing spots.

THERAPIST: You were very specific. That was excellent. Could you tell how I, as your dad, was reacting to your suggestion?

CSO: I thought you were a little interested. But you kept coming up with excuses, and I wasn't sure how to handle them.

THERAPIST: You're right. I *was* interested. You made it sound tempting. But since we think your dad is somewhat depressed, I figured he wouldn't agree right away to do it. That's where the excuses came in. What else did you like about your conversation this time?

CSO: I didn't start out with that negative comment about alcohol.

THERAPIST: John, you certainly did a lot better in that area this second time around, but I noticed that you still referred to my drinking in a somewhat negative way. Maybe it's a minor point, but I felt myself reacting when you said you *weren't* going to mention how I drank too much. I know you meant *while* we were fishing you weren't going to mention it, but it already felt like you were getting a dig in right there. You were already mentioning it. But like I said, it *was* much better than your first attempt.

Note: The therapist uses the sandwich technique for offering feedback.

CSO: But how do I offer to help if I don't say that I'm not going to do that?

THERAPIST: That's a real good question. I think you can keep it positive by saying what you *will* talk about, instead of what you're trying to avoid. For example, you could say you promise to keep the conversation "light", or that you're only going to discuss sports—something along those lines.

CSO: That's cool. I can do that. I just have to think about it at the time.

Note: The therapist points out John's violation of guideline 2: to be positive. Although this particular communication problem is not John's most serious one, it is still one that could affect his father's reaction to his invitation.

THERAPIST: How about the other points you were going to add? Did you give an understanding statement and accept partial responsibility?

CSO: I meant to. I thought I did it right along with the offer to help. At least, I did when I told you about it a few minutes ago.

THERAPIST: You seemed to say it a bit differently this time, which is fine. Earlier you said you wouldn't blame him if he didn't want to go— which is an understanding statement—and you tied that understanding in with accepting partial responsibility by saying that you usually brought up his drinking. These points got a little blurred this time, and you went straight to your offer to help. That's fine, though. As I said before, you don't need to add *all* of these suggested comments. I just want to make sure you recognize what you *are* and *are not* saying in here, so that you can decide if it's what you want to say out there, when you actually face your dad. By the way, you gave multiple offers to help: You also told him you'd help him find his equipment or you'd lend your own.

CSO: I suppose I did. Ya know, I just got nervous and forgot some of the stuff we talked about.

THERAPIST: That's why we need to keep practicing it. You're less likely to leave out important parts if you've gone over the points repeatedly in here. It sometimes helps to go home and practice it with somebody else first, as well. How about your wife? Could you explain to her what you're trying to do, and then do some role plays with her?

CSO: Sure. She'd go along with it. She's worried about my dad, too.

THERAPIST: Good. Let's try it once more here. Then we'll come up with an assignment that involves practicing with your wife, before you try it out on your dad. And we still have to talk about the best time to actually have this conversation with him.

The therapist did not conduct a reverse role play because John seemed to know how his dad would respond, and he was not worried about his father having any type of exaggerated reaction to the new communication. However, if the CSO continued to insert negative drinking remarks into his role-played conversations, the therapist would have asked John to play his father's part so he could experience the impact of those negative comments. The need to modify the communication would be apparent at that point.

POSITIVE COMMUNICATION ASSIGNMENTS

How would you develop a communication homework assignment and what would it sound like for the CSOs in these two cases just discussed? The process of constructing the assignment would differ slightly, depending on whether you had already shown your client the Goals of Counseling form (Chapter 8, pp. 224–225) and its basic guidelines for formulating behavior change strategies. If not, *and* there was insufficient time remaining in the session to do so, then you would simply help the CSO narrow down an assignment that adhered to the Goals of Counseling rules without explaining them at the time.

For example, John's therapist had already decided, on the basis of John's anxiety and skill level, that the first step of the positive communication homework assignment would be a trial run with John's wife. John would set aside a time when he could explain role plays and the value of their feedback to his wife. He would then run through the same kind of scenario as was practiced in the session, with his wife playing the role of his father. She would be asked to supply constructive, supportive feedback after each role play. After rehearsing the scene (with varied endings) at least three times, John would visit his father at a predetermined time, when he was most apt to be sober and in a pleasant mood. If his father was indeed sober, John would begin the practiced conversation about a fishing trip. The final step would be to take the father on the trip. If the father refused to go, this last step instead would be to generate a list of alternative enjoyable activities for John and his father.

In the earlier case of Tassie and her newly acquired assertiveness skills, the specifics of the assignment would depend on what she hoped to accomplish by the assertive communication, and her skill level. The simplest option would be for Tassie to sit down with her husband and revisit the topic she had been rehearsing in the session; namely, responding to his sarcastic remarks about her therapy. In this case a lead-in line that referred back to the prior day's conversation, would need to be added to the already rehearsed segment. Since Tassie determined that Marcello's mood had a sizeable impact on how he reacted to her comments, she first would be asked to assess Marcello's mood after dinner that evening (or some specific time later that week). If he was not irritable, she would ask him whether it was a good time to discuss something. If he agreed to listen, she would offer her rehearsed, assertive response while referring to the earlier interaction. Alternatively, if he said it was an inopportune time to talk, she would ask him to commit to a specific time in the next day or two for the conversation.

Assume Tassie decided that she did not want to resurrect the earlier conversation and instead wished to respond to her husband's *next* sarcastic comment about her therapy. In this case you would rehearse additional role plays to prepare Tassie to generalize her assertive response to other mocking comments her husband might make. If she were quite certain that Marcello would make a critical comment about her therapy in the upcoming week, for example, Tassie's assignment would be to give her assertive response the next time this verbal onslaught occurred. On the other hand, if the frequency of these sarcastic comments were low, conceivably she might not have the opportunity to complete her assignment. In this case the back-up plan might be for Tassie to offer to tell him about her therapy some time before her next session. Naturally, you would rehearse this conversation in advance in role plays as well, and the timing for delivering this message would be discussed. As with all assignments, you would inquire about the outcome in the next session and resolve any problems (as described in Chapter 7).

SUMMARY

This chapter presents the reasons for teaching CSOs communication skills and offers guidelines to follow in doing so. The importance of conducting role plays to allow CSOs the opportunity to practice the skills is stressed, as is the need to offer feedback in a supportive and informative manner. Sample homework assignments that emphasize applying newly learned positive communication skills are supplied. Later chapters draw upon these same communication skills when describing how to teach CSOs more advanced procedures.

FIGURE 5.1. SAMPLE INDEX CARD FOR COMMUNICATION ASSIGNMENTS

Guidelines for Positive Communication Skills

1. Be *brief.*
2. Be *positive.*
3. Refer to specific *behaviors.*
4. Label your *feelings.*
5. Offer an *understanding* statement.
6. Accept *partial responsibility.*
7. Offer to *help.*

CHAPTER 6

POSITIVE REINFORCEMENT OF CLEAN AND SOBER BEHAVIOR

According to behavioral principles, an activity or behavior that is positively reinforced or "rewarded" will be repeated. Unfortunately, a prime example of this learned behavior, for some individuals, is drinking or using drugs. Many IPs continue to engage in this behavior because it is experienced as positive. This positive experience may take the form of enjoyable physical sensations or emotions or involvement in gratifying social situations that go hand-in-hand with the using behavior. Theoretically, positively reinforcing the IP's *non*drinking or *non*-drug-using behavior should increase it—which is precisely one of the objectives of CRAFT. And as these non-substance-abusing behaviors increase, they tend to compete with the old unhealthy (substance-abusing) ones for time in the IP's schedule.

PRESENTING THE CONCEPT
OF POSITIVE REINFORCEMENT TO THE CSO

Any object or behavior whose presentation increases the behavior that it follows is a positive reinforcer (Malott & Trojan Suarez, 2004; Spiegler & Guevremont, 2003). You would modify this definition slightly for a CSO and instead state:

> "A *positive reinforcer (a reward)* is something that is experienced as pleasurable by an individual, thereby making the individual interested in repeating the behavior that got him or her the reward in the first place."

Often it is helpful first to mention a universal reinforcer, such as money. Explain how a paycheck strengthens peoples' resolve to go to work each day, because daily work is required in order to earn that paycheck. Then introduce the idea of the abused substance (alcohol, drugs) as an example of a positive reinforcer (albeit, an unhealthy one). Point out that alcohol or drugs are rewarding to some people simply because of the way they make them feel, and consequently these individuals keep using them. Remind the CSOs that you touched upon this idea earlier when you did the functional analysis (Figure 3.1, column 4). Ask the CSOs to try to remember the already covered positive (i.e., rewarding) aspects of the alcohol or drug use for their IP that appear responsible for maintaining those abusive behaviors. Encourage CSOs to guess about additional rewards. As noted, in response, clients sometimes mistakenly list the negative consequences of their IP's use, since these are prominent in the CSOs' minds. If this occurs, explain that while all of those negative consequences may be accurate, IPs definitely find positive aspects to the alcohol or drug use, or it would not be repeated so often. Ask the CSOs to imagine what *their IP* would say in response to the question about the rewards associated with substance use. If additional prompting is required, you might give several common examples:

- Pot makes him feel mellow, relaxed.
- Alcohol increases her sex drive.
- A few drinks make him feel more skilled in a social setting.
- Heroin allows her to feel an immediate and intense euphoria.

It is not unusual for CSOs to mix in examples of what are technically the *negatively* reinforcing aspects of drugs; namely, drugs serving to *remove* something *aversive*, such as feelings of sadness, guilt, or physical pain (Monti et al., 2002; Pierce & Epling, 1995; Spiegler & Guevremont, 2003). Although you are going to focus on positive reinforcement practices, there is no reason to point out this distinction, as long as the CSOs basically understand that a reinforcer increases a behavior. If the issue has not already been raised, discuss how the substance-using behavior is often rewarded in ways other than its direct chemical reaction, such as by getting other people to take care of temporarily incapacitated IPs. Then introduce the idea of a loving CSO rewarding the IP's *non*drinking/*non*-drug-using behavior and demonstrate how the same principles apply. Remind the client that a positive reinforcer increases the occurrence of the behavior it follows and therefore it should increase the frequency of clean and sober behavior if delivered properly.

"BUT ISN'T THIS 'ENABLING'?"

It is fairly common for CSOs to express some initial concern about, or even outright opposition to, the idea of rewarding the IP's nonusing behavior. Inevitably, clients think back to all the times they have been criticized by others for doing nice things for their IP. Directives to "stop being an enabler" ring loudly in their ears. Point out that you are not asking them to "enable" their IP to use; on the contrary, you only want them to reward the IP's *non*-substance-using behaviors. This distinction between which types of behavior should and should not be rewarded is extremely important and it is wise to devote a fair amount of time to covering it. Sometimes CSOs who understand the distinction are still uncomfortable with the notion of positively reinforcing the IP's nonusing behavior. They argue that they have already gone out of their way, time and again, for the IP, and that it has not helped. Furthermore, they do not see why they must continue being the ones who "give," since the IP has been "taking" for so long. It is essential for you to be supportive at these times and to acknowledge these feelings. At the same time, remind the clients that the objective is *not* to prod them to deliver additional random acts of kindness, but instead, to use carefully planned and systematically executed rewarding acts in response to *non*-using behavior. Also, simply ask the CSOs if they would be willing to "sample" these new reactions to the IP for a short time, since the ultimate payoff is what the clients want: an increase in the nonusing behaviors and a decrease in the using behaviors. CSOs tend to agree to at least a trial period.

GENERATING A LIST
OF REASONABLE POSITIVE REINFORCERS

Once CSOs have agreed to provide positive reinforcement for non-substance-using behavior, it is important to help them generate a list of reasonable, effective reinforcers. Preface the procedure by telling CSOs that *they* know their loved one better than anyone else does, and consequently, they are in a unique position to do this. Since CSOs often assume that the reward must be a store-bought material gift of some sort, it is useful to offer examples of social or activity rewards (Spiegler & Guevremont, 2003):

- Relaxing with the IP while listening to the IP's favorite music.
- Doing one of the IP's chores.
- Expressing warm feelings for the IP.
- Agreeing to watch a TV show that the IP wants to see.
- Making an effort to talk about topics that the IP enjoys discussing.
- Complimenting the IP.
- Preparing the IP a special meal.
- Gently squeezing the IP's hand.

Next present the guidelines for the reinforcer listed in Table 6.1 (Spiegler & Guevremont, 2003). After presenting and discussing these guidelines, encourage the CSO to begin the list, keeping in mind that the rewards will be delivered *only when the IP is clean and sober.* Once the preliminary list is completed, glance through the Guidelines for Reinforcers to be sure that these potential rewards meet the necessary requirements. For example, item 1 states that the reward should be experienced as pleasurable by the IP. A common error is for CSOs to assume that their IP's reinforcers are the same as their own reinforcers. You can check on this point by asking clients to rate each "reward" for its reinforcing value in the manner they believe their IP would rate it. Using a scale with instructions is often helpful the first time you introduce this concept:

"Read down the list of reinforcers you came up with and think about each reward the way you think your loved one would. Using the scale below, rate each item on your list the way you think _____ [IP] would rate it for *pleasure.*"

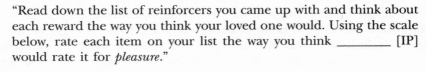

1 ——————— 2 ——————— 3 ——————— 4 ——————— 5
Very little pleasure   Moderate pleasure   Tremendous pleasure

The main point of the exercise is to assure that the CSO has truly considered whether the suggested "rewards" are, in fact, reinforcing to the IP. This is a critical issue because if they are not reinforcing, then they certainly are not going to increase the nonusing behavior they will be scheduled to follow (Spiegler & Guevremont, 2003). Quickly review the ratings and discuss with the client whether those with low pleasure ratings are apt to work well. If a large number of the "reinforcers" is rated low, modifications may be required. For example, if a CSO's highest rating is a '3,' ask what it would take to make that reward a "5" to the IP. Rather then checking for adherence to the remaining reinforcer guidelines (i.e., items 2–4) for the CSO's entire list of proposed reinforcers, ask the CSO to narrow down the list to one or

---

TABLE 6.1. GUIDELINES FOR REINFORCERS

The list of reinforcers should contain objects/ behaviors/comments/activities that are:

1. *pleasurable* for the IP.

2. *inexpensive*, if not free.

3. *available* to deliver immediately.

4. *comfortable* for the CSO to deliver.

two rewards to use in the upcoming week. Only for these selected rewards would you fully explore their appropriateness.

ILLUSTRATIVE CASE OF A CSO SELECTING AN APPROPRIATE IP REINFORCER

The dialogue that follows illustrates how a therapist might discuss a reward's value and overall suitability, and why it is important to do so. The conversation takes place between a therapist and a female CSO at the time of her final selection of a reward for her husband (IP):

THERAPIST: Good job, Denise. You've come up with a long list of possible rewards for Bernard, and you've narrowed it down to one that you want to use this week. Now I'm going to check it against those Guidelines for Reinforcers that I showed you earlier. You say that you are going to join Bernard in the living room to watch a TV show at 8:00 on the nights that he doesn't smoke pot this week. You said that about twice a week he skips his pot-smoking hour in the garage after work and instead lifts weights in the basement, with music blaring. So you'll really be rewarding him for choosing weightlifting over pot smoking, and from what I gather, he enjoys the workout, so that will help. Excellent. Now, you're pretty sure he'll want you to join him to watch TV?

Note: The therapist checks on item 1 of the Guidelines for Reinforcers: that the "reward" is truly a reinforcer for the IP. Items 2 and 3 will be addressed next.

CSO: Yes. He's always trying to get me to watch TV with him at night, but I don't like to sit there with him if he's high.

THERAPIST: Good. That sounds like something that will stand out as special. Now as far as the other characteristics of a good reward, it's definitely free. And I bet it's readily available when you need to use it, because you already said that you're both home most evenings. I guess my only concern is that it's not being given right after the workout. It might work better if it is.

Note: Rewards usually are more effective when presented immediately after the behavior being reinforced. When practical constraints prevent this contiguity, a verbal explanation of the reason for the reward becomes even more important.

CSO: But our son doesn't go to bed before 8:00, so that would be impossible.

THERAPIST: OK. We'll track this point to see if the delay in delivering the reward turns out to be a problem. It means you'll probably end up having to tell him relatively soon what you're doing, so that he definitely sees the connection. But you would have done that eventually anyway. We'll practice that conversation in here first though.

CSO: Phew! I'm relieved. I'm not exactly sure how I'd tell him what I'm up to.

THERAPIST: Don't worry. We'll go over that. And as I mentioned before, we'll also talk about how you'll want to make sure he's not high before you deliver the reward.

Note: These two issues are addressed later in this chapter.

THERAPIST: Let's see. Item 4: How would you feel about offering this as a reward? Would you be comfortable watching TV with him?

CSO: I really don't like watching TV that much. Is that what you mean by "being comfortable"?

THERAPIST: That's part of it. *Comfortable* means that you don't feel uneasy, for any reason, as you imagine yourself delivering the reward. Part of this process also involves picking a reward that you're not opposed to in some big way. For one thing, I'm trying to get you to respond to his nonsmoking behavior with activities that the two of you might want to keep doing together in the future. So if you already know that you aren't going to enjoy it, it's probably best not to introduce it now. You're not going to want to keep doing it, if it's not fun for you too, right?

Note: If the behavior is not at least minimally reinforcing for the CSO, she is not likely to repeat it. Furthermore, she is more apt to feel resentful if she does not enjoy the activity, and this resentment could interfere with a positive presentation of the reinforcer.

CSO: I see what you're saying. TV is not my favorite thing, but I think it's mostly because I associate it with having to deal with Bernard when he's high. I mean, when he's sitting in front of the TV stoned, he tries to talk to me about . . . nonsense. Maybe that's the part I don't like.

THERAPIST: Can you think of any times when you've watched TV with Bernard when he wasn't high? What was that like?

Note: The therapist decides to further pursue the TV watching as a potential reward, because it seems to be a good reinforcer for the IP in other ways.

CSO: I've definitely watched TV with him when he wasn't high. I'm sure it was OK. I wouldn't mind trying it. I think the real problem is him going on and on while I'm sitting with him.

THERAPIST: So there were probably *some* decent times when you watched TV with him, and those were times when he wasn't bothering you by talking nonsense. Well, since now you'd only be watching TV with him if he hadn't been smoking, do you think there's a good chance that he wouldn't be talking nonsense?

CSO: Probably. He only gets that way when he's high.

THERAPIST: OK. So it's still worth a try. Let's talk next about when and how to do it.

Although it did not occur in this case, in the course of discussing reinforcers it is common for CSOs to report that they already had tried a specific potential reinforcer, and that it did not work. In exploring such a conclusion, in most cases you discover that the CSO did not systematically deliver the reinforcer in the way that was necessary for it to be effective. For example, if Denise insisted that she already tried joining her husband for television viewing and it did not "work," it is likely that the IP was not "clean" each time she did this. Or, the content and style of her communication during those times may not have been positive and therefore were not experienced by Bernard as reinforcing. It is also possible that the husband did not make the connection between being "clean" and getting a reward. These crucial features of reward delivery must be highlighted for the CSO in advance.

Prior to concluding the discussion of a reward, it is worthwhile to encourage CSOs to select one "backup" reinforcer in the event that obstacles are encountered when attempting to deliver the chosen reward (explained in "Potential Complications When Delivering Reinforcers" later in this chapter). For example, assume Denise anticipated an occasional "emergency" at her mother's house that would prevent her from reinforcing her husband by watching television with him on a day when he had worked out. The CSO could plan to deliver a substitute reinforcer when she returned home (e.g., a cold glass of iced tea, a back-rub, a caring word) while explaining the link between the kind act and the IP's abstinence that day.

IDENTIFYING ONGOING NONUSING ACTIVITIES TO REWARD

In most cases it is difficult for a CSO to decide upon a specific reinforcer for the IP without some consideration of the IP behavior to be reinforced.

Naturally, it goes without saying that the IP's behavior must be alcohol/ drug-free. And although almost any drug-free behavior is suitable to reinforce, it is highly preferable to reward one that the IP finds pleasurable, since there is a greater chance then that the IP will choose it over the substance use in the future. This healthier behavior is also much more likely to be chosen if it directly competes with the substance use in terms of when it occurs and the function it serves. Additionally, the identified behavior should already be occurring sufficiently often so that the CSO has the opportunity to selectively reinforce it in the course of a week. Finally, if the behavior chosen for reinforcement is an activity that the CSO plans to participate in, along with the IP, it should be one that the CSO enjoys as well, because it is then more apt to be supported consistently by the CSO.

Some CSOs cannot decide upon a behavior to reinforce because they are never sure whether or not their loved one has been using. In response to this problem, you would work with the CSO to become aware of signs of IP use ("Recognizing Signs of Substance Use" is presented later in this chapter). Other clients state that it is extremely difficult to find a time when their IP is not under the influence. These CSOs are given the assignment of carefully monitoring their loved one's behavior for a few days, so that they can detect even small periods of time when he or she is drug free. Yet another complication occurs when CSOs cannot think of any *ongoing,* enjoyable IP activity. Although it is easier to increase the frequency of an already ongoing activity, as opposed to persuading an IP to try a new one, the latter is attempted, if necessary.

More often, CSOs are able to volunteer an IP behavior to reinforce, but the behavior is not ideally suited for a variety of reasons. In collaboration with the CSO, routinely check the suggested behavior against a list of characteristics for an ideal reinforcing behavior (see Table 6.2). Emphasize that *ideal* characteristics comprise the list and that there are acceptable IP behaviors to reinforce that do not necessarily satisfy *all* of these conditions.

In regard to the case just presented, Denise automatically identified a healthy *behavior* for which she could reward her husband in the process of deciding upon a *reinforcer.* She knew that Bernard opted to lift weights instead of getting high after work approximately twice a week, and so she planned to reinforce his workout in the basement by joining him to watch TV those evenings. The weight lifting appears to be a good choice, because it meets the first three criteria for Selecting Alcohol/Drug-Free IP Behaviors to Reinforce (Table 6.2). First, the IP apparently gets some enjoyment out of weight lifting, and thus there is a reasonable chance he will choose it over pot smoking if it is properly reinforced. Second, the weight lifting competes with the marijuana smoking in terms of the time they both occur. The question of how well weight lifting can satisfy the

TABLE 6.2. SELECTING ALCOHOL/DRUG-FREE IP BEHAVIORS TO REINFORCE

The alcohol- and drug-free IP behavior (activity) to reinforce should be one that:

1. The *IP enjoys.*
2. *Competes* with the substance-using behavior in terms of time and function.
3. *Occurs* fairly *often* currently, or can occur often in the future.
4. The *CSO* also *enjoys* (if applicable).

---

function of the pot smoking is unknown. At this point it is unclear why the IP chooses to lift weights instead of smoke pot on those two evenings each week. The therapist could decide to conduct a functional analysis of the healthy behavior (i.e., weight lifting) to address the issue of the function served by this nonusing recreational behavior (see next section).

The third favorable aspect of reinforcing the husband's weight lifting is that it occurs fairly often: twice a week. Not only is this an ongoing activity, but its relatively high frequency of occurrence will increase the chance that the CSO will be able to "catch him in the act" of being drug free, thereby allowing her to reward him. At this point the fourth criterion for an ideal behavior to reinforce is not applicable, given that the CSO does not participate in the weight lifting. However, the client eventually might decide that joining her husband in the basement to work out could be yet another way to support his choice of a healthy behavior. At that point it would be important to have Denise monitor her own (and, of course, her husband's) reactions to determine their level of enjoyment with this revised plan.

FUNCTIONAL ANALYSIS OF INCREASING A HEALTHY, ENJOYABLE BEHAVIOR

In the process of discussing a healthy IP behavior to reinforce, sometimes it becomes apparent that it would be useful to obtain more information about the exact circumstances under which the IP normally selects the healthy behavior over the unhealthy (substance-abusing) one. Or, as noted earlier, perhaps you are unclear about the function of the healthy behavior and whether it can compete with the purpose served by the unhealthy behavior. These are occasions for conducting a functional analysis of the healthy, enjoyable behavior, with the objective of helping the CSO find ways to attempt to *increase* it. To suit this new purpose (i.e., increasing a behavior as opposed to decreasing it), the CRAFT Functional Analysis of a Loved One's Drinking/Using Behavior chart is modified accordingly. The most salient change involves the last two columns, wherein the negative consequences of the behavior are addressed before the positive consequences (Figure 6.1, end of chapter). The intent is to end the interview on an upbeat, motivating note.

Knowledge of the healthy behavior's current triggers or consequences can stimulate ideas regarding the manner in which CSOs can best influence their IP's decision to engage in that healthy behavior. Some therapists concentrate exclusively on the functional analysis of the healthy behavior to accomplish this goal, whereas others find it valuable to contrast these CSO responses with those contained in the client's substance abuse functional analysis. For the sample case just presented, imagine that Denise (CSO) outlined her husband's enjoyable, healthy weight lifting behavior after work (see Figure 6.2, end of chapter) and compared the results with those of its main competitor for time: pot smoking in the garage. How could she use this information in her effort to increase the weight lifting behavior? Certainly, many unspoken aspects of the case would need to be considered before finalizing any choices; possible examples are listed below.

EXTERNAL TRIGGERS

In general, if CSOs want to capitalize on the identified *external* triggers for the *non*using behavior, they could attempt to increase their IP's contact with these antecedents (or similar triggers) or make the antecedents more prominent. This would set the stage for the healthy behavior to be chosen more often. In Denise's case, assume she discovered a difference in location (i.e., basement vs. garage) as the immediately preceding external trigger for her husband's weight lifting and pot-smoking behaviors.

Sample External Trigger and Plan

• *Basement.* Denise could make the basement more appealing so that the IP is automatically drawn to it more than to the garage (e.g., encourage him to upgrade his sound system there, paint it bright colors, suggest that he totally take over the room for his own use, keep the son out of the basement when the husband is down there, leave the IP high-energy snacks in the basement each day after work). *Note:* These last two suggestions address negative consequences 1–3 (column 4 in Figure 6.2) as well.

INTERNAL TRIGGERS

As far as *internal* triggers, CSOs would guess the main themes in their IP's thoughts and feelings that precede the healthy activity, and would then attempt to strengthen the link between these antecedent thoughts/ feelings, *whenever* they occur, and the healthy behavior. In the sample case, Bernard's dominant themes prior to choosing to lift weights were anger and stress (Figure 6.2, column 2). How could the CSO use this information?

Sample Internal Triggers and Plan

- *Anger and stress.* The CSO might (1) watch for subtle signs of anger/stress and suggest that the IP work out (especially if he is heading toward the garage at the time); (2) point out evidence of the IP's exercise regimen effectively reducing his stress (e.g., he may be more patient with his son and sleep better on the days he exercises); (3) tell her husband how pleasant he is to be around when he is managing his stress in such a healthy way; (4) share personal instances of alleviating her own stress through a physical workout.

NEGATIVE CONSEQUENCES

Short-term *negative* consequences for a healthy behavior are viewed as obstacles that might interfere with the IP choosing that behavior in the future. CSOs should determine which negative consequences are the most serious threats and should try to remove them so it is easier for the IP to choose the healthy behavior. Assume Denise has heard her husband register a number of complaints about his workout (see column 4 in Figure 6.2).

Sample Negative Consequences and Plan

- *Bored.* The wife could (1) join the IP so he has company working out; (2) occasionally buy him a new CD to listen to while exercising; (3) offer suggestions for varying his workout.
- *Son bothers him.* The CSO should keep the son out of the basement when the IP is down there exercising.
- *Tired; hungry.* She could (1) leave out a high-energy snack for him; (2) encourage him to do shorter but more frequent workouts.
- *In pain.* The wife might (1) join him in stretching before and after the workout; (2) suggest that he vary his exercise (e.g., take a brisk walk with her?) so as to reduce the risk of overexerting certain muscles; (3) recommend that he see his doctor; (4) suggest he take a prophylactic dose of ibuprofen (if appropriate).
- *Feeling unfit.* Denise could comment on the progress he has made toward getting fit.
- *Thoughts of job stress.* She might suggest that he distract himself from job thoughts until later, when he can discuss them with her.

POSITIVE CONSEQUENCES

The long-term *positive* consequences of the healthy behavior are those factors that are maintaining the behavior already. Sometimes they can be
made more powerful by supporting and enhancing them (verbally or otherwise) (see column 5 in Figure 6.2).

Sample Positive Consequences and Plan

• *Improved CSO–IP relationship.* Denise could (1) comment on positive aspects of their relationship that are primarily apparent on the days
he works out (e.g., better communication, desire to spend time together);
(2) continue to socialize with the IP in a pleasant manner when he has
chosen weight lifting over pot-smoking.
• *Improved IP health.* The CSO might (1) compliment the IP's
improved physique and his efforts to be healthy; (2) further support his
overall efforts to be healthy by cooking healthier meals.
• *Reduced job stress.* She could create new occasions on which she
could talk with him about job stress, such as while taking a walk with their
son after work.

ANTICIPATING POSSIBLE NEGATIVE REPERCUSSIONS FOR OFFERING A REINFORCER

As noted previously, whenever some type of behavior change is planned
by the CSO that will affect the IP, it is always critical to anticipate and prepare for potential negative reactions. This preparation is necessary even
in the current low-risk situation being outlined, in which a CSO is preparing to offer the IP a reward—a reward that will be given at a time when the
IP is not under the influence of alcohol or drugs. Regardless, some individuals have difficulty dealing with the implied message about their problem, or adjusting to change of any sort, and thus may show signs of resistance. As always, the biggest concern is for the CSO's safety; therefore,
the planned reward episode first must be reviewed for any potential violent reactions by the IP. If triggering violence is a possibility, the administration of the reward should be reconsidered. If a decision to proceed
appears reasonable in spite of this possibility, then the CSO's safety plan
must be revisited and updated (see Chapter 4).
    One of the most common reactions from IPs who notice that their
CSO is doing something nice for them is suspicion. This is not surprising,
since often the relationship between CSOs and their loved ones has dete-
riorated into one marked by tension and anger. In many cases the CSO
has not offered a kind word or act to the IP in a long time, so this occa-

sion stands out and raises questions when it occurs. But although IPs apparently often notice the reinforcer and become suspicious, typically they do not question it initially. Some of them confess later that they knew precisely why they were being treated in a special way, but that since they had no interest in instigating a discussion of the topic, they said nothing. Thus, in these situations, any acknowledgment of the act and its meaning probably will not take place until the CSO specifically makes a point of communicating directly on these matters. Since you cannot be sure if or when an IP will inquire about the purpose of a planned reinforcer, you should teach the client from the outset how to respond (as outlined in the section "Verbally Linking Rewards with Clean and Sober Behavior" in this chapter). These communications are role-played in several ways, and a number of them include provisions for responding to an angry, upset IP. Problem-solving methods are sometimes used to generate options for a response (see Chapter 7).

RECOGNIZING SIGNS OF SUBSTANCE USE

Given the fact that positive reinforcers increase the behavior they follow, it is extremely important for the CSO to deliver these rewards when the IP is clean and sober and *not* suffering from a hangover (Meyers & Smith, 1997; Meyers et al., 1996). Consequently, the CSO must become adept at identifying these opportune periods. Although frequently the IP's substance use will be obvious, on certain occasions it may not be. Therefore, you should devote time to evaluating the client's ability to recognize whether the IP is under the influence of alcohol or drugs, and if necessary, teaching the CSO how to improve this skill.

You typically begin by reminding the CSO about the functional analysis of the IP's using behavior that was completed earlier, in which common drinking or drug-using situations and people were identified (Chapter 3). Since these likely occasions for substance use have been defined, advise the CSO to be particularly wary of them. Unfortunately the picture is much more complex, because the IP certainly can resort to using at other times as well. Also, if an IP did *not* use substances during one of his or her common drinking or using occasions, then it would be extremely helpful for the CSO to be cognizant of a positive circumstance like this so that the nonusing behavior could be reinforced.

Continue by asking the CSO to describe the most obvious signs of substance use demonstrated by their IP. Specifically, inquire about any changes in the loved one's speech, mood, and behavior that are associated with substance use. Sometimes changes in appearance are noted as well. Occasionally clients will have difficulty identifying even these more obvious signs and may report that they are confident claiming IP use only when they actually *see* their IP using. In these cases you would give an assignment for the CSO to carefully observe the way the IP's behavior changes the next time the CSO sees the IP using. This new focus will help the CSO to recognize the signs of use in the future without having to observe the using behavior, per se. As a starting point, you may also review with the CSO some of the common signs of use for the IP's drug of choice (see Figure 6.3, end of chapter). Once a client can identify obvious signs of use, ask about the more subtle cues. Remind the CSO again to think of the functional analysis that outlined the IP's common triggers for substance use, particularly the internal triggers (i.e., feelings, thoughts), since, in all probability, they will be associated with early behavioral signs of use. End the exercise by reiterating the reason why it is so important for CSOs to be able to distinguish between substance-using and nonusing times: so that they reward only nondrinking/non-drug-using behavior.

VERBALLY LINKING REWARDS
WITH CLEAN AND SOBER BEHAVIOR

The decision regarding whether it would be in the CSO's best interest to actually explain to the IP why he or she is being reinforced is one that should be made by you and the client after a discussion of the pros and cons of doing so. Many CSOs initially prefer to reward the nonusing behavior without offering their IPs a rationale. Some of these CSOs are curious as to whether their IP will even notice the change, and importantly, whether they will respond to it. Other clients are reluctant to inform their IP specifically about their objectives, because they sense it will lead to revealing the fact that they are in therapy—information they may not yet be ready to divulge. For those CSOs who are eager to verbally link their reinforcing acts with the IP's nonusing behavior, therapy time is devoted to identifying the best times to do this and rehearsing this conversation. To select an optimal time, ask CSOs to focus on occasions in which both they and the IP are likely to be in positive moods. In many cases mutual good moods naturally coincide with the occasion of delivering the reward itself.

In order to begin the rehearsal of verbally linking rewards with nonusing behavior, a CSO must have already received some basic communication training (Chapter 5). First review the basic rules for a good conversation:

1. Be brief.
2. Be positive.
3. Refer to specific behaviors.
4. Label your feelings.

5. Offer an understanding statement.
6. Accept partial responsibility.
7. Offer to help.

This communication training is now expanded to cover the manner in which CSOs can explain to their IP the connection between nonusing behavior and the rewards they are receiving.

ILLUSTRATIVE CASE OF A CSO VERBALLY LINKING A REWARD WITH HER BROTHER'S CLEAN/SOBER BEHAVIOR

A sample dialogue follows in which a CRAFT therapist works with a young woman (CSO) to incorporate a number of the positive communication components into a conversation with her brother (IP). The objective of the planned conversation is for the CSO to point out the connection between a reinforcer she is offering her brother and his clean, sober behavior:

THERAPIST: All right, Samantha. Since you want to tell Nicholas exactly why you went out of your way to cook one of his favorite meals, and it seems like a good time to do it, we should practice how you are going to tell him.

CSO: I think that's a good idea, because I'll probably be a little nervous when the time comes.

THERAPIST: And that's understandable. That's also why I started the session today by reviewing the characteristics of a good conversation. I thought maybe we could use some of those points in this particular conversation with your brother. Now, remember, you shouldn't feel pressured to use all seven parts. Just include a few that seem to fit. Go ahead and just try to get started.

Note: The therapist would have already shown the CSO a card with the communication rules listed, or would have written them on a board so that the CSO could refer to them.

CSO: OK. I invited him over to dinner at 5:30, so if all goes as planned, he'll actually get there on time. I don't think I'll bring up the drinking until we're enjoying the meal. And I know I'm not going to make a big deal of it. I'll just mention it.

THERAPIST: Excellent plan. You don't want to bring it up the minute he steps foot in your house. It usually works best if the person has had a chance to relax a little and enjoy himself first. And as we've discussed before, you don't want to be confrontational about it. Just like you said; you want to mention it. Oh . . . and don't forget to make sure, as best you can, that he's sober when he arrives.

Note: The therapist reinforces the CSO's good ideas whenever possible and offers reminders about using CRAFT's nonconfrontational style and making sure that the IP is sober when the rewards are delivered.

CSO: Coming on strong will definitely not work with him. And I'll be able to tell if he's been drinking, so you don't have to worry about that.

THERAPIST: OK. Now let's do a role play where I play the part of your brother. Assume we're halfway through the meal. I'll start. (*As brother*) Sammy, what a feast!

CSO: (*In role-play*) Thanks. Ya know, Nicholas, I'm really glad that you were able to come over tonight.

THERAPIST: (*As brother*) I'm the one who's glad! When you told me yesterday that you were going to grill fresh salmon with vegetables—well, I couldn't resist! Thanks for this delicious meal.

CSO: (*In role-play*) My pleasure. Actually, one of the reasons why I told you ahead of time about the salmon, which I know you love, is because I was hoping it would get you to come straight over here after work, without stopping for a drink first.

THERAPIST (*As brother*) Well, I noticed that you'd planned dinner sort of early.

CSO: (*In role-play*) Yes, I did that on purpose. You see, I love having dinner with you, Nicholas, and spending time with you, in general, but only when you're sober.

THERAPIST: (*As brother*) You *had* to say that, didn't you? Ya know, I'm not *always* out of control when I drink. And some people even think I'm fun to be around after I've had a few.

CSO: (*To therapist*) Help! This is where it will all fall apart for me. I don't know what to say to him. And I'll end up feeling like I wrecked the dinner.

THERAPIST: Well, let's review the positive parts of the conversation so far, and that will give us some ideas about how to continue. We're assuming that you picked a good time: midway through the meal. Now as far as what you've said, what do you think?

CSO: I know I was brief and specific. And I expressed my feelings, too. I'm not sure if I did anything else.

THERAPIST: You also stated things positively by saying what you *liked* to do—spend time with him when he is sober—as opposed to saying what you *didn't like* to do.

CSO: I didn't even realize I did that. Hey, I guess I'm doing OK so far.

THERAPIST: You're doing better than OK. But he still got defensive, didn't he? And that caused you to panic and freeze up. But we can work on that. In the meantime, don't lose sight of the fact that you did an excellent job.

Note: The therapist played the role in a challenging manner so that this rather skilled CSO could work on her response in a supportive setting. The client responded well to the challenge and used the first four components of a positive communication. Still, there was room for improvement. Also, she did not realize that she had used an important component (to be positive). The therapist pointed this out so that she could make an effort to include it again. Note the therapist's use of the sandwich technique for offering feedback.

CSO: Well, the conversation was pretty realistic. I could imagine him saying those things.

THERAPIST: Good. That's what we need to practice, then. How about trying to use one or two of the last three parts of a good conversation? What would it sound like, for example, to say something understanding, or maybe to accept partial responsibility? Remember, ultimately you are more likely to get what you want—namely, that your brother cuts down on his drinking—if you say things in such a way that he can *keep listening*.

Note: The therapist recommends that the CSO add communication points 5 or 6, and reminds the CSO about *her* reason (i.e., her reinforcer) for trying to enhance her conversation in the first place. Although the client had already utilized four positive communication items, the additional components were suggested as a way to respond to the IP's likely defensive reaction. The CSO had sufficient social skills to successfully master this advanced conversation.

CSO: I could give it a try.

THERAPIST: Let's pick up from where we left off. (*As brother*) I'm not always out of control when I drink, and some people even enjoy being with me then.

CSO: (*In role-play*) Nicholas, I'm sure it must seem like I'm getting after you for being "out of control" all the time. I really don't mean to. And I know I don't always say things to you in the nicest way when I'm upset. What I want to say is that I like our time together when you haven't been drinking. And I'm trying to show you this by having you over to dinner when you're totally sober.

Note: The CSO has used an understanding statement and has accepted partial responsibility.

THERAPIST (*As brother*) Sammy, I always like our time together. I didn't mean to get so nasty. It just seems like people have been bugging me to death lately about my drinking.

CSO: (*To therapist*) Now that he's calmed down, should I bring up the topic of therapy?

THERAPIST: There's no way to know for sure when it's the best time to mention therapy. I'd probably suggest that you take it slowly with him. After all, this is the first time you've even tried linking a reward with his sober behavior. Maybe we should just stick with that for a while. Eventually he'll ask what you're up to, or where you got the idea to do that. That's often a good time to mention you're in therapy, and why.

CSO: Yes, that feels better to me.

THERAPIST: Good. Hey, you used almost every good communication rule in that last role play! Why don't you point them out first, and then we'll do the whole conversation again. I'll change my reaction a little, so that you can practice some different responses. We'll make sure we discuss your feelings, too.

As noted in Chapter 5, CSOs should rehearse several variations of an upcoming encounter, including some that involve negative IP reactions, such as anger. This kind of thorough rehearsal enables clients to practice responding safely and appropriately to a wide variety of scenarios and enhances their confidence overall. It also affords an opportunity to discuss the feelings evoked during the role plays, which tend to be quite similar to those experienced in real-life encounters. In this particular example, the therapist would want to process the fact that the sister anticipated feeling guilty if the outcome for the evening were less than perfect. In terms of the question raised about whether it was the right time to mention therapy, you normally would devote considerable session time to discussing this factor with the CSO (as outlined in Chapter 9). Given that this was going to be Samantha's first effort at both linking a reward with nonusing behavior *and* explaining it to her brother, the therapist cautioned her against moving too quickly by bringing up therapy.

ILLUSTRATIVE CASE OF A CSO VERBALLY LINKING A REWARD WITH HIS WIFE'S CLEAN/SOBER BEHAVIOR

Another example of a CSO's attempt to verbally link a reward with clean and sober behavior follows. This time the CSO is a husband and the IP is his wife. Her drugs of choice are Ativan and Xanax. Al (CSO) has decided to reward his wife for a tranquilizer-free day by taking her shopping for an hour after dinner. The therapist begins by commenting on the appropriateness of both the reward and the behavior selected for reinforcement:

THERAPIST: Al, based on everything you've said, it seems like taking your wife shopping for an hour is an excellent choice of a reward for her. As you mentioned, she seems to truly enjoy these trips, they're readily available, and you feel comfortable using this type of reward. But do these shopping trips get expensive?

CSO: No. She's a bargain hunter. And half the time she just likes to look.

Note: As usual, the therapist scans the Guidelines for Reinforcers (Table 6.1, p. 138) to be sure that the "reward" selected by the CSO is one that satisfies the first four basic criteria.

THERAPIST: OK. Now you said that when you took her shopping last week, you weren't sure that she saw the connection between her being drug-free and being taken shopping.

CSO: Maybe she noticed, but I doubt it. I want to make sure she knows why I'm doing it.

THERAPIST: Sounds reasonable. Before we talk about how you can explain this connection to her, let me first check on the behavior you're going to reward. Usually we try to keep it to a simple behavior. You're planning to reward Joan if she doesn't use for an entire day. That's not a simple behavior to monitor, but maybe we can narrow it down. I just need to make sure that you'll be able to tell if she's used pills on that day.

Note: The therapist is concerned that it might be difficult for Al to know whether his wife has used, since he will not be home to monitor her behavior throughout the day.

CSO: I don't have to worry about the whole day. If she takes pills, it's always late in the afternoon, like around 4:00. And I can definitely tell if she's had any. She can't even get up off the couch if she's started in. On the days that she hasn't popped any pills she's usually outside gardening when I get home.

THERAPIST: It helps to know that. So maybe we can say that you'll reward her with a shopping trip on a day that she's outside gardening when you arrive home—because then you *know* she hasn't used, right?

CSO: I think it's safe to say that.

THERAPIST: Good. And does your wife enjoy the gardening? How often does she do it?

Note: The therapist now starts to assess whether the behavior possesses any of the characteristics of an ideal behavior to reinforce, since essentially the husband will be rewarding his wife's choice of gardening over using pills. These are items 1 and 3 on the list for Selecting Alcohol/ Drug-Free IP Behaviors to Reinforce (Table 6.2, p. 143).

CSO: Oh, she definitely likes it. I'd say it's her hobby. She's probably out in the garden three days a week. I wish she'd do it everyday, though. I hate to come home and find her on the couch.

THERAPIST: And it seems like the gardening occurs at about the same time of day that she chooses to take pills some of the time. Later we might decide to look into how she decides which one to do.

Note: The therapist determines whether the gardening behavior can compete with the using behavior as far as time is concerned (item 2). The various functions of the gardening could be evaluated in a functional analysis later, if the desired behavior change does not occur, and the findings could be contrasted with the function of the pills.

CSO: I sure don't get how she decides on one over the other. I've tried to figure it out.

THERAPIST: Let's not worry about that for now. Instead, let's talk about how and when you're going to tell her. When is a good time to tell her?

Note: The therapist skips item 4 on the behavior list. At this point it is inconsequential whether or not the CSO enjoys gardening, as he is not currently engaging in the activity with his wife.

CSO: She seems to be in a really good mood on the way home after she's shopped for a little while and found a good bargain. So maybe I should tell her then.

THERAPIST: Good idea. But would you tell her even if she didn't find a bargain that night? Would she still be in a good mood? And what about you?

Note: The therapist makes sure that Al has selected a time when both he and Joan are likely to be in a good mood. Additionally, the therapist tries to get the CSO to anticipate obstacles to carrying out the plan so that solutions and backup plans can be generated in advance.

CSO: If she doesn't find anything on sale to buy, our trips tend to be shorter, so I could stop at the Dairy Queen for ice cream cones on the way home. It may sound silly, but that puts both of us in good moods.

THERAPIST: There's nothing silly about it. Good. Let's rehearse it now. I'll play your wife's part. Let's pretend we're driving home after shopping, and Joan is in a good mood. (*As wife*) Thanks for taking me tonight.

CSO: (*In role-play*) Joan, I don't know if you realize it, but I took you shopping tonight because you weren't strung out on your old pills today.

THERAPIST: (*As wife*) What? What does shopping have to do with my pills? I felt better today so I didn't need them.

CSO: (*In role-play*) Yea, well *I'm* going to end up needing them if I have to keep worrying about you. Anyway, that's why I took you shopping. I hope you liked it.

THERAPIST: Let's take a break right here and review how it's going. Al, which of the pieces of a good conversation did you use? Do you remember them? [Shows CSO the list of seven basic rules for good communication.]

CSO: Oh, those. I guess I was brief . . . and specific. I told her exactly what I was doing and why.

THERAPIST: You sure did. Good job. And you even mentioned your feelings when you said that you worry about her.

Note: Always search for ways to compliment the CSO's attempts, regardless of how much refinement they require. Here the CSO used positive communication components 1, 3, and 4, but since there was a negative tone to the communication, the therapist will encourage the CSO to add at least item 2 yet.

THERAPIST: All right, Al. So far you've made it real clear to Joan why you took her shopping. And that's precisely what we're practicing: verbally linking her reward with her drug-free behavior. But I bet you can make it sound even better, because in playing Joan's role, I noticed that some of your message came across with a negative edge to it. And if *I* felt it, I bet she would too. Do you know which part I'm referring to?

Note: The therapist again reinforces the CSO's efforts. The therapist also tests the CSO's awareness of his negative tone and offers a reasonable reaction to it. The CSO is more likely to get a positive response from his wife if he communicates in a positive manner.

CSO: Hmmm. Ya mean the part where I said I was going to end up needing pills?

THERAPIST: That statement could use a little work. Actually, in Joan's role I reacted more to your earlier comment about me not being "strung out" on my "old pills." It hurt my feelings, and since I don't think you gained anything by saying it, it might be better to work around it. What do you think?

CSO: You think that would bother her? I say stuff like that all the time. OK. Whatever.

Note: The role play has afforded the opportunity for the therapist to give specific feedback about how some of the CSO's comments may be unnecessarily angering his wife, thereby triggering a defensive reaction from her.

THERAPIST: I think it would bother her, but I also think you are more likely to get what you want out of this if you reach out to her in a gentle, supportive way. Remember how we've talked about not coming on too strong or being confrontational?

Note: The therapist reminds the CSO that he is more likely to get his reinforcer—namely, getting his wife to change her drug-using behavior—if he communicates in a positive manner.

CSO: Confrontational? I thought we were just talking. Well, you know best! What should I say then?

THERAPIST: For starters, how about just sticking with the positive things that are going on now, instead of referring back to those negative times? I bet she's heard you talk about those times a lot already.

CSO: Sure, I can do that. Let me try it again.

THERAPIST: Make believe that we're halfway home again. (*As wife*) Thanks. That was fun.

CSO: (*In role-play*) Joan, I took you shopping tonight because it seemed like you had a real good day; I mean, it seemed like you didn't take any pills today.

THERAPIST: (*As wife*) I did have a good day. But what does that have to do with us going shopping?

CSO: (*In role-play*) I wanted to show you how happy I was that you didn't take any pills.

THERAPIST: (*As wife*) Well, I'm happy when I don't need any pills, too.

CSO: (*To therapist*) So now what do I say? She's making it sound like it's just dumb luck that she didn't *need* to take pills today. What am I supposed to do with that?

THERAPIST: OK. Let's stop the role play a minute. First of all, Al, you're doing terrific! Let's review. This time it felt much better to me. Do you know why?

Note: The therapist wants to make sure that the CSO realizes *why* his conversation was improved, so that he can repeat it in the future.

CSO: I tried not to say anything negative, like about her being strung out and about me needing pills, too.

THERAPIST: Yes, and you also simply told her how you felt when she didn't use pills. You said you felt happy when she didn't use pills. That came across real nice. And as far as responding to her comment about not *needing* any drugs today, I'd probably just leave that one alone for now. She's not going to change dramatically after one reward and one conversation about it. Let's take it slowly. What's important right now is that you've made the connection between the reward and the drug-free day. It's a first step, and we'll build on it later.

In this situation, the therapist made several decisions. The first decision was *not* to push the CSO to enhance his conversation by adding even more components of a good conversation, such as items 5–7. Given the modest skill level of this particular CSO, the therapist believed that Al might feel overwhelmed if he were asked to focus on anything else new besides keeping his tone positive. And since this simple change in his normal conversation would probably be quite noticeable to his wife, it appeared worthwhile to start with that change alone. The therapist also decided not to have the CSO address his wife's comment about not needing pills—a statement that seemed to abdicate all responsibility for her drug use. Issues such as this would best be addressed by a therapist and ideally would be "shelved" until the wife began therapy herself. In the meantime the therapist would ask the CSO to continue to work on linking (verbally and otherwise) appropriate rewards with his wife's nonusing behavior.

POTENTIAL COMPLICATIONS
WHEN DELIVERING REINFORCERS

In the course of doing role plays with CSOs about how they will verbally link the chosen reward with their IP's nonusing behavior, it is not uncommon for potential problems to become apparent. In actuality, this development is considered another benefit that results from the in-session role plays, because solutions can then be generated in advance. One of the frequently anticipated problems is the situation in which a client has carefully planned a reward for what appears to be a drug-free occasion, only to discover that the IP has used. The ideal solution would be for the CSO to withhold the reinforcer, if at all possible, and to deliver it at a later date. In many circumstances, the reinforcer can be withheld without complications, because the IP is not aware of the impending reward and consequently does not realize that it has been withheld. However, if the IP knows about and is looking forward to the upcoming reinforcer, in some cases withholding it could cause more harm than good. An obvious example of such an exception would be if withholding the expected reinforcer (e.g., a special dessert) was likely to cause the IP to become violent toward the CSO. Certainly you would encourage the CSO to give the reinforcer in this case and to choose a safe time to discuss it later with the IP.

Even without the potential for violence, there are some situations in which a CSO might still appropriately decide to offer the reward despite the fact that the IP is under the influence. Take the case of Samantha noted previously, in which she was going to prepare her brother's favorite salmon dinner. She purposefully scheduled the dinner for early in the evening, since she surmised that this would make it difficult for Nicholas to stop at the bar after work. Nevertheless, conceivably he could have managed to stop for a quick drink anyway. So what would be the best course of action if Samantha suspected that her brother had been drinking when he arrived for his "reinforcer"? Sometimes the reasonable course of action is not obvious to the CSO, because you would have told the CSO repeatedly that it is extremely important for the reward to be paired with *non*using behavior. In this case, a rather uncomfortable conflict between Samantha and her brother could result if she refused to feed him when he arrived. Consequently, the therapist would advise her to go ahead with the meal, and to plan on discussing the situation with her brother at a later date when he was sober.

There are several methods for preparing CSOs for the possibility that their IP may drink or use drugs just prior to the supposedly drug-free reinforcement period. One is to routinely practice a role play in which the IP is already under the influence, and then discuss suitable reactions. In the absence of a role play, the potential problem should at least be discussed. Additionally, have the client select at least one backup IP behavior and reinforcer for the week. Importantly, if the original reinforcer plan involves a fair amount of work for the CSO, as it did in Samantha's case, encourage the CSO to make this second reward extremely easy to set up and deliver. If too many complex reinforcers, requiring an extensive time commitment from the CSO, are decided upon, the CSO is at great risk for becoming discouraged if the scenarios do not unfold as planned. In Samantha's situation, an example of a reasonable backup reinforcer is a brief, pleasant phone call to her brother during the workday. Assume that Samantha has reported that

Nicholas never drinks until after work; consequently it should be easy for her to "catch him in the act" of being sober early in the workday. Delivering the reinforcer would not be complicated; it could simply be a compliment about some ongoing drug-free behavior of Nicholas's. An example would be for Samantha to comment on her brother's sharp wit when he is alert in the morning. Although she implicitly would be referring to his wit in a drug-free state, she may or may not make this connection explicit, depending on her progress in therapy.

THE CSO'S READINESS TO DELIVER A REINFORCER

Although you cannot know with certainty when a CSO is ready to deliver a positive reinforcer, problems should be minimized if you utilize the techniques and guidelines presented in this chapter. These procedures and the skill level recommended for the CSO are outlined in Table 6.3.

TABLE 6.3. THE CSO'S READINESS TO DELIVER A CONTINGENT POSITIVE REINFORCER

A CSO is ready to deliver a positive reinforcer contingent upon the IP's clean and sober behavior when the CSO:

1. *Understands* the concept of a positive *reinforcer*.

2. Recognizes the *difference between rewarding* clean/sober behavior and *"enabling."*

3. Has had the opportunity to *express resentment* regarding rewarding a loved one who has caused a lot of pain.

4. Has generated a *list of potential reinforcers* that satisfy the Guidelines for Reinforcers.

5. Has identified an *ongoing nonusing activity or behavior to reward* while considering the criteria for an ideal behavior.

6. Has *anticipated possible negative consequences* upon introducing the positive reinforcer, and has developed an appropriate plan to deal with them.

7. *Recognizes the signs of substance use* for her or his IP.

8. Has demonstrated the *ability to verbally link a reward* with nonusing behavior through behavior rehearsal.

9. Has *discussed the feelings evoked* by the role plays.

10. Has decided upon *a plan for safely handling common problems* that arise when attempting to administer reinforcers for sober behavior.

SUMMARY

This chapter covers the concept of a positive reinforcer: what it is and how it can be used effectively by the CSO to increase the occurrence of the IP's alcohol- or drug-free behavior. The importance of CSOs using positive reinforcement will be emphasized during the discussion of other CRAFT procedures as well, such as when CSOs are taught to positively reinforce themselves (e.g., Chapter 8). Finally, as noted in Chapter 2, CRAFT therapists continually watch for opportunities to use verbal positive reinforcement with their clients. Additional examples of how this reinforcement can be delivered frequently and effectively by therapists will also be highlighted throughout the remainder of the book.

FIGURE 6.1. CRAFT FUNCTIONAL ANALYSIS OF A LOVED ONE'S ENJOYABLE, HEALTHY BEHAVIOR

External Triggers	Internal Triggers	Enjoyable, Healthy Behavior	Short-Term Negative Consequences	Long-Term Positive Consequences
1. *Who* is your loved one usually with when (*behavior*)?	1. What do you think your loved one is *thinking* about right before (*behavior*)?	1. *What* is your loved one's enjoyable, healthy behavior?	1. What do you think your loved one dislikes about (*behavior*) [*with whom*]?	1. What do you think are the positive results of your loved one's (*behavior*) in each of these areas: a. Interpersonal:
		2. *How often* does he/she engage in it?	2. What do you think he/she dislikes about (*behavior*) [*where*]?	b. Physical:
2. *Where* does he/she usually (*behavior*)?	2. What do you think he/she is usually *feeling* right before (*behavior*)?		3. What do you think he/she dislikes about (*behavior*) [*when*]?	c. Emotional: d. Legal:
3. *When* does he/she usually (*behavior*)?		3. *How long* a period of time does it last?	4. What unpleasant *thoughts* do you think he/she has while (*behavior*)?	e. Job:
			5. What unpleasant *feelings* do you think he/she has while (*behavior*)?	f. Financial: g. Other:

FIGURE 6.2. **CRAFT FUNCTIONAL ANALYSIS OF A LOVED ONE'S ENJOYABLE, HEALTHY BEHAVIOR: COMPLETED**

External Triggers	Internal Triggers	Enjoyable, Healthy Behavior	Short-Term Negative Consequences	Long-Term Positive Consequences
1. *Who* is your loved one usually with when (*weight lifting*)? Nobody usually Sometimes our son	1. What do you think your loved one is *thinking* about right before (*weight lifting*)? I can't let my job get to me so much They're a bunch of jerks	1. *What* is your loved one's enjoyable, healthy behavior? Lifting weights while listening to loud music	1. What do you think your loved one dislikes about (*weight lifting*) [*with whom*]? Boring sometimes Son gets in his way	1. What do you think are the positive results of your loved one's (*weight lifting*) in each of these areas: a. Interpersonal: We're nicer to each other (argue less) b. Physical: Good for his overall health Looks better
2. *Where* does he/she usually (*weight lift*)? Basement	2. What do you think he/she is usually *feeling* right before (*weight lifting*)? Angry at boss, coworkers Stressed	2. *How often* does he/she engage in it? 2 x/wk	2. What do you think he/she dislikes about (*weight lifting*) [*where*]? Son comes downstairs and bothers him	c. Emotional: Decreases his anger & stress
		3. *How long* a period of time does it last? 45 minutes	3. What do you think he/she dislikes about (*weight lifting*) [*when*]? Tired sometimes Hungry	d. Legal: It's not illegal
3. *When* does he/she usually (*weight lift*)? Right after work			4. What unpleasant *thoughts* do you think he/she has while (*weight lifting*)? This hurts I'm not as fit as I'd like to be My job is going to kill me	e. Job: Reduced job stress due to our evening talks about his stressors
			5. What unpleasant *feelings* do you think he/she has while (*weight lifting*)? Physical pain Distressed	f. Financial: Doesn't cost anything (except if buying music) g. Other:

FIGURE 6.3. **COMMON SIGNS OF ALCOHOL AND ILLICIT DRUG USE**

Depressants (e.g., alcohol, barbiturates, benzodiazepines)

Speech	*Mood*	*Behavior*	*Appearance*
Slurred	Agitated	Unsteady gait	Bloodshot eyes
Odor on breath*	Labile	Impaired judgment	Poor hygiene
	Depressed	Impaired motor skills	Flushed skin
	Irritable	Drowsiness	
	Elated	Confusion	
	Passive	Memory lapses	
		Nausea	
		Blackouts	
		Tremors	

Marijuana

Speech	*Mood*	*Behavior*	*Appearance*
Talkative	Silly	Relaxed state	Dilated pupils
Loud	Passive	Enhanced sensations	Bloodshot eyes
Outbursts	Withdrawn	Impaired coordination	Dry mouth
Smoky breath	Labile	Slowed reflexes	Smoky-smelling clothes
		Increased appetite	
		Inappropriate laughter	
		Impaired attention	
		Impaired memory	
		Lack of energy	
		Low motivation	
		Flashbacks	
		Increased heart rate	

Hallucinogens (e.g., LSD, PCP)

Speech	*Mood*	*Behavior*	*Appearance*
Slowed	Labile	Blending of senses	Dilated pupils
Loud	Anxious	Confusion	Bloodshot eyes
Outbursts	Depressed	Impaired coordination	Dry mouth
Garbled		Flashbacks	Poor grooming
		Visual distortions	
		Hallucinations	
		Agitation	
		Disorientation	
		Delusions	
		Increased heart rate	

(cont.)

* = alcohol only

FIGURE 6.3. *(cont.)*

Stimulants (e.g., cocaine, crack, methamphetamine, Ecstasy)

Speech	*Mood*	*Behavior*	*Appearance*
Accelerated	Violent	Increased breathing	Dilated pupils
Lacks continuity	Erratic	Increased mental	Dry mouth
Frequent change	Anxious	alertness	Runny nose
of subject	Elevated	Confusion	Extreme weight loss
		Paranoid thinking	
		Restlessness	
		Insomnia	
		Loss of appetite	
		High energy	
		Elevated blood pressure	
		Increased heart rate	
		Distorted perceptions	
		Teeth grinding**	

Opiates (e.g., heroin, morphine, Percocet, OxyContin)

Speech	*Mood*	*Behavior*	*Appearance*
Slurred	Sullen	Nodding off	Constricted pupils
Slowed	Flat affect	Drowsiness	Needle tracks
	Withdrawn	Lethargy	Scars
	Euphoric	Slowed breathing	Droopy eyelids
		Chronic constipation	
		Nausea	
		Decreased blood	
		pressure	

** = Ecstasy only
Data from Falkowski (2003) and Schuckit (1995).

CHAPTER 7

THE USE OF NEGATIVE CONSEQUENCES

Positively reinforcing sober IP behavior is a decisive step in the CSO's efforts to address the substance abuse problem, but it is rarely sufficient to effect appreciable change. Techniques that actively and directly pair negative consequences with the IP's drinking or drug use are often required in addition. This chapter presents two such techniques: (1) a time-out from positive reinforcement, and (2) the allowance of natural consequences for substance-using behaviors. As the descriptors imply, neither one involves asking CSOs to introduce novel, harsh punishments. Instead, the procedures highlight their current reactions to using behavior so that CSOs can learn to refrain from responding in a manner that is experienced by the IP as positive—and therefore reinforcing. Although the notion of a CSO *stopping* certain positive behaviors may sound too simplistic to have much of an impact, the results can be profound. Typically, CSOs have engaged in these "caretaking" behaviors for a long, long time, and their absence is definitely noted. However, the removal of these reinforcers often creates unique problems for CSOs. Since many of them feel overwhelmed and ill-equipped to handle these problems, a problem-solving procedure is needed.

Persuading CSOs to think about, and then implement, the negative consequences techniques outlined in this chapter is usually considerably more difficult than convincing them to introduce positive reinforcers for sober behavior. In part, this added challenge is due to their apprehension about acting in a way that may upset their IP. Perhaps more importantly, though, the very rationale given for using these techniques is an uncomfortable message for CSOs to hear. Specifically, CSOs are told that they have been unintentionally rewarding the IP's using behavior at times, and these occasions are precisely the focus of the negative consequences interventions. Suggestions for presenting and discussing this message are pro-vided at several points in the chapter.

TIME-OUT FROM POSITIVE REINFORCEMENT PROCEDURE: RATIONALE FOR WITHDRAWING REWARDS

A straightforward procedure for applying negative consequences involves CSOs withdrawing a reward from their IP during a substance-using epi-sode, thereby creating a time-out from positive reinforcement. Since just one specific reinforcer is removed, as opposed to removing all of the rein-forcers present at the time, this particular type of time-out procedure dif-fers from the time-out that is commonly recognized as a behavioral strat-egy (Spiegler & Guevremont, 2003). Given that your client already has learned how to positively reward sober behavior, she or he has imple-mented variations of several techniques that are relevant to the current time-out technique. For example, regardless of whether CSOs are *giving* rewards for sober behavior or *removing* rewards on substance-abusing occasions, they must be able to distinguish between using and nonusing times. Furthermore, the strategies employed for selecting the appropriate behaviors and reinforcers to target for the time-out procedure are similar to the techniques already mastered when learning how to properly use positive reinforcement (see Chapter 6).

Since CSOs know how to link new rewards with sober behavior at this point in treatment, it is helpful to remind them of an ongoing example of this connection in their home as a means of introducing the new time-out procedure. For instance, if a CSO now routinely compliments his wife (the IP) about how well she takes care of the house and the children on those evenings when she is sober, point out that by *not* complimenting her on evenings when she is drinking, the CSO is already practicing the appropriate withdrawal of positive rewards. In an effort to introduce posi-tive rewards for clean and sober behavior, one of the CSOs in Chapter 6 decided to spend time watching television with her husband (the IP) on those days when he had chosen to work out instead of smoke pot. Impor-tantly, the IP enjoyed having his wife watch TV with him, and conse-quently he experienced her company as reinforcing. Once the husband became accustomed to the CSO joining him in the evening, he would be disappointed if she did *not* join him—which would occur if he were high. This absence would then serve as a time-out from positive reinforcement, and it would provide a link between the using behavior and the loss of something valued by the IP.

Tell your clients that your objective now is to teach them how to iden-tify additional substance-abusing occasions that lend themselves to the active removal of rewards. State that although you believe that they never intended to reward their IP's drinking or drug use, this reinforcement sometimes happens accidentally. Inform CSOs that upon carefully examining the types of things they do after their IP has been using, they might be surprised to realize that their behavior could be perceived as positive by the IP. If so, the CSOs' responses could unintentionally support and help to maintain the substance use. Assure them that this pattern of behaving is common for CSOs, and that the behavior can be changed. Finally, discuss the CSOs' reactions to this information.

APPROPRIATE OCCASIONS AND REINFORCERS FOR THE TIME-OUT PROCEDURE

As reported in Chapter 6, it is difficult to select an occasion (i.e., a time and behavior) for a reinforcement procedure without also considering the relevant reward—which, in this case, will be withdrawn. Start by examining an ongoing situation in which the IP is either drinking or using drugs in the CSO's presence, or is under the influence. That the situation should be ongoing is necessary so as to allow the CSO to respond immediately, thereby linking an IP (using) behavior more effectively with a CSO (withdrawing) response (Spiegler & Guevremont, 2003; Wilson & O'Leary, 1980). In scrutinizing the particular using scenario, determine whether the CSO currently is reacting in what could be construed by the IP as a positive manner. If so, the occasion is probably a suitable choice point for intervening, since if the CSO restrained from responding in that manner, the IP would experience the changed behavior as a time-out from something rewarding. If the CSO is perplexed about which episode to address, you might refer to an occasion outlined in a completed functional analysis. Alternatively, ask the CSO to describe either the most recent or a familiar episode. In either case, look for relevant reinforcers that are introduced *after* the IP's use and are under the CSO's control.

In determining whether a suitable occasion has been chosen, first check to see that the "reward" is, in fact, a reward for the IP. In other words, is it something of value that the IP will miss once it is no longer available? This reward should also be easy and safe for the CSO to withdraw. If the reward is not easy to remove, the CSO will have difficulty following through consistently. In testing the safety factor, discuss the IP's probable reaction to a time-out from this reward that he or she is accustomed to receiving. If there is a potential for violence, then a different reward should be chosen for removal. Furthermore, the reward needs to be one that the CSO is willing to reinstate whenever the IP is *not* using, so that the distinction between reward-meritorious and reward-unmeritorious behavior is clear. Finally, the reward should be one that can be withdrawn close in time to when the substance use occurs, because otherwise the strength of the pairing is diminished (Spiegler & Guevremont, 2003; Wilson & O'Leary, 1980). The guidelines for helping a CSO choose a reward to remove are outlined in Table 7.1.

EXAMPLES OF REINFORCERS TO WITHDRAW

Initially, CSOs require considerable assistance in selecting a reward to withdraw. Because each case is different, it is not possible to cite standard reinforcers that all CSOs can routinely withdraw for this time-out procedure. Examples of small, reasonable rewards that appear eligible for such an exercise follow. The removal of reinforcers with longer-lasting consequences that are not as readily reversed is discussed later. In reviewing the list below, assume the following: (1) The guidelines are satisfied for each act before it is approved by the therapist, (2) the CSO can distinguish between using and nonusing occasions, and (3) a rationale for the change in behavior is given to the IP by the CSO while employing positive communication skills.

- Parents (CSOs) who routinely allow their teenage son (IP) to use the family car on weekends explain that he will only be entitled to that privilege when he has not used drugs the preceding night.
- A father (IP) enjoys attending the Saturday matinee with his family each weekend. Usually his wife (CSO) says nothing when he is either already drinking that day or is sick with a hangover. She decides to tell him that she would love for him to continue participating in the Saturday outing, but only if he is sober.
- An older sister (CSO) typically goes out to lunch on Friday with

TABLE 7.1. GUIDELINES FOR SELECTING A REINFORCER TO WITHDRAW

The reward being taken away should be one that the CSO:

1. Believes the *IP values* and will miss when it is withdrawn.
2. Is *willing to reintroduce* when the IP is clean, sober, and not hungover.
3. Finds *easy* to take away.
4. Feels *safe* withdrawing.
5. Can *withdraw close in time* to when the alcohol or drug use occurs.

coworkers, and she always invites her younger sister (IP) to join them. However, for some time now the younger sister has been showing up high. The CSO informs her sister that she is only welcome to join them for lunch if she has not smoked marijuana that day.

- A 35-year-old son (CSO) bowls in a league. Most weeks he asks his dad (IP) to substitute for someone on the team. The dad gladly does this, as he likes bowling and spending time with his adult son. However, the IP typically has already had a few beers before arriving, and he continues to drink throughout the evening. The CSO tells his dad that he will only invite him to bowl in the future if he does not drink before or during the activity.

- A 70-year-old woman (CSO) hosts a bridge game with her female friends every other Tuesday. Her husband (IP) loves to tease and joke with the women during their visit, but his pain medication use has become a noticeable problem. The wife tells him that he is welcome to socialize with them on Tuesdays only if he refrains from abusing his medication that day.

- A mother (CSO) traditionally asks her older sister (IP) to join her and her two daughters for several back-to-school shopping excursions that everyone loves. This year the CSO tells the IP that the trips will include her only if she has not been drinking that day.

- After consulting with his wife, a 28-year-old Little League coach (CSO) tells his brother-in-law (IP) that he will be asked to serve as the assistant coach only on nights when he does not show up high.

- The parents (CSOs) of a 13-year-old girl (IP) inform her that she will be allowed to keep her cell phone for the evening whenever she comes home from school free of the smell of pot.

- The 62-year-old mother (CSO) of a drug-addicted son (IP) tells him that she will only drive him to do his shopping and other appointments on days when he is clean and has not used the preceding night.

- A wife (CSO) tells her husband (IP) that in the future, she will only grant his request and accompany him to a company function if he remains sober throughout it.

USING POSITIVE COMMUNICATION TO EXPLAIN THE REMOVAL OF A REWARD TO AN IP

In teaching CSOs how to withdraw positive reinforcers in response to IP drinking or drug use, you should devote time to discussing *when* and *how* they will explain their actions to the IP. With regard to the former, many clients feel more comfortable informing the IP in advance about the proposed action so that it is not experienced as a surprise, and so that the IP has the opportunity to decrease the substance use in response to the "warning." In line with other CSO–IP communications, the timing of the message is at least as important as the words used. As a reminder, the communication ideally should be delivered when the IP is not using substances or hungover, and when both the IP and CSO are in reasonably good moods (Sisson & Azrin, 1986).

For those CSOs who are interested in explaining their new behavior to the IP, the positive communication skills emphasized throughout Chapter 5 play a critical role. As a starting point, remind CSOs about the seven positive communication skills listed in Figure 5.1 (p. 134). See if they remember practicing and using these conversational skills when explaining the link between the IP's sober behavior and the introduction of positive reinforcers. Invite them to do a role play in which they explain to the IP the reason for the withdrawal of a reward. Reinforce all efforts, provide clear feedback, and repeat the role play, as needed (Monti & Rohsenow, 2003).

Below are examples of polished communications regarding removing reinforcers in two of the CSO–IP scenarios given as illustrations above. References to the positive communication components employed from Figure 5.1 are included in brackets. The CSO in the first example is the 70-year-old wife with a medication-abusing husband (IP) who likes to socialize with her bridge group:

> "Nate, I think you know how much me and the gals love having you around on bridge night. But my favorite nights are those when you act like your old sweet self [making a positive statement], when you haven't overdone the pain pills [referring to a specific behavior]. I probably should have brought this up long ago [accepting partial responsibility], but I was afraid you'd take it the wrong way [identifying feelings]. Anyway, I get embarrassed for you when I hear you slurring your words or when I see you nodding off in the corner [identifying feelings; referring to a specific behavior]. Lately I've been thinking that if I wasn't going to speak up, I shouldn't expect you to change [accepting partial responsibility]. So, Honey, from now on I only want you to join us Tuesday evenings if you haven't taken more than your prescribed dose for the day. With that said, is there anything I can do to make it easier for you to join us Tuesday nights [offering to help]?"

The CSO in the second example is the Little League coach who has decided to take away from his brother-in-law (IP) the privilege of serving as the assistant coach for the evening if he arrives at the game high:

> "Teeny, I just wanted to let you know how much I appreciate your help during the games, especially when you're straight [making a pos-

itive statement]. But I'm worried [identifying feelings] about the kids figuring out that you're high on the nights that you're real talkative and distractible [referring to a specific behavior]. I know these games can get pretty nerve-wracking, so it doesn't surprise me that you're looking for a way to relax ahead of time [making an understanding statement]. But there must be another option. Maybe I can help you figure one out [offering to help]. I feel strongly about us being good role models for the kids, so from now on I'm only going to ask you to be my assistant if you come to the game straight. What do you think?"

ILLUSTRATIVE CASE OF A CSO
SELECTING A REINFORCER TO WITHDRAW

Assume that a CRAFT therapist has explained the rationale for the time-out procedure and reviewed the guidelines noted above to a male CSO. The CSO volunteers his attendance at a Sunday morning church service as a possible intervention point for withdrawing a reward. He explains that his wife (the IP) drinks heavily every Saturday night and then attends church Sunday mornings with a hangover. Since the wife believes church attendance is important to them as a couple, the CSO acquiesces and accompanies her, despite his firm desire to stay home. The CSO states that many heated discussions have centered on what he sees as a hypocritical practice of hers. The dialogue that follows shows a CRAFT therapist attempting to discover if the nominated reward and occasion are appropriate.

THERAPIST: OK, Tim. Let's make sure this is a good place to start. As you know, it's real important that the "thing" you decide to take away is something Shirley values.

CSO: Oh, it *is*. She always twists my arm to go to church with her. I could care less about going.

THERAPIST: That's good, then. Since you said you didn't particularly like going, I wanted to be sure you didn't just select it because you didn't want to go anymore.

CSO: (*Laughing*) Well, I won't miss it, if that's what you mean!

THERAPIST: That's OK. But, remember, if you're going to choose it as the reward to withdraw when Shirley has a hangover, then it means you're prepared to *go* to church with her when she *doesn't* have a hangover. That would be critical. Are you willing to do that?

CSO: Sure. I usually do it anyway.

Note: The therapist makes sure of several things: the reward picked to be withdrawn is truly valued by the IP; the CSO is prepared to reintroduce the reward at alcohol-free times; and the act is something easy for the CSO to carry out (items 1–3 on Table 7.1, Guidelines for Selecting a Reinforcer to Withdraw, p. 168). Safety concerns (guideline 4) are addressed next.

THERAPIST: I think I know the answer, but I still like to get people into the habit of reviewing safety issues before they try anything new. Is there a chance that Shirley will get violent in some way when you don't go to church with her the next time she's got a hangover?

CSO: She'll have a few choice words, but that's about it. And then she'll hold a grudge.

THERAPIST: So it might be uncomfortable for a while?

CSO: Yup, but I can't leave things the way they are. It'll be worth it if it works.

THERAPIST: The only thing we haven't covered is guideline 5. What do you think about the link between *when* the drinking is taking place and *when* you're withdrawing the reward?

CSO: I know you said they should be close together. I don't know what to take away Saturday nights. I guess I could sleep somewhere else. That would upset her. But I don't really want to sleep on the couch. Why should *I* be uncomfortable when *she* drinks?

THERAPIST: Good question. But remember, Tim, sometimes it's necessary to make some changes that temporarily make you uncomfortable so that you get what you want in the long run; namely, Shirley beginning treatment. I don't think you need to sleep on the couch, though. You *are* linking the removal of a reward with her hangover. I think the connection will be clear. But to make sure, it would make sense to tell her ahead of time exactly what you plan to do and why.

Note: The therapist reminds the client about his long-term goal as a means of increasing his motivation to follow through, and then suggests verbally linking his new behavior with the wife's hangovers.

Normally, several role plays are conducted at this point. An ideal time for initiating the conversation at home is discussed and together you agree on an assignment. At the next session you see if the assignment was completed correctly and what its impact was. Depending on the outcome, you decide if the assignment needs to be modified or if additional reinforcers need to be targeted and planned for removal.

THE WITHDRAWAL OF REINFORCERS LINKED
WITH MORE SERIOUS NEGATIVE CONSEQUENCES

The reinforcers discussed for withdrawal thus far are relatively small ones, associated with discrete using episodes, and which could easily be reinstated if the IP had a clean and sober day. Unfortunately, at times the removal of small reinforcers proves to be inadequate in terms of having a significant, lasting impact on the IP's problematic behavior. In such a case, you might suggest that the CSO choose a more powerful reinforcer to withdraw, such as one that has more serious or long-term consequences. The objective remains the same: to stop reinforcing or maintaining the substance-using behavior. CSOs usually struggle with the notion of increasing the reward to be removed. Although most of them realize such an act is necessary, they anguish over the thought of their IPs actually experiencing some of the negative consequences that will directly or indirectly result. The situation is even more complicated by the fact that a time-out from these powerful reinforcers for the IP frequently results in fresh challenges for the CSO. Upon carefully reviewing the entire array of likely consequences, it often becomes apparent that a problem-solving strategy is needed to sort through these issues. Such a procedure is introduced later in this chapter.

Changes in the Guidelines for Selecting a Reinforcer to Withdraw when considering the removal of these more potent reinforcers involve *when* the reinforcer will be withdrawn and *if* it will be reintroduced. With regard to the former, the CSO does not typically wait until the next substance-abusing episode occurs but instead removes the reinforcer as soon as there is an opportunity to explain the plan to the IP. In regard to reinstating it, the intent is *not* to do so as soon as the drinking or drug use subsides—and, in fact, reinstatement may never occur. The change is being instituted because *the old style of interacting appears to be making it easier for the IP to continue using.* Sample scenarios describing the withdrawal of this caliber of reinforcer follow, as do initial concerns raised by CSOs about following through on the change in behavior, and their eventual justification for proceeding.

- A father (CSO) has been loaning the family car to his 25-year-old polydrug-abusing son (IP) in the evenings. The father wants to tell his son that he cannot borrow the car anymore. He is hesitant to do so, however, because one of the reasons the son uses the car is to get to his part-time job. The CSO is worried that his son will quit his job, as opposed to finding another mode of transportation. The father decides to tell the IP that he can use the car for another 6 weeks, but only to drive to and from work. Ideally, this restriction would pressure the son to secure full-time work, so that, among other things, he could buy a used car. In turn, the extra hours at work will compete with his using behavior.

• A 70-year-old mother (CSO) wishes to ask her 45-year-old son (IP) to find his own place to live because his drug use has become intolerable. However, she is worried that if she tells him to leave, she will rarely see him. Furthermore, she cannot bear to imagine him homeless or living in a substandard dwelling. After much discussion, she proceeds to ask him to move out. In order to still maintain contact (in part, so that she can continue implementing the CRAFT procedures with him), she invites him to join her for dinner several times a week if he is clean and sober. She decides not to worry about her son becoming homeless, realizing that it is not apt to happen; instead, the threat of it will force him to get a job.

• A 55-year-old woman (CSO) has been babysitting her granddaughter several evenings a week so that the daughter (IP) can pick up additional hours at work. Although the IP *does* work those extra evenings, she immediately spends most of the money she makes by going out afterward with friends to drink. Whenever the CSO tries to discuss the problem with the IP, the daughter says she needs time to have fun. The CSO is afraid that if she stops babysitting, the IP will get angry and stop bringing the granddaughter to see her. Nevertheless, the CSO decides to go ahead and tell her daughter she is no longer willing to babysit in the evening. The CSO believes that the IP will respond by cutting back her drinking for financial reasons, as she will now have to pay a sitter if she wants to work or socialize evenings. The CSO also thinks that although her daughter may "punish" her temporarily by keeping the granddaughter away, eventually she will bring her to visit again.

• An older brother (CSO) hired his sister (IP) as his receptionist 3 months ago. The IP's ongoing marijuana problem has regularly resulted in her late arrival to work and her lack of initiative or energy when there. The brother has given her feedback about the problem numerous times but has seen no significant improvement in her behavior. Although he is worried about her ability to keep another job, he knows that he needs to fire her. He decides to give her 4 weeks' notice, so that she can pass a drug test and find another job in the meantime. He believes that she will be forced to cut back on her smoking in order to hold her next job, as any nonrelative would not tolerate her poor work performance.

• An ex-wife (CSO) was granted full custody of the couple's son, primarily due to the ex-husband's (IP's) drinking and marijuana smoking. The IP was awarded unsupervised visitation rights. Given that the IP's substance use has not only continued but escalated, the CSO is worried about the son's safety and the effect of such a poor role model on the boy. Still, the ex-wife knows how much the father and son love spending time together, and she is reluctant to take that pleasure away from her child. After much consideration she decides to request that the court order only supervised visitation for her ex-husband. She hopes this substantial change will pressure him to get his addiction under control.

Despite the best conceived plans, there is no guarantee that the anticipated outcomes will occur when CSOs withdraw reinforcers. At times, situations actually appear to degenerate, at least for a period of time. Therefore, it is imperative to prepare CSOs for a wide range of possibilities. Stress the need for patience and consistent adherence to the plan, since the desired IP response may not be immediate. Then only assign the time-out procedure when you are certain the CSO can handle the gamut of possible outcomes. Problem solving may be introduced to address any anticipated dilemmas. When later reviewing a supposedly ineffective time-out assignment, never assume that the procedure was properly implemented. Ask clients to give exacting details regarding how they executed their homework and what the IP's response was at every point. It is common to discover that an improper execution of the task is at the root of the failed procedure.

THE "NATURAL CONSEQUENCES" PROCEDURE

The second procedure that relies on the pairing of negative consequences with substance-using behavior is one that simply allows the natural consequences of the IP's substance use to occur. In essence, this means that CSOs do not intervene in any way to "fix" the IP's problem or prevent a problem from impacting the IP *when the problem results directly from the IP's drinking or drug use.* As noted, the popular term for the act of fixing or preventing a substance-related problem is "enabling," because the behavior inadvertently makes it easier for the IP to continue abusing substances. For the most part these acts entail CSOs stepping in and, with the best of intentions, blocking the negative consequences that normally would be experienced by the IP upon abusing substances. Importantly, these consequences, were they experienced, *could* act as external controls or deterrents for the problem behavior. However, this is *not* to suggest that enablers *want* their IP to continue using. Many of them honestly do not realize that a fair number of their responses to the IP's using behavior actually render it more likely to happen in the future. Others feel helpless and hopeless, for they see no alternatives for handling the situation in question.

Getting CSOs to understand the role they play in maintaining substance-using behavior is a critical part of CRAFT. The objective is *not* to make CSOs feel guilty and ashamed for their reactions to their IP's use but instead to help them recognize and appreciate the connection between the two so that their own behavior can be modified. Ordinarily, you will have touched upon this notion early in treatment, such as during the overview of CRAFT in the first session. Similarly, if you already have taught CSOs how to withdraw positive reinforcement, you will have raised this issue. CSOs who enter treatment with some awareness of this dynamic often respond to the observation with frustration, because they do not know what to do about the seemingly unsolvable dilemma in which they find themselves. Among the CSOs who are surprised or embarrassed by the observation, many respond with a determination to take steps to alter their behavior. Finally, some clients become angry and defensive at what they perceive to be an accusation that they are not invested in their IP's recovery. Although the likelihood of this third type of response is minimized when you use a nonjudgmental, matter-of-fact style in presenting your findings, sometimes it cannot be avoided. Regardless, it is critical to normalize the enabling behavior, and to tell CSOs that no one is routinely "schooled" in how to respond properly to a substance abuser.

A brief illustration follows in which a therapist asks a CSO to consider how her response to a specific drinking episode is affecting the IP, and what it would be like to allow the natural consequences to take over instead. Assume that 36-year-old Sarah (CSO) has just reported that her partner, Brenda (IP), returns home inebriated one or two nights each week and typically proceeds to vomit in the bathroom. Although the IP makes a feeble attempt to clean up her mess at the time, the CSO invariably does most of it for her. The therapist addresses the CSO:

> "Sarah, I'd like to go back a minute to the situation you've just outlined. Let's see. Despite your requests for Brenda to stay home with you, she chooses to go out with her friends one or two nights a week to drink. When she arrives home, she throws up in the bathroom pretty regularly. You end up doing the bulk of the cleanup while she sleeps off her hangover. Interesting. What would happen if you didn't clean up after her? I'm wondering whether having to clean up the bathroom regularly *herself* the next morning would act as a deterrent for drinking excessively. I bet it would be quite a negative consequence for Brenda to have to deal with the vomit around noon the next day. And I wouldn't be surprised if the seriousness of her drinking problem became more apparent if she had to tackle the mess when she was sober. It would also illustrate how earnest you are about wanting Brenda to change her behavior. Of course, we'd have to consider how the mess that next morning would affect you."

Obviously there are numerous considerations before proceeding with an assignment to allow the natural consequences in this situation and all others. Upcoming sections of the chapter provide guidelines for implementing this technique and illustrations of how the CSO can share the plan with the IP. As an aside: It is useful to remind CSOs that one intervention alone, such as the one outlined above, is not expected to solve their IP's substance-abuse problem. It is considered but one step in the implementation of the comprehensive CRAFT package.

FINDING A SUITABLE NATURAL CONSEQUENCE TO TARGET

The process of selecting an occasion on which to allow the IP to experience the natural consequences of substance use typically begins informally. Although you should be alert to signs that a CSO is interfering with the occurrence of a negative consequence, you usually would not set out looking for them. Instead, these occasions become obvious in the course of discussing the various using scenarios—for example, sometimes while conducting a functional analysis of substance use. Recall that one segment of this interview inquires about the short-term positive consequences of a substance-using episode. Since these positive consequences appear to be at least partially responsible for maintaining the behavior, you should ascertain whether any of the CSO's own actions were among those reinforcing consequences mentioned. Normally, CSO involvement is only indirectly implied, so probing is used to gain a clearer picture. For example, assume that a CSO reported believing that her 20-year-old son (IP) liked to party on Friday nights, in part, because he rarely got called in to work an extra shift on Saturdays. An obvious follow-up question to ask is, "And what would happen if he did get called in to work?" You might discover that the mom makes up excuses to the boss if her son is too hungover to go in to the office. This is a prime example of a CSO preventing the natural consequences of the problem behavior from occurring, thereby limiting the potential control these negative consequences could exert over the substance use.

If there is not even an allusion to the CSO's response to the drinking or drug-using episode in the positive consequences section of the functional analysis, you could ask specifically about the CSO's immediate and delayed reactions to it. This question can also be posed if the episode under scrutiny is not the one that was used in the functional analysis, or if you simply prefer to directly test the client's awareness of her or his actions. Watch for evidence of CSOs unwittingly blocking the negative consequences, thereby clearing the path for their IP to keep using. To illustrate, assume that our CSO above only reported on the functional analysis chart that she believed her son enjoyed drinking on Friday nights because he did not have to worry about getting up early the next day. You might ask, "So there's nothing he ever has to get up and do on Saturday mornings?" A broad question such as this could open the way for a number of responses, such as, "Occasionally a study group for the one course that he takes at the community college gets together to work on a project," or "Sometimes he gets called in to work, but he doesn't go." Both responses suggest that the CSO is probably stepping in and addressing a potential problem by offering an excuse for the IP. If the excuse is that the IP is sick, the natural consequence of the drinking is prevented, because the other students let him remain in and benefit from the study group, or the boss does not become upset with the IP for being unavailable. Perhaps the CSO answers your question about Saturday mornings by stating that it is reserved for yard work. You might guess that the work is not being done—that the CSO is doing it herself or is paying someone else to take care of it.

Why are the outcomes in each of these scenarios problematic? To begin with, the IP is being protected from the natural, negative consequences of his drinking, thereby increasing the chance that he will drink (with impunity) again the next week. At the same time, there are repercussions for others as well. There is extra work for the other students in his study group, or the mom's supplemental income from her son is jeopardized (i.e., he could lose his job), or the CSO is doing more than her share of the yard work or using precious financial resources to have it done. In turn, the IP eventually would be affected by most of these outcomes, because his relationships would grow increasingly strained.

GUIDELINES FOR ALLOWING THE NATURAL CONSEQUENCES

Once you have identified a specific CSO behavior that is blocking the natural, negative consequences of the IP's use and discussed the CSO's feelings about this observation, you should cover several additional points before agreeing on a task for changing the behavior. An important question to ask the CSO is what will likely happen if she or he stops engaging in the behavior that typically interferes with the negative consequence. What will the IP do? How will the change impact the CSO and other loved ones? In part, you are looking for signs that the change in CSO behavior has a high probability of decreasing the IP's use. Given that this decreased use typically does not occur immediately, remind the CSO that the change in question may come only after consistently and repeatedly allowing the natural consequences to unfold. You also need to know that the proposed change has a low probability of causing physical harm to the CSO. Furthermore, when asking the client to anticipate the outcome of the new behavior, listen for reports of novel problems created for the

CSO in the process. Since it will be essential for the CSO to have the skills to address these new problems, you may need to introduce a problem-solving strategy, such as the one outlined later in this chapter. Finally, discuss *when* and *how* the CSO should describe the natural consequences plan to the IP. The material included earlier in the chapter, "Using Positive Communication to Explain the Removal of a Reward to an IP" serves as a useful framework for CSOs to use when explaining to their IPs both of the negative consequences procedures introduced in this chapter. Table 7.2 summarizes the components for selecting an appropriate natural consequence to target.

ILLUSTRATIVE CASE FOR ALLOWING NATURAL CONSEQUENCES

A segment of a therapy session follows in which a therapist discovers that a CSO is blocking the natural consequences of the IP's drinking. When the therapist gently offers this observation, the CSO responds in an angry, defensive manner initially. The therapist further inquires about the behavior in question, to determine if it is an appropriate one to target in the natural consequences exercise. Notice that he covers each of the steps in the guidelines presented in Table 7.2:

THERAPIST: Barbara, I have a pretty clear picture now of what goes on Friday nights as far as Lance's drinking and smoking. I guess I'm just not sure how you respond to it.

CSO: What do you mean? I scream at him, of course. I can't stand it. I'm waiting for him at the back door when he finally drags his butt home.

TABLE 7.2. GUIDELINES FOR ALLOWING THE NATURAL CONSEQUENCES

1. The consequence being allowed to occur is a *result of the substance use*.
2. The *CSO's feelings* (e.g., guilt, anger, shame) about previously blocking the consequence are discussed.
3. The *consequence* will be perceived by the IP as *negative*.
4. Allowing this natural consequence will likely serve to *decrease the use*.
5. It is *safe* to allow the consequence.
6. Other *problems* that arise for the CSO as a result can be *resolved*.
7. The CSO knows how and when to *explain the plan*.

THERAPIST: OK. So you scream at him when he first comes home. What do you do next?

CSO: I remind him that he's supposed to be reading to the kids and putting them to bed. He *wanted* Friday nights to be his night. But I know he doesn't have the energy to do it, so I put the kids to bed myself. They get upset, though, especially when I'm so pissed at him that I skip their bedtime story. It takes them forever to settle down then.

THERAPIST: So Friday nights are rough on everybody in your household, except maybe Lance?

CSO: That's the way I see it.

Note: The therapist inquires about the CSO's immediate *and* delayed reactions to her husband's using episode. As shown here, the CSO's delayed reactions are often the ones that are helping to maintain the using behavior. The therapist also shows empathy for the CSO's predicament. In an attempt to determine whether this situation is a good candidate for teaching the CSO how to stop blocking the natural consequences of the IP's use, the therapist inquires about the likely outcome if the CSO did not take over the IP's duties.

THERAPIST: No wonder you want to see what we can do about Friday night episodes! It's quite a hardship on you to have to step in there and do your husband's job. What do you think would happen if you simply didn't do it?

CSO: Didn't do it? Who would put the kids to bed? Somebody has to!

THERAPIST: You're absolutely right. Somebody has to. But what if it wasn't you?

CSO: I suppose if I didn't do it, they'd be up real late. Eventually he'd get around to it; maybe after he'd taken a big nap. Great (*Sarcastically*). Is that what this program is about . . . keeping the kids up late?! They'd be unbearably cranky the next day. At least I wouldn't be around to deal with it. I have my appointments first thing Saturday morning.

Note: The therapist will further investigate the use of this situation as a viable option for the natural consequences exercise, because it seems ideal in a number of ways. The problematic outcome that will result if the CSO does not prevent it is definitely due to the IP's substance use (Table 7.2, guideline 1). Furthermore, it will be experienced as negative by the IP (guideline 3), both Friday night and Saturday morning. The therapist next gently suggests that the CSO's behavior might be impeding the occurrence of negative consequences, thereby accidentally supporting the IP's continued use.

THERAPIST: So eventually Lance would put the kids to bed, if you didn't. And they'd be real cranky the next day, but you wouldn't be around to deal with it. Hmmm. So, in some ways, if you didn't step in and take care of things, Lance would have to. And he'd have some real consequences to pay if his drinking made him sleepy enough for a long nap, because the kids would get to bed late, and as a result he'd have to deal with their crankiness the next morning. What do you think?

CSO: (*Angrily*) Are you saying that what I've been doing all along has been wrong? I thought I was being a good mother by doing those things!

THERAPIST: Oh, you're definitely being a good mother. But let's think about the effect your behavior might be having on Lance and his drinking. Remember how we talked a little bit the first session about how sometimes we take such good care of the people we love that it makes it a little easier for them to continue drinking or using drugs? Of course, that's never our intention. It just works out that way.

CSO: So now you're saying that I'm helping him drink?! I *hate* his drinking, and he knows it. I just told you how I blast him even before he has a chance to get through the door.

THERAPIST: Yes, I heard that. I have no doubt that you hate his drinking; that's why you're here. And I'm sure *he* knows you hate it, too. I'm just trying to help you come up with a different way of responding to it besides blasting him and then taking over his child-care duties for him. You've been doing both of these things for some time now, and he's still drinking, right? So maybe it's time to try something else.

CSO: Well, I could see trying something else, but I don't see what *not* putting the kids to bed has to do with him stopping drinking.

THERAPIST: It might not have anything to do with it, but I think it's worth "sampling" as part of a bigger plan. You can always stop doing it if you don't like the outcome, right?

Note: The therapist reassures the client that the issue is not whether she disapproves of the drinking, but whether there might be a more effective way of handling it. He refers to her current practice of blocking the negative consequences as a normal act motivated by love. He then introduces the concept of sampling a new, foreign behavior to test *its* consequences.

CSO: I'm not opposed to trying new things, but I still don't get the connection. I'm supposed to just wait until he puts the kids to bed, right? OK. I guarantee that he'll only do it after a big old snooze. Even then, he'll have a hard time because he'll be half awake *and* half drunk. And he won't read to them, so they'll be mad.

THERAPIST: Who will they be mad at?

CSO: Him. Oh . . . I get it. At least they won't be mad at me for not reading their story.

THERAPIST: That's right. *He's* the one having to pay the consequences for his drinking. And it will be a burden for him to have to rally himself to put them to bed once he's been napping. Also, since he's putting them to bed late, they'll be cranky the next morning . . .

CSO: But *I* won't have to deal with it because I'm not home. *He* will. OK. So then what?

THERAPIST: Tell me what you think will happen? Here are the normal consequences for him staying out and drinking: (1) He has to rally himself to put the kids to bed when he'd really rather just sleep, (2) The kids are mad at him because they didn't get their story, and (3) He has to deal with their cranky moods Saturday morning because they didn't get enough sleep. What will happen?

Note: The therapist is making sure the client sees the connection between the drinking and all the natural consequences. Next he evaluates several things: whether this scenario is likely to affect the IP's drinking, whether there is cause for concern about a violent reaction, and whether the CSO can handle other problems that might arise once this change in the normal routine is introduced (guidelines 4–6). Another safety consideration is whether the husband will be too incapacitated to care for the children.

CSO: He'll be in a bad mood, for sure. He'll ask me why I didn't put them to bed.

THERAPIST: If you decide to go ahead with this plan, we'll need to think carefully about the chance that he'll get really mad at you and lash out physically. I know he doesn't have a history of that, but you'd be acting very differently from how you usually do. So is he apt to hurt you either that night, when he realizes you aren't putting the kids to bed, or when you get home from your appointments on Saturday?

CSO: No. If anything, he'd give me the icy stare and go huffing around for a while.

THERAPIST: OK, so there's no safety issues. What about other problems that might spring up in the process of carrying out this plan? Picture yourself actually holding back and *not* putting the kids to bed for him Friday night. What do you see happening?

CSO: It will just be hard for me *not* to take over. The kids will just sit watching TV till all hours. Eventually they'll fall asleep on the floor.

THERAPIST: So the only real problem is keeping yourself from stepping in and putting them to bed. How will you handle that?

CSO: Oh, I can do it if I have to. I'll just watch TV with them or read a magazine. If I know it's for a good reason, I can hold back.

THERAPIST: Sounds good. Can you think of any difficulties when he gets home that night, or maybe Saturday morning? Or how about Saturday afternoon when you return?

CSO: Not really. He won't be happy, but he'll put the kids to bed. The only problems on Saturday morning will be *his*. Like I said before, he'll be upset with me, but that's about it.

THERAPIST: That's fine, then. Now, the purpose of all of this is to eventually get him to decrease his drinking. This should be a first step toward that goal. What do you think? Is this change in your behavior likely to point things in that direction?

CSO: It sure won't hurt things. I don't know. Maybe. I'm curious to see what he'll do. It might be a start.

Note: The therapist decides not to resort to the official problem-solving procedure here, because there do not seem to be unresolved problems. Next he checks with the CSO about her feelings before raising the issue of informing the IP about the plan (guidelines 2 and 7).

THERAPIST: I want to take a moment to check in with you about how you're feeling. You reacted pretty strongly when I first brought up the topic today of not stepping in and taking care of things for Lance on Friday nights.

CSO: Maybe I overreacted a little. At first I thought you were saying I was doing everything wrong, but it doesn't seem that way now. I know you're right. I'm just sensitive about it. I'm never really sure if I'm doing what's right. I feel OK now. I want to do it.

THERAPIST: I'm glad to hear that. I'll check back with you periodically about your feelings, because this topic of natural consequences tends to be tough for people, in general. Now we need to decide whether you'll tell Lance in advance about the plan, or whether you'll explain it to him the next time the situation arises. What do you think?

CSO: I'm not sure. I think I'd rather give him some warning.

THERAPIST: Probably a good idea. Remember what we said before about picking an ideal time to have conversations such as this one?

CSO: Yes. It should be a time when he's not drinking or hungover, and when we're both getting along.

THERAPIST: Excellent! So what do you think?

CSO: I always have the most courage right after my sessions here. And he's kind of curious about what goes on. He might even ask.

THERAPIST: That's a good sign. When we discuss inviting him to treatment, we'll probably make the offer at a time when he asks about your sessions. But that will come later.

Note: The technique of responding to an IP's curiosity about treatment with an invitation to attend a session is presented in Chapter 9. In the current situation, notice that the therapist does not let the CSO rely exclusively on this one opportunity for the conversation but requests a backup. The positive communication components being referenced are discussed in Chapter 5 and summarized in Figure 5.1.

THERAPIST: OK. So if he doesn't ask about your therapy tonight, will you be able to bring up the topic anyway? And what will you say? Pretend I'm Lance. I'll start it off. I'm just arriving home from work. And don't worry if I don't say exactly what he would. It should be close enough for our purposes here. Try to use some of the pieces of a good conversation that we've practiced. (*Points to a chart with them listed.*) Here I go. (*As husband*) So how'd your talk with "the good doctor" go today? My ears were ringing again.

CSO: (*In role play*) I'm not surprised. We *did* talk about you. I've got a new plan that I'm going to try.

THERAPIST: (*As husband*) Uh-oh! Here we go again. What's it this time?

CSO: (*In role play*) It has to do with Friday nights. Ya know how you said you wanted to read the kids their story and put them to bed on Fridays, but how I usually end up doing it?

THERAPIST: (*As husband*) Well, it's not *my* fault if you butt in and do it. I said I would.

CSO: (*In role play*) Yes, and I think you have good intentions, but it gets so late that I worry about the kids being up still. And you know how cranky they are Saturday mornings if they haven't had enough sleep.

THERAPIST: (*As husband*) I can't argue with that. So what's the plan?

CSO: (*In role play*) I'm not going to step in anymore. I'm going to let you put them to bed, even if it's late.

THERAPIST: (*As husband*) What's this supposed to accomplish?

CSO: (*In role play*) I'm going to stop making it easier for you to drink.

THERAPIST: (*As husband*) *What*?!

CSO: (*In role play*) Maybe if I stop taking care of things for you, you'll think twice before overdoing it next time. If you have to deal with the kids being up late and getting upset with you for not reading to them, maybe you'll make an effort to get home earlier.

THERAPIST: (*As husband*) Fine. So I'll come home early and drink *here*. So much for your plan!

CSO: (*To therapist*) He's right. What then?

THERAPIST: Sure, he could do that. But it would be a disruption of his normal routine; maybe enough to make him think twice about his drinking. And from what you've said before, he drinks less at home than he does when he's out. So it's a start. Also, he'd see that you're real serious about things changing at home, since you'd be changing your own behavior. Now let's review how your conversation went. Then we'll practice a scene in which Lance hasn't brought up the therapy topic at all, so that you'll be ready if you end up having to bring it up yourself.

Next, the therapist would compliment the CSO's description of the purpose of her plan, as it was clear that she understood what she was doing and why. Together they would review other positive aspects of the communication and generate ideas for improving it. In subsequent role plays the therapist might portray the husband as more critical or, as noted, would leave the initiation of the topic entirely to the CSO.

SAMPLES OF POTENTIAL SITUATIONS TO TARGET FOR ALLOWING THE NATURAL CONSEQUENCES

Listed below are additional examples of occasions on which it might be reasonable for CSOs to step aside in order to allow the natural consequences of a substance-abusing episode to emerge fully. Caution must be exercised, as all the factors of the case would need to be considered thoroughly before determining whether the situation is, in fact, suitable. As mentioned, new problems for the CSO are often created in the process of allowing the natural consequences of IP using behavior. Naturally the CSO would need to judge whether any hardships created by these "complications" would be worth the potential gain if the procedure succeeds. Some of the obvious problems triggered by the proposed acts are noted. Assume that the seven Guidelines for Allowing the Natural Consequences are met in each scenario:

• A mother (CSO) typically spends about 45 minutes each Sunday morning trying to get her older son (IP) awake and out of bed so that he can attend his little brother's 10:00 soccer game. The IP's marijuana use the night before is responsible for his morning's difficulty. The IP insists that his mother perform this ritual, because he hates to miss the games and disappoint his brother. However, the duty is time consuming and frustrating for the CSO. The natural consequence for the IP's drug use is to let him sleep through his brother's game, if a brief, normal attempt by the CSO to rouse him does not work. The main problem created for the CSO in executing this plan is dealing with her younger son's sadness when his big brother misses the game.

• A 70-year-old alcoholic father (IP) has been living with his daughter (CSO) since his wife died suddenly 2 months ago. The IP has a long history of staying late at bars, where his wife would appear, around midnight, with the car to drive him home. The daughter begrudgingly followed in her late mother's footsteps initially. The natural consequence of the IP's drinking would be for him to take responsibility for getting himself home at that late hour. The daughter realizes that this is a complicated issue. Although he rides the bus during the day, he cannot do so at night because they do not run after 8 P.M. Since he no longer drives and abhors asking anyone at the bar for a ride, he would have to call a cab. However, he is opposed to spending money on cabs; he firmly believes that "family members should watch out for each other." The CSO's main problem is guilt.

• The wife (CSO) of a drug-abusing husband (IP) has gotten into the habit of calling her parents for financial help as it nears the end of the month. Although the husband's salary used to be sufficient to cover expenses, much of it now is being used to purchase drugs. The natural consequence for the IP would be to let him pay the bills late. Eventually, this practice could result in a variety of negative consequences for the IP, such as receiving a bad credit rating or finding the utilities turned off or the car repossessed. The dilemma facing the CSO is that *she* would be affected by many of these consequences, as well, and would need to be prepared to deal with them if she decides to proceed.

• An older sister (CSO) has been colluding with her brother (IP) to deceive his parole officer. One of the conditions of the IP's parole is that he not go in the vicinity of the drug-dealing section of town. Nevertheless, he frequents that location and continues to sell and use drugs. The CSO shares an apartment with her brother and is typically home when his parole officer stops by for an unannounced visit. The brother expects his sister to alert him via his cell phone and then to detain the officer long enough so that the IP can slip in the back door. She has grown tired of this arrangement and her brother's drug problem. She has no safety fears.

The natural consequence for the IP's drug use begins with the CSO *not* phoning him whenever the parole officer visits. Since the officer is likely to proceed downtown, conceivably he will come upon the IP selling and using. This violation of his parole could land the brother back in jail. The problems created for the CSO by this plan include the wrath of her brother and possibly that of other family members, and the loss of someone with whom to share apartment expenses.

• A wife (CSO) routinely covers for her husband (IP) by calling the boss and making excuses every time the IP misses work due to his drinking. Allowing the natural consequences for the drinking entails not calling the boss and letting the husband face the job problems that ensue. The CSO's own difficulties created by this move might include an angry husband, a demotion for her husband, or even the loss of his job and income.

As illustrated by these cases, when CSOs stop running interference between IPs and their substance-related problems, the range in the seriousness of the anticipated negative consequences for IPs varies tremendously. It should also be apparent that it is virtually impossible for CSOs to witness major consequences for IPs without the fall-out of the problems also affecting the CSOs. It is important for CSOs to consider all potential outcomes carefully, so that they can make an informed decision about proceeding. During this discussion you should assess whether they possess the requisite problem-solving skills to manage the various possibilities. At times, CSOs decide that, although the natural consequences plan appears appropriate and necessary, they are not prepared to face the consequences that will likely result. If problem-solving procedures do not present a satisfying solution and assuage their fears and guilt, a different plan should be selected, at least temporarily.

PROBLEM-SOLVING PROCEDURE

In this chapter *problem solving* is referenced in the context of having a strategy for handling new dilemmas created by the negative consequences procedures. The ability to solve problems is a skill that most people rely on daily (Monti & Rohsenow, 2003). Yet many clients regularly become overwhelmed by their problems and report not knowing where to turn or what to do next (D'Zurilla, Chang, Nottingham, & Faccini, 1998). Applying a standard problem-solving procedure can be extremely helpful in these situations. The procedure outlined below is included as part of the Community Reinforcement Approach (Meyers & Smith, 1995). A variation of it was introduced much earlier by D'Zurilla and Goldfried (1971). The steps are as follows:

1. Define the problem narrowly. Clients often present problems that initially appear to be complex, because in reality, they represent a number of problems as opposed to just one. Most individuals find it easier to tackle a series of smaller problems than one large complicated problem. Not only are the solutions to smaller problems more obvious and manageable, but clients feel more optimistic as they face them. So help CSOs narrow down their complex problems into one or more specific problems, and ask them to select just one to address first. Often solving the first problem obviates the need to even address the secondary, related problems that originally were identified.

2. Brainstorm possible solutions. Brainstorming is supposed to be the fun part of problem solving! The objective is to have clients generate many potential solutions to the problem, so that a variety of alternatives are available from which to choose. The ideas need to be recorded; generally it is preferable to use a whiteboard or a large easel during group sessions, but you may opt to use the Problem-Solving Worksheet (Figure 7.1, end of chapter) or a blank piece of paper when working one-on-one. When introducing brainstorming in a group setting, it is important to convey the message that *all* suggestions are welcome and that criticisms are not appropriate. The rationale is straightforward: If individuals are immediately criticized upon offering a solution, they will be less likely to offer additional ones. You should highlight the point that all suggestions are welcome even when you are conducting an individual session, as CSOs often need encouragement to speak up and participate in this phase. To emphasize the nonjudgmental quality of the procedure, some therapists start the brainstorming process by suggesting some obviously wild or funny solutions. Finally, since most CSO problem-solving attempts occur during individual sessions, it may be necessary for you to assist by generating serious alternatives if the CSO falls short on ideas.

3. Eliminate unwanted suggestions. This step entails asking the client to eliminate any of the potential solutions that are unappealing for virtually any reason. Instruct the CSO to read each suggestion, erasing or crossing out those that she or he cannot imagine doing in the upcoming week. Furthermore, state that it absolutely is *not* necessary to explain why an item is being eliminated. Offering explanations adds significantly to the time required to complete this step of problem solving without providing any substantial benefit. It also detracts from the overall positive emphasis of CRAFT, given that it instead focuses on things that presumably will *not* work. Nevertheless, many CSOs automatically mention the reason for excluding an item. One of the most common reasons given is that they already have tried something similar, and it did not help. Additional reasons include the suggestion being (1) too difficult to carry out (emotionally, financially, or both), (2) unappealing, given the client's or

IP's personal likes/dislikes, (3) too complicated, or (4) potentially dangerous. Occasionally a client might eliminate every suggestion that was made. If this happens, simply repeat the brainstorming step.

4. Select one potential solution. Ask your client to examine the remaining potential solutions and to select one that appears worth trying. Then have the CSO describe exactly how the task will be enacted. The degree of detail should allow you to determine whether the client is carefully evaluating whether the act is feasible, under the circumstances. Sometimes eager CSOs want to select more than one solution. Depending on the skills of the client and the complexity of the initial solution selected, this course of action might be acceptable. If so, the remaining steps would need to address each solution being attempted.

5. Identify possible obstacles. In the process of completing step 4, various obstacles to carrying out the new solution often become apparent. If obstacles do not become apparent, ask CSOs to imagine attempting the solution in the upcoming week and to describe any foreseeable problems that could interfere with completing the task. Based on your knowledge of them and their situation, you should be able to identify problems as well. Not only are you trying to help clients anticipate problems so that they can be resolved in advance, but, in essence, you are also asking them to list the excuses they might otherwise present at the next session. Discussing these "excuses" tends to have a paradoxical effect: It lessens the chance they will use them (Akillas & Efran, 1995; Ascher & Turner, 1979).

6. Address each obstacle. Every identified obstacle must be addressed and usually this is accomplished by developing a simple backup plan after a brief discussion. For example, assume a CSO states that she might not have the opportunity to initiate a planned conversation with her husband during dinner, because he might be intoxicated each evening that coming week. The backup plan could be to settle upon another precise time to have the conversation, or to ask the husband, in advance, to set aside a (sober) time so that something important can be discussed. Sometimes obstacles are best addressed by using an abbreviated problem-solving procedure. Importantly, if the obstacle cannot be resolved in advance, advise the CSO to select another solution.

7. Decide on the assignment and do it. Once the plan has been mapped out and foreseeable obstacles have been addressed, ask the CSO to verbalize the assignment and its time frame for completion. If the client has elected to attempt two solutions, be sure the plan for each is clear (e.g., sequence, circumstances). Set an expectation for the assignment to be completed by the next session.

8. Evaluate the outcome. As with all assignments, it is critical to inquire about the outcome of the plan in the next session. It is best to avoid the question "Did you do the assignment?", since you do not want clients to know you are even considering the possibility that they did *not* do it. Instead, ask something general, such as, "How did the assignment go this week?" This wording still allows them to tell you if they did not attempt it, while, at the same time, opening a discussion of the positive and negative aspects to an assignment if they did complete it. If the assignment was not attempted, consider it an ideal opportunity to conduct a problem-solving procedure around that very issue. In other words, you should problem solve the reason why the client did not do the assignment.

If the assignment was attempted, ask CSOs to describe what happened in terms of both the process and the outcome. If it was carried out as planned, did it work? Was the outcome satisfactory? Is it worth doing again? The plan may have been perfectly executed but the outcome unexpected and undesired. If so, a modified plan might be required. Or perhaps the client faced some unanticipated difficulty in doing the assignment, and a revised plan is now needed. Either of these scenarios could entail reviewing the options generated previously in the brainstorming step or redoing the problem-solving procedure altogether.

The basic problem-solving steps, which are summarized in Table 7.3, can easily be written on an index card and given to a client for easy reference during the week. Alternatively, the Problem-Solving Worksheet in Figure 7.1 can be provided.

ILLUSTRATIVE CASE USING THE PROBLEM-SOLVING WORKSHEET

A case follows in which the problem-solving procedure is demonstrated via use of the Problem-Solving Worksheet. For instructional purposes, a

TABLE 7.3. PROBLEM-SOLVING GUIDELINES

1. *Define* the problem *narrowly*.
2. *Brainstorm* possible solutions.
3. *Eliminate* unwanted suggestions.
4. *Select one* potential solution.
5. Identify possible *obstacles*.
6. *Address each* obstacle.
7. Decide on the *assignment* and do it.
8. *Evaluate* the outcome.

sample worksheet provides likely client comments. If this information would not normally appear on a client's worksheet, it is placed in brackets. The case involves a wife (CSO) and her alcohol-dependent spouse (IP). The assumption is that the CSO has learned the procedure for allowing the natural consequences of the IP's using behavior, and she is ready to apply it. Her plan is to refrain from calling her mother-in-law with an excuse as to why they cannot attend Sunday dinner, when the truth is that her husband has a hangover and is too sick to go. At some level the CSO believes that her mother-in-law knows about her son's drinking problem. Regardless, the CSO thinks that her plan will present a natural consequence for her husband: He will have to deal with his mother directly about the issue. However, in the course of thinking through this plan, the CSO stumbled on a problem that the therapist is concerned might jeopardize the client's ability to complete her natural consequences task. The identified problem is an example of the fall-out that often affects a CSO when allowing the natural consequences for an IP. The therapist immediately resorts to the problem-solving procedure.

SAMPLE PROBLEM-SOLVING WORKSHEET

1. *Define the problem narrowly.*

   If I don't call my mother-in-law with an excuse about why we can't come to dinner the next time Miguel is sick with a hangover, she'll get really upset and blame me for putting her through the trouble of unnecessarily preparing dinner.

2. *Brainstorm possible solutions.*

   - Don't call; the possible payoff justifies me letting her get upset.
   - Leave the house so Miguel has to deal with her when she calls.
   - Call her but tell her the truth about the drinking.
   - Ask Miguel to call her.
   - Call her but hand the phone over to Miguel, so he has to make the excuse.
   - Refuse the dinner invitation in the first place.
   - Tell Miguel before he starts to drink that I'm not making excuses to his mom for him again.
   - Next time she invites us over, insist that she come to our house instead.
   - Ask Miguel to attend counseling now so we can work on the problem.
   - Call her and say that we can't come, and that Miguel will explain it to her tomorrow.

- Walk out on Miguel once and for all.
- Take some Valium and forget about it.

3. *Eliminate unwanted suggestions.*

- ~~Don't call; the possible payoff justifies my letting her get upset.~~ [Would make me too nervous to wait and do nothing, and I'd feel guilty for possibly creating unnecessary work for her.]
- Leave the house so Miguel has to deal with her when she calls. [Maybe; feels mean though; plus he'd get really angry.]
- ~~Call her but tell her the truth about the drinking.~~ [He should probably tell her.]
- ~~Ask Miguel to call her.~~ [I've already tried this; he won't call.]
- ~~Call her but hand the phone over to Miguel, so he has to make the excuse.~~ [I've done this before, too; it really makes him mad.]
- ~~Refuse the dinner invitation in the first place.~~ [I'd still have to give an excuse.]
- Tell Miguel before he starts to drink that I'm not making excuses to his mom for him again. [Maybe; but then if he drinks anyway, what do I do?]
- Next time she invites us over, insist that she come to our house instead. [This could work some of the time, because he drinks less if he knows she's coming over, but we'll still get invited to her house another time.]
- ~~Ask Miguel to attend counseling now so we can work on the problem.~~ [He won't agree to come.]
- Call her and say that we can't come, and that Miguel will explain it to her tomorrow. [Maybe; I'd have to get off the phone really fast because otherwise she'll ask questions, and I'll end up giving an excuse after all.]
- ~~Walk out on Miguel once and for all.~~ [I'm not ready to do this.]
- ~~Take some Valium and forget about it.~~ [Sometimes I do, but the problem doesn't go away.]

4. *Select one potential solution.*

- Call her and say that we can't come, and that Miguel will explain it to her tomorrow. [I feel like it would be really mean if I didn't call his mom and let her know we wouldn't be coming. So I like the idea of speaking to her briefly just to say we won't be coming, and then leaving it up to Miguel to explain the next day.]

5. *Identify possible obstacles.*

- I might have trouble getting off the phone; what if she keeps asking me what's wrong?

- Miguel might not call his mom the next day to explain; she'd get a hold of me instead, and I'd be in that same awkward position of having to explain it anyway.
- Miguel could get really mad at me for springing this on him without any warning, and I'm not sure I want to deal with that reaction.

6. *Address each obstacle.*

- [I might have trouble getting off the phone; what if she keeps asking me what's wrong? *Solution?*: If I plan ahead of time what I'm going to say and I keep it short, I can probably do it.]

Note: The therapist would have the CSO role-play the phone conversation several times, and would make appropriate suggestions. For example, she would be advised to immediately assure her mother-in-law that there is not a medical emergency of any type.

- [Miguel might not call his mom the next day to explain; she'd get a hold of me instead, and I'd be in that same awkward position of having to explain it anyway. *Solution?*: I could say that he really needs to be the one to talk to her about it. But I'm afraid that I'd avoid her in the meantime.]

Note: Again, the therapist would role-play this conversation with the CSO in advance. She also would discuss her concern about the perceived need to avoid Miguel's mom. If these uncomfortable feelings were strong and appeared to be a serious obstacle to carrying out the solution, the therapist would label it as a problem needing resolution. For example, the CSO might be advised to extend her initial phone conversation with her mother-in-law by adding a comment about feeling uncomfortable being caught in the middle between Miguel and his mom. Alternatively, the client simply might be asked to monitor her feelings during this potentially uncomfortable time to see whether additional action is required.

- [Miguel could get really mad at me for springing this on him without any warning, and I'm not sure I want to deal with that reaction. *Solution?*: I'll just have to live with it. He gets mad at me all the time anyway.]

Note: The therapist would not leave this response as the solution, but would treat it as a solvable problem. She would suggest that the CSO take another look at the list of potential solutions already generated to see if another one could be added. For example:

- Tell Miguel before he starts to drink that I'm not making excuses to his mom for him again.

Note: The CSO originally considered this one as an option. If the therapist rehearsed this conversation and discussed the best time to deliver it, it might effectively address the obstacle raised about the husband being upset when he was not "warned" in advance.

7. *Decide on the assignment and do it.*

- Miguel is always sober and in a good mood Friday mornings, so I'll tell him during breakfast this Friday about my plan to stop making excuses to his mom. She's already invited us to Sunday dinner.
- If he's drunk or hungover Sunday afternoon but doesn't call her to cancel, I will. I'll simply tell her we can't come, and that Miguel will explain it to her tomorrow. I'll mention that there's no emergency, so she shouldn't worry.
- If she tries to talk to me the next day because Miguel didn't call to say why we didn't come, I'll tell her that Miguel needs to be the one to talk with her about it.

Note: Before finalizing the assignment, the therapist would make sure that the client (1) had the skills to effectively deliver the messages, (2) had selected the best time for the conversation with her husband as well as a backup time, and (3) had ruled out the potential for any violent reactions.

8. *Evaluate the outcome.*

Assume that the following dialogue occurs at the start of the CSO's next therapy session. It begins with the therapist inquiring about the status of the assignment that resulted from the problem-solving procedure outlined above.

THERAPIST: I'm anxious to hear how your assignment went this week.

CSO: Oh, the one about not making excuses to Miguel's mom anymore? I don't know. Not too good, I guess.

THERAPIST: You had come up with a really good plan, but even the best plans don't always work out. Can you tell me exactly what happened?

Note: The therapist first determines whether the plan was executed as outlined, since a deviation from the original plan is often the reason for a "failed" assignment.

CSO: Well, I did what we talked about. I told him that I wasn't going to make excuses for him anymore. He got really pissed and said that he didn't care if we *never* went to his mom's again. I didn't call her, though. I stuck to my guns. But then she called when we didn't show up, and so I ended up saying he was sick again. I'm still making excuses for him. And now she's probably really mad at me for not letting her know we weren't coming.

THERAPIST: Actually, that's exactly the problem we tried to problem-solve. You anticipated that one perfectly. Hmmmm. According to what's written on your worksheet, the plan was for you to go ahead and call his mom if he didn't, but for it to be a different type of phone call this time. Remember? You were going to avoid making excuses; you simply were going to say you weren't coming.

CSO: Oh, that's right.

THERAPIST: OK. So let's see. You *did* speak to Miguel. That was part of the plan. Ya know, it would help me understand what went wrong here if you started by telling me *how* and *when* you told Miguel that you weren't going to make excuses anymore.

Note: The therapist speculates that something went amiss in the delivery of the message to the IP: perhaps either the wording used or the timing of the communication. Regardless of the type of difficulty encountered by the CSO in executing the task, it is important for her to recognize what went wrong so that she can correct the problem when she attempts the next assignment. The therapist also gently pointed out that the plan was not, in fact, executed as intended as far as the CSO calling the mother-in-law in advance.

CSO: I know I said that I was going to tell him Friday morning, but he was in such a good mood that I didn't want to spoil it by bringing this stuff up. I guess I just hoped he'd stay in a good mood and not need to drink so much that weekend. But he went out Saturday night, just like he always does, and so then I had to tell him Sunday afternoon when he finally got up.

THERAPIST: OK. And can you demonstrate how you told him? Can you use roughly the same words you used?

CSO: He was yelling at me to bring him cream for his coffee. I don't know. I guess I was kind of upset, because I sort of yelled back that I was sick of doing things for him when he had a hangover, like calling his mom and making excuses for him. That's when he said he didn't care if we ever ate over there again. It just made me feel sorry for his mom.

THERAPIST: At least you told him how you felt about making excuses for his behavior. That's something new for you. But I still think your original plan, including *when* and *how* to tell him, could work. Do you see what you did differently from what we'd outlined about discussing the issue with Miguel, and do you know why you made the decision to do it this way instead? By the way, lots of people have trouble the first time they try out something new at home, so don't get down on yourself.

Note: It is clear that the client did not follow some of the crucial details of the assignment involving the timing of the message to the IP and the use of positive communication. By waiting and responding out of anger, the message was delivered in a negative tone to an IP who was feeling poorly (i.e., hungover). Next the therapist determines whether these obstacles can be overcome or if a new solution will need to be adopted and tested.

CSO: I know we've talked about *not* having these important conversations when either of us is upset, so I probably should have stuck with the original time. It's hard, though. The words don't always come out when you want them to.

THERAPIST: You're right. It's *real* hard to wait until you're both calm. That's why it helps to have the conversation *before* you're in a situation where either of you is upset. That's why you picked Friday morning at breakfast.

CSO: I know I did. And I didn't forget. I just didn't want to spoil things. And I convinced myself that he was already changing, that his drinking wouldn't be a problem this week. I know better than that, though.

THERAPIST: Well, it's good to be hopeful . . . but at the same time, to be realistic, too. It's still early in your own therapy. There's lots of time to work toward influencing Miguel's behavior. You also said that you didn't want to spoil things. Can you think of a way to have that conversation during Friday's breakfast so that you don't have to be afraid it will spoil things?

Note: The therapist conveys support and then moves on to detect other obstacles that interfered with the CSO's ability to bring up the topic.

CSO: There wasn't anything wrong with the conversation we practiced. I guess I just had to see, once again, that he's not going to change on his own.

THERAPIST: OK. But let's go ahead and rehearse that conversation one more time. I'll play Miguel's role again. Last time you told me he'd act annoyed. Does that still seem to fit?

CSO: Pretty much. Nothing worse, really.

Note: The therapist wants to play the role as realistically as possible because the client's concern about the IP's reaction was an obstacle to carrying out the assignment as planned. In turn, the outcome affected the CSO's decision to notify the mother-in-law in advance.

THERAPIST: I'll start it off. (*As husband*) Friday, at last! What a week it's been. Boy, am I ever looking forward to a few days of relaxing!

CSO: (*In role play*) Me, too. Don't forget that we're supposed to go to your mom's on Sunday.

THERAPIST: (*As husband*) That's right. I hope she makes pot roast again. Man, was that ever tasty.

CSO: (*In role play*) I bet she would if you asked her to. Hey, Miguel, I'm worried that you're going to be sick again, and that we'll have to cancel. You know what I mean?

THERAPIST: (*As husband; sarcastically*) No, I'm stupid. Of course, I know what you mean. Why don't you just come right out and say it: I'll have a hangover!

CSO: (*In role play*) I hate to see you sick. And it's gotten really hard for me to keep making excuses to your mom. It makes me feel bad. I don't want to keep lying to her.

THERAPIST: (*As husband*) Then don't. Tell her that her son is a drunk and leave it at that.

CSO: (*To therapist*) Yup. That's what he'll say. I hate to start the day off like that if we don't have to. It seems like we have so little pleasant time together as it is.

THERAPIST: I can understand that, but let's think about two things. First, if you don't change how you interact with Miguel, the problem of having to make excuses to his mom will still be there, right?

CSO: I know. You're right. I *do* want to try to fix that. It really bothers me.

THERAPIST: Second, it's good to remember the big picture. In other words, it's important to keep in mind that you're taking small steps toward getting Miguel to cut down his drinking and get into therapy. We're hoping that he will cut down on his drinking because he doesn't want to have to face his mom about having a hangover on Sunday, right? If he does this in response to you doing your assignment, then you've taken a big step toward helping him reduce his drinking. Does that make sense?

CSO: Yes. I just need to remind myself of that when I'm finding it hard to bring up the topic.

Note: To enhance motivation, the therapist reminds the client about what she may potentially gain, both short- and long-term, if she follows through with the planned intervention.

Next the therapist would examine the communication to see if it could be made more positive, and therefore easier, for the IP to hear. Perhaps the CSO could have introduced a more positive tone by mentioning what she likes about Sundays when Miguel is feeling good and has not been drinking. The last three components of a positive communication were missing as well. As her understanding statement, the CSO could have said: "I know it's hard to be planning for Sunday dinner at your mom's when you're out having a good time with your friends on Saturday . . . " As far as accepting partial responsibility, the CSO might have stated: "I guess I kind of got myself into this uncomfortable situation when I took charge of making excuses to your mom months ago." The wife's offer to help could sound like, "Is there something I could do to make it easier for you to come home earlier Saturday nights?" Finally, although the therapist thinks that the unsettling conversation with the IP was largely responsible for the CSO deciding *not* to call the mother-in-law to cancel Sunday dinner, this issue would still be raised directly.

SUMMARY

This chapter presents two procedures that CSOs tend to find difficult to implement; ones that if properly executed result in the IP experiencing negative consequences. Importantly, negative consequences are the intended outcome because they are linked with the IP's substance-abusing behavior. A strategy that is theoretically similar to the practice of giving positive rewards for sober behavior is described first. However, instead of bestowing rewards, it entails removing reinforcers of substance-abusing behaviors. Procedures for teaching CSOs to refrain from stepping in and either "fixing" or preventing problems that IPs would normally have to face as a result of their drinking or drug use are described as well, as is a sound problem-solving procedure for CSOs to use in dealing with the fallout from the newly allowed negative consequences.

FIGURE 7.1.	PROBLEM-SOLVING WORKSHEET

1. *Define the problem narrowly.* [Just one . . . and keep it specific. Write it out below.]

2. *Brainstorm possible solutions.* [The more, the better! Let yourself go here! List below.]

3. *Eliminate unwanted suggestions.* [Cross out any that don't seem practical/helpful.]

4. *Select one potential solution.* [Which one looks really good to start with? Circle it.]

5. *Identify possible obstacles.* [What might get in the way of this working? List below.]

6. *Address each obstacle.* [If you *can't* solve each obstacle, pick a new solution; restart with #5.]

7. *Decide on the assignment and do it.* [List below exactly when/how you'll do it; then do it!]

8. *Evaluate the outcome.* [Did it work? If it needs some changes, list them below and try again.]

CHAPTER 8

HELPING CONCERNED SIGNIFICANT OTHERS ENRICH THEIR OWN LIVES

Thus far this book has focused explicitly on various ways to influence the IP's behavior through changes in the CSO's behavior. Some of these procedures involve direct attempts to elicit change, whereas others are more subtle. All of the procedures are geared toward the two CRAFT goals that focus specifically on the IP: (1) influencing the IP to reduce substance use, and (2) successfully encouraging the IP to enter treatment. It is certainly the case that many CSOs reap "rewards" in the process, either through an improved CSO–IP relationship, or as a result of learning valuable skills (e.g., communication, problem solving). A subset of clients automatically are happier, whatever the state of their IP, because they feel empowered. But the CRAFT program does not stop here in working with CSOs to enrich their own lives. As noted previously, CRAFT's third major goal is to help CSOs improve their own psychological functioning and the overall quality of their lives, regardless of whether their IPs ever begin treatment. Many of the behavioral techniques for accomplishing this goal come from the Community Reinforcement Approach—the program that is used directly with treatment-seeking individuals who have substance abuse problems (see Meyers & Smith, 1995).

PSYCHOLOGICAL FUNCTIONING ISSUES OF CSOs

Chapter 1 outlines some of the many stressors that CSOs face on a daily basis as a result of their relationship with an individual who chronically abuses substances. To review, these stressors include physical violence, verbal aggression, emotionally empty relationships, financial problems, social embarrassment, sexual relationship problems, and disrupted relationships with the children (Jacob et al., 1991; O'Farrell & Birchler, 1987; Romijn et al., 1992; Velleman et al., 1993). The point was made in Chapter 1 also that, not surprisingly, these CSOs frequently exhibit symptoms of depression, anxiety, anger, and somatization (Brown et al., 1995; Collins et al., 1990; Kirby et al., 1999; Meyers et al., 1999; W. Miller et al., 1999). If you are familiar with this profile, you may already know how to help CSOs deal with their own personal therapy "issues" that may or may not be highly associated with their IP's alcohol or drug problem. What follows is a description of the CRAFT approach to addressing this third goal of the program: helping CSOs enrich their own lives.

ASSESSING THE CSO'S OVERALL DEGREE OF HAPPINESS

In working with CSOs, it is important to determine which particular issues in addition to the CSO–IP relationship should be addressed in order to enhance their quality of life. Conceivably you evaluate this area formally at the Intake. Regardless, CRAFT therapists conduct a brief assessment of clients' satisfaction across a variety of life areas at the time that the therapy is ready to focus specifically on aspects of CSOs' happiness. The Happiness Scale (Azrin et al., 1973), which is part of the Community Reinforcement Approach program, is the instrument typically used (see Meyers & Smith, 1995). This individualized version of the already mentioned (Chapter 2) Relationship Happiness Scale for couples focuses on clients' satisfaction with themselves, as opposed to their partners. Use of the Happiness Scale serves several purposes within the CRAFT program: (1) to send the message that all areas of the CSO's life are worth examining, not just those associated with the IP; (2) to identify CSO life areas that appear to require attention and possibly intervention; (3) to establish a baseline with which to later contrast the CSO's feelings during the course of treatment; and (4) to lay the foundation for goal setting and treatment planning regarding CSO issues.

In introducing the Happiness Scale to a CSO, you should provide an abbreviated account of its general purpose (just noted). For example, you might state that the purpose of the Happiness Scale is to:

1. See how the CSO feels about a variety of life areas outside the realm of a substance-abusing loved one.
2. Gather information that is useful for treatment planning and for monitoring the CSO's satisfaction.

The Happiness Scale is a 10-item, clinician-friendly tool that inquires about an individual's current degree of happiness in 10 different categories: substance use (the CSO's), job or education progress, money management, social life, personal habits, marriage/family relationships, legal issues, emotional life, communication, and general happiness (Figure 8.1, end of chapter). Supplemental categories can be added to suit a particular client's situation. The individual is instructed to ponder each category, asking her- or himself, "How happy am I with this area of my life?" Responses to this question range from 1 (completely unhappy) to 10 (completely happy).

Hand the client a copy of the Happiness Scale to follow while explaining its format and instructions. Answer any questions and then ask the CSO to complete it. Invite the CSO to comment on the experience and together discuss what the completed form suggests about the CSO's satisfaction with various parts of her or his life. For those areas that received low ratings of happiness, ask the CSO explain the reason for the dissatisfaction if it is not already obvious. For instance, assume that a female client has rated the Emotional Life category a "2," suggesting a high degree of unhappiness. You would want to know what she had in mind when she gave the rating: What aspects of her emotional life was she referring to, and precisely what about them causes her discontent? One example would be a CSO who said she felt depressed all the time, and who knew that the depression was *not* solely in response to her husband's drinking. She further clarified the problem area by adding that she had struggled with depression, on and off, her entire adult life.

Learning about this particular CSO's dissatisfaction with her emotional life serves several purposes, as outlined already for the Happiness Scale, in general. First, it let the client know that something of importance to her which is quite separate from her relationship with the IP (i.e., her ongoing struggle with depression), is being taken seriously in the CRAFT program. Second, it draws attention to the significance she attributes to this life area as compared to other areas. Third, it establishes a baseline happiness rating for her emotional life (i.e., her level of depression) that can be contrasted with subsequent sessions' ratings, as the problem is addressed. Fourth, it serves as an impetus for goal setting and treatment planning in this area of concern.

ESTABLISHING GOALS
AND A STRATEGY FOR ATTAINING THEM

How should this information from the Happiness Scale be used to set goals? The standard way to proceed in the Community Reinforcement Approach is to ask clients to select the category from the Happiness Scale they want to work on in the upcoming week. If clients select an area for which they gave extreme ratings of unhappiness, you might encourage them to instead choose a category that received at least a moderate rating of happiness. The intent here is to begin the goal-setting process with a problem area that offers a reasonable chance of early success, as opposed to tackling the most difficult problems first. Alternatively, you could allow the client to proceed with goal setting for even the most burdensome problem area, but only after you have helped narrow down the problem to something manageable. For instance, assume that the CSO who rated Emotional Life a "2" was invested in working on that area first. Since doing so makes good clinical sense as well, it would be reasonable to begin with this category, despite the extremely low happiness rating. But you would make sure that the depression problem, which could be experienced as overwhelming, was approached incrementally—by breaking it down into small, clearly defined "subproblems" with modest goals that a depressed person has a good chance of successfully achieving.

Once a CSO selects an area on which to begin working, and you have clarified the reasons behind the unhappiness in that category, it is time to present basic guidelines for behavioral goal setting (see Table 8.1). (Most cognitive-behaviorists will already be familiar with some variation of this procedure.) Guidelines 1–3 are similar to the first three positive communication "rules"; namely, be brief, state things positively, and refer to specific, measurable behaviors. As part of being brief, the first point also stipulates "uncomplicated." In other words, complex goals and strategies should be broken down into discrete steps in order to make them more manageable and to minimize confusion. In essence, carefully defining goals/strategies is a process comparable to the first step of the problem-solving procedure, in which the problem is narrowed down. The use of positive wording for a goal or strategy ensures that CSOs state what they want and will do, as opposed to what they do *not* want and will *not* do. Not only is this subtle difference in line with the positive emphasis of the

---

TABLE 8.1. GUIDELINES FOR BEHAVIORAL GOAL SETTING

1. State goals/strategies in a *brief* and *uncomplicated* manner.

2. Use *positive* wording, indicating what *will be done*.

3. Use only specific, measurable *behaviors*.

4. Design goals/strategies that are *reasonable* and achievable.

5. Select goals/strategies that are under the *CSO's control*.

6. Rely on *skills the CSO possesses* or is learning.

CRAFT program, in general, and with positive communication training, in particular, but it also provides a specific plan of action. Clients often can readily name the things they are going to *stop* doing, but they have difficulty selecting behaviors with which to replace them. Setting goals that involve specific and measurable behaviors minimizes any uncertainty regarding precisely which behavior is supposed to be changed, thereby increasing the chance that the behavior change will be attempted. Selecting observable behaviors is essential for monitoring progress.

The remaining three guidelines center around the establishment of goals and strategies that are both reasonable and under CSOs' control, and which incorporate skills the CSOs possess or are learning. CSOs may set themselves up for failure if they choose goals that are overly ambitious or rely on somebody else's behavior. And assignments will not be achievable if the CSOs do not have the necessary skills to carry them out, and no provision is made to teach them.

It is not necessary to go into great detail when initially presenting these guidelines. They will become meaningful as their application is demonstrated when you aid the CSO in formulating the first goal and strategy. Be prepared to model how to put clients' verbal descriptions of goals into a format that adheres to the guidelines. Shaping the CSO's behavior is an expected step in the procedure, as is reinforcing her or his efforts throughout. The Goals of Counseling form from the Community Reinforcement Approach program (see Meyers & Smith, 1995) is typically used to record the client's goals and strategies (see Figure 8.2, end of chapter). The form lists the nine specific problem categories from the Happiness Scale in its first column. There are blank spaces on which to list goals and the strategies for obtaining them in each category, as well as a column to note the time frame for their completion.

ILLUSTRATIVE CASE OF A CSO SETTING A GOAL AND A STRATEGY USING THE GOALS OF COUNSELING

A dialogue follows between a CRAFT therapist and a CSO who selected the Personal Habits category (i.e., the fifth category on the Goals of Counseling form) as the area on which she wanted to work first. Assume that she indicated a moderate degree of unhappiness for the category. Upon inquiry, she tells the therapist that she is dissatisfied with her weight. The therapist asks her what she considers to be the basis for her unhappiness with her weight, and which personal habit she had in mind when selecting this category. It is important to hear the problem described fully by the client before devising the treatment plan. The client may be unhappy with her level of physical activity, or with binge eating or compulsive overeating, or with all three. Alternatively, the CSO might be expressing body dissatisfaction because the IP no longer acts interested in her sexually. Each of these suggests a different treatment goal and strategy.

The conversation below picks up with the therapist commenting on the appropriateness of the CSO's choice of a goal area:

THERAPIST: OK, Katie, so you want to take a look at ways to increase your happiness in the Personal Habits area. That's a good place to start, because you rated it as causing you a medium amount of unhappiness. It's best not to pick the hardest area first. So can you tell me what you had in mind when you rated Personal Habits a "5"?

CSO: The main thing is my weight. Every time I lose a few pounds I put them right back on. My doctor said I'm about 25 pounds overweight, and it could create health problems down the road. Plus, I'm just not happy at this weight.

THERAPIST: That seems like a reasonable area to work on. Can you say a little more about what you think is contributing to your weight problem?

CSO: Sure. I don't eat all that badly, but I never exercise.

THERAPIST: So you think it's mostly a problem of not exercising enough, as opposed to eating poorly. Did you want to do something as far as exercise?

CSO: Yes, I'd like to start walking. I'm actually trying to walk 30 minutes every day. I heard you're supposed to do it four times a week just to be healthy, so I figured I'd better do it every day if I want to lose weight.

THERAPIST: So your goal has been to walk 30 minutes every day. And when you said that you never exercise, does that mean you aren't currently walking?

Note: First the therapist narrowed down the client's perception of her weight problem to one of insufficient exercise, and then gathered information in order to determine whether the CSO's original goal had been reasonable (guideline 4 from Table 8.1).

CSO: I walk once in a while, but I never keep it up for more than a few days. It's too boring, and it's hard to fit it in sometimes. I don't know. Maybe I'm just good at finding excuses.

THERAPIST: It's frustrating to have trouble following through with something that's important to you. But, you know, it's perfectly normal to have trouble sticking to an exercise plan. Can you think of any other people who've had trouble following through with their exercise plans?

CSO: Most of my friends don't even try to exercise. I've asked them to come with me because I thought it would be more fun, but I have trouble getting any takers. I guess you're right. It's not just me.

Note: The therapist finds a way to normalize the CSO's problem in the hope that she will not feel so discouraged.

THERAPIST: You mentioned that you'd like company on your walks. That sounds like it would help, both in terms of making it more fun and in regularly making room for it in your schedule. But you've had trouble getting takers. So, there's nobody available to take walks with?

Note: The therapist agrees that a walking partner is generally a good idea. However, given that this solution has not worked in the past, it might not be the best choice on which to focus. The therapist pursues this line of questioning briefly before deciding whether to consider other solutions. If the latter appears necessary, the therapist would likely utilize the standard problem-solving procedure (outlined in Chapter 7).

CSO: Nobody from work will go with me. There's one neighbor I've seen walking sometimes, but I'm not sure I want to ask her.

THERAPIST: You're not sure you want to ask her?

CSO: No . . . well . . . actually, I guess I'm embarrassed to talk to her.

THERAPIST: Embarrassed?

CSO: I'm sure she's heard lots of yelling coming from our house at times when my husband's been really drunk. I don't know. It's hard to face the neighbors.

THERAPIST: Katie, I remember you telling me during our first session that one of the reasons why you came to the CRAFT program was because you were tired of your husband's drinking interfering with your life. Not being able to face the neighbors sounds like one of the ways the drinking has interfered, especially if it means that you can't ask a neighbor to go for walks.

CSO: But what would I talk with her about?

THERAPIST: My impression is that you're a good talker under normal circumstances.

Note: The therapist suspects that the CSO is less concerned about running out of things to say, and more about the effect of her husband's drinking on the relationship with the neighbor.

CSO: I *am* a good talker. I don't know. I guess I'm more worried that she might not want to go with me because of what she thinks about my husband . . . and me.

THERAPIST: Well, we *don't* know what she thinks about you, but I'm not sure she'd hold it against you if she knows about your husband's drinking. Still, we don't know if she'll agree to go for a walk. There's no guarantee. So the question is, do you want to risk asking her, or would you prefer to work on a different solution to your exercise problem?

CSO: I think I should ask her first. It would be silly not to, because we live near each other and she seems to have about the same work schedule as I do.

THERAPIST: Shall we practice when and how to approach her?

CSO: No, I know what to say. I just need to go and do it.

Note: A therapist might normally rehearse the upcoming encounter in a role play to ensure that the client had adequate communication skills (guideline 6). Here, assume that the therapist was confident about the CSO's conversational skills, and thus did not insist on practicing them in the session.

THERAPIST: OK, then. Let's go ahead and set an exercise goal. Here's a quick review of the guidelines I mentioned before, which are helpful when planning goals: State your goal briefly and in positive terms, and stick with specific behaviors. Pick something that's not too hard to do, that's under your control, and that involves skills you already possess. But don't worry about remembering all of these things. Just start it off, and I'll help.

CSO: Maybe I can use the goal I've been trying to do all along—the one about walking 30 minutes every day.

THERAPIST: As far as following the guidelines, it's quite good. It's a briefly stated and uncomplicated goal, you're saying what you *will* do, and it's a specific behavior. Those were the first three guidelines I covered. It's also something that's under your control, and you probably don't need to learn any new skills to do it. Those were guidelines 5 and 6. I have one concern, though.

CSO: That I didn't say anything about doing it with my neighbor?

THERAPIST: No, that part is OK. We can list her as part of your strategy for reaching your goal. I'm wondering if it's too hard. Planning to walk every single day sounds like a lot, and it doesn't allow for an emergency. I don't want you to set yourself up to fail.

CSO: Oh. I get it. You're probably right. Maybe I should set a goal of 4 days a week. I can always do more if I feel like it.

THERAPIST: Excellent idea. How about you write it on this Goals of Counseling form (see Figure 8.3, end of chapter, for a sample of a partially completed form; category 5 pertains to this goal).

Note: The therapist reinforces the CSO for adhering to most of the guidelines for stating a goal, but determines that the goal is too ambitious, given the CSO's inability to achieve it with any consistency in the past. Another "failure" right now could adversely affect her motivation. He next asks the CSO to break down the strategy into steps that can be recognized and dealt with accordingly (guidelines 4 and 1, respectively).

THERAPIST: Now we need to state exactly what your strategy will be for reaching this goal. You mentioned walking with your neighbor as an extra incentive. But it sounded like there was a preliminary step, because you've got to ask her first, and that isn't easy. Let's break this strategy down into all of its steps. What's first?

CSO: First I have to get the nerve up to go over to Julie's house and invite her to walk with me. If I say I'm going to do it, I will.

THERAPIST: Good for you. I'll write this down under "Strategies." But before you leave here today, we should talk about what it will feel like if she says no . . . for whatever reason. It helps to be prepared. Now, what's the next step once you've asked her.

CSO: It depends on whether she agrees to go with me. If she does, we'll set up a day and time. Oh. But I doubt she'll be able to go with me 4 days a week, like I've planned.

THERAPIST: Good thinking. Even if Julie agrees to go, chances are she won't be available four times a week when you are. So you should have a strategy for the days she can't go, or in case she can't go at all. And it would be best if the strategy was different from some of the things you've tried in the past that haven't worked so well.

CSO: So you mean I can't tell myself, "Just Do It"? (*Laughs.*)

THERAPIST: Only if it's worked pretty regularly when you've used it before. (*Smiles.*) And remember, we want it to be a solution that satisfies guideline 5: It's under your control. We could do problem solving to come up with ideas.

CSO: I remember most of the problem-solving steps, so I don't think we need to go through it. Let's see . . . I still think I'd like to plan on going with somebody else, but I'm not sure who. Hmmmm. I could have my son come along on his bike. He loves riding on the trail behind our house, and since he's not allowed to do that alone, he's always trying to get someone to take him. If I told him ahead of time that I was going to take him certain nights of the week, he'd get after me to go. I'll figure out which nights to tell him, once I've talked to Julie about her schedule. That might actually work.

THERAPIST: Your strategy sounds like a good, solid plan that satisfies all of the guidelines here. It's definitely worth trying. Here, go ahead and write it on your form. What do you want to put for the time frame for reaching your goal?

CSO: I'd like to say I can do it right away—this week—but maybe I should give myself some time to get things set up. How about 2 weeks?

THERAPIST: Two weeks it is, then. Mark that down too. I'll check on your progress toward the goal next week. If you're running into any problems, we'll address them right away.

The primary clinical issue involved highlighting the connection between the IP's drinking and his wife's vanishing social support system. This issue is addressed later in the chapter (see "Broadening the CSO's Support System"). As far as procedural points, in the course of devising a strategy to obtain a goal, the question of whether additional skills training was needed for the CSO in order to adopt the strategy arose twice, once in terms of communication skills, and then for problem-solving ability. If the therapist had determined that the training was necessary, it would have been included in the "Strategies" section. Typically brackets are placed around strategies that require therapy time, because they are more the therapist's responsibility than the client's.

SHAPING CSOs' DESCRIPTIONS OF THEIR GOALS AND STRATEGIES

Several difficulties that frequently arise when assisting a CSO in developing goals and strategies were illustrated in the case just presented: setting a goal that is overly ambitious, devising strategies that are not under the client's control, and using strategies that have yet to be broken down into manageable steps. Additional examples of goals and strategies for the same CSO are included below; goals or strategies that are initially problematic because they do not adhere to important guidelines are given first, and improved versions follow. (The improved versions also appear on the sample Goals of Counseling form in Figure 8.3.) For instance, assume that Katie next decided to go back and set a goal in the Social Life category (i.e., the fourth category on the Goals of Counseling form) because she agreed that she should reestablish contact with some old friends:

- *Problematic goal.* "To stop refusing invitations to socialize just because I'm afraid my husband's drinking will come up."

The positive aspects of this goal are that it is brief and uncomplicated (guideline 1 from Table 8.1), measurable (guideline 3), not overly ambitious (guideline 4), and probably does not demand any skills training (guideline 6) for this CSO. The first problematic aspect of this goal is the use of negative terms (guideline 2): It states what the CSO will *stop* doing. Although it implies what Katie will *start* doing (i.e., accept invitations), this feature of the goal raises the second problem with its wording: The goal is not entirely under the CSO's control (guideline 5). If the week passes without the client receiving any invitations to socialize, she will not have the opportunity to meet her goal despite her willingness to comply. Rather than passively wait for invitations to arrive, a better goal for accomplishing the same objective would be for Katie to state that she would initiate a specific social event:

- *Improved goal.* "To have coffee with a girlfriend (Amy, Penny) late Tuesday afternoon."

The goal is now worded in positive, active terms, and it is under the CSO's control. The goal assumes, of course, that Katie has several girlfriends from whom to choose. If the client has but one close friend to invite, the goal should be modified slightly:

- *Improved goal.* "To *invite* Stephanie to coffee late Tuesday afternoon."

This wording allows the CSO to be successful regardless of whether Stephanie meets her for coffee, because the goal is simply to extend the offer. The larger goal of building a support system would be tackled in small steps.

If the therapist asked Katie to describe her *strategy* for achieving her goal of having coffee with one of her (several) girlfriends, the CSO might respond with something along these lines:

- *Problematic strategy.* "I'll just get one of them to go with me."

One drawback of this strategy, as stated, is that it is not specific and measurable (guideline 3), because it is not clear whether the client plans to call a friend on the phone or hopes to simply run into one of them by chance. This vagueness makes it easier for the CSO to do nothing. Furthermore, the CSO is more likely to follow through and make the contact if she plans in the session exactly *who* she is going to contact and *when*.

- *Improved strategy.* "I'll call Amy tonight to see if she can have coffee Tuesday. If she's not available, I'll call Penny tomorrow at work and invite her."

Formulated in this manner, the strategy appears to satisfy the six guidelines. The time frame for the goal would be 1 week (see Figure 8.3). You would then decide whether it appeared beneficial to add another strategy in order to maximize the CSO's chances of accomplishing her goal. Given the straightforward goal and the fact that a backup plan was built into the existing strategy, this would not be necessary in this situation.

Imagine that next, Katie wants to jump forward and set a goal in category number 6: the Marriage/Family Relationships category, because she is unhappy with her relationship with her 7-year-old son. If she has not already received a fair amount of training in goal setting, she might start with a vague goal:

- *Problematic goal.* "To improve my relationship with my son."

This goal mentions no specific behavior and therefore is not measurable (guideline 3). It also refers to a complex undertaking, and so should be broken down into manageable steps (guideline 1). Finally, the outcome is not entirely dependent on the CSO's behavior and thus is not under her control (guideline 5). With shaping, the client could narrow her focus to the time she spends interacting with her son:

- *Improved goal.* "To spend more quality time with my son."

Although improved, this goal could still be made more specific and measurable:

- *Improved goal.* "To help my son with his homework 30 minutes each weeknight."

The *strategy* for achieving this objective would vary, depending on the particular CSO and son. A reasonable series of steps for a CSO who is concerned that her son might not cooperate during this time would be the following:

1. "Tell my son that we are going to start working on his homework together each night after dinner but before dessert."

2. "Allow him to earn a star every night that he sits and works the full 30 minutes, and help him make a chart for the stars."

3. "Take my son to Target to pick out a $2 prize, once he's earned 5 stars."

This third step is critical not only in terms of the success of the contingency, but it also is congruent with the CSO's initial objective, which is to spend more time with her son (see Figure 8.3).

Two general problems in the goal-setting area are worth mentioning. The first entails assigning too many goals in one week. For the illustrative CSO case, sample goals were set in three different categories: Personal Habits (category 5), Social Life (category 4), and Marriage/Family Relationships (category 6). Each individual goal was reasonable, but the combination would be overwhelming, given the time requirements, if they were all started during the same week. Conceivably Katie could be attempting to have coffee with a friend, take a half-hour walk, and help her son with homework for 30 minutes all on the same day. Although the CSO might actually want to do all of these activities, she would need to gradually adjust to such a change in schedule. In the meantime, she automatically would be working on more than one problem category simultaneously, since she would be addressing her social life (as well as her personal habits) whenever she walked with a friend. And she would be addressing her relationship with her son on those days that she took him on her walks when she "technically" was working on her personal habits area.

The second general problem in goal setting involves the failure of therapists to establish a mechanism for regularly evaluating progress toward goals, despite the time frame column on the Goals of Counseling form that serves as a reminder. Not only should reviewing goals and strategies be a standard part of CRAFT sessions, but you should also have clients develop their own plan for continuing the practice once therapy ends.

ADDITIONAL EXAMPLES OF CSO GOAL SETTING

If behavioral goal setting is part of your standard practice, you probably will not need the supplemental examples provided below. The additional examples illustrate common CSO goals and strategies, presented here in the context of a second case. Imagine that the CSO (Liz) is a single mother, and that the IP (Emily) is her 28-year-old daughter who abuses marijuana and alcohol. These individuals live in the same household, and while the CSO works full time, the IP holds down a job only sporadically (refer to Figure 8.4, end of chapter, for a sample completed Goals of Counseling form for categories 1–3 and 7–9 for this CSO.)

CATEGORY 1: DRINKING/DRUG USE

The CSO stated that she drank only one glass of wine with dinner each evening, but she was concerned that it was giving her daughter the message that alcohol was a standard part of supper. Liz first set a goal of "not drinking at home anymore." When reminded to use positive and specific terms, she rephrased the goal as "to drink sparkling water with dinner at home instead of wine." Her strategy for achieving this goal was twofold. First, she enjoyed sparkling water but refused to pay high prices for it, so she planned to make it a priority to pick up a case at a discount warehouse store. Second, she decided it was not necessary to avoid drinking alcohol at home altogether. Liz simply wanted to show Emily that alcohol was not an automatic part of every dinner for her. So her strategy, at least for the next month, involved allowing herself an occasional glass of wine at home in the evening (approximately two per week) but not with dinner.

CATEGORY 2: JOB/EDUCATIONAL PROGRESS

Liz was very interested in setting an education-related goal, because she had been debating about finishing her nursing degree for quite some time. She verbalized her goal as "to finish my BS degree in nursing." The goal was positively worded, specific/measurable, mostly under her control, and probably within her skill level. But since Liz needed almost 2 years of coursework to achieve this goal, it had two major pitfalls: being complicated and overly ambitious (guidelines 1 and 4). The therapist advised her to set a short-term educational goal that would put her on the path of obtaining her long-term goal of finishing her bachelor's degree. The goal became "to finish one course toward my nursing degree," and the time frame was based on the semester.

CATEGORY 3: MONEY MANAGEMENT

Liz said that her money worries were constant. She decided that she wanted to ask Emily to contribute a substantial payment to the household funds or to move out. Liz was reminded that she should word the goal in a way that put it under *her* control, as opposed to having it depend entirely on her daughter's behavior. So the goal was listed as, "to find a source of an additional $200/month." Upon the therapist's suggestion, Liz reduced the amount to $100/month as a preliminary goal.

Since the CSO was not confident that she could achieve this goal (either by relying on her daughter or otherwise) and was having trouble coming up with concrete ideas, the therapist conducted a problem-solving exercise to assist her. The stated goal became the defined problem. The resulting strategies were added to the Goals of Counseling form. The first involved a contingency plan for Emily that essentially required her to work on a more regular basis. Importantly, it was stated such that it was under the CSO's control. The second strategy entailed Liz advertising her clothing alteration skill. The plan appeared reasonable, as she could schedule the sewing jobs around her regular job and her coursework. The third part of her strategy was advertising her pet-sitting services again. She had done this fairly recently, but she wanted to put up fresh notices. After praising Liz for her ideas, the therapist expressed concern that she might be taking on too many new jobs. In response, Liz agreed to start by asking Emily for the money. If she refused to comply or did not contribute the $50 at the end of the first month, then Liz would post the flyers about the clothing alterations. If there was only a minimal response to these flyers, she would post the pet-sitting flyers the following month (strategies 1–3).

CATEGORY 7: LEGAL ISSUES

Liz did not have any legal problems, but her daughter had a minor one that she had never handled. The client knew it would not be healthy for her to simply straighten out Emily's legal dilemma, so she set the goal of providing her daughter with the name and phone number of the contact person to call in order to start sorting out the problem. Liz planned to call the county court house to get this information. She would then inform her daughter that this would be the extent of her assistance, and she would encourage her to follow through with the call.

CATEGORY 8: EMOTIONAL LIFE

Liz said that she felt emotionally stressed much of the time, and so for her goal she wanted "to be less stressed." The therapist complimented the CSO for coming up with a goal that was brief, reasonable, and at least somewhat within her control and ability. He then pointed out that it was not specific/measurable, as worded, and it was somewhat negatively phrased because it stated what would *not* happen anymore rather than what *would*. After clarifying Liz's stressed feelings, the goal was restated as, "to have 1 hour of relaxation (e.g., hiking, swimming, napping) each weekend." The strategies included (1) reminding herself that she did not need to feel guilty about taking a little time off on a regular basis, (2) gathering information about hiking trails and pool hours and costs, and (3) calling two friends to see if they wanted to join her. The goal and strategies for this Emotional Life category were ideal, as they mostly addressed Liz's Social Life category as well.

CATEGORY 9: COMMUNICATION

The CSO knew immediately what she wanted to work on in this category: "to stop criticizing Emily every time I talk to her." But she realized that she had used negative terms, so she reworded it as "to say something nice or even neutral to Emily whenever I talk to her." When questioned whether *nice* was specific enough and whether her goal was too ambitious, she modified it: "to give a small compliment or be neutral toward my daughter during the majority of our conversations." Liz wanted to leave the "neutral" piece in because she thought it might sound too superficial to compliment Emily every time they spoke. In order to accomplish this goal, she knew she needed some communication training, particularly for those situations in which she typically "blew up" at her daughter. Therapy time was scheduled for this purpose and placed on her Goals of Counseling form in brackets, since the step was largely the therapist's responsibility. Liz then decided she had better spend time developing a list of reasonable compliments for her daughter, since they did not occur to her automatically.

BROADENING THE CSO'S SUPPORT SYSTEM

As mentioned previously, most CSOs who spend a considerable amount of time with their substance-abusing IP are subjected to shrinking social support systems. The process is a gradual one, in which the CSO sometimes plays a direct role by refusing more and more invitations for social activities. The refusals are the result of their concerns that the event could easily become a fiasco if their IP resorted to aggressive or obnoxious behavior in public while under the influence of alcohol or drugs. Or if the social event does not include the IP, CSOs may instead dread the thought of their IPs' substance use being raised in the course of a social conversation. The consequence of these refusals, over time, is that the invitations cease coming, and the CSOs do not replace these lost activities with other forms of recreation. Essentially, they find it safer to stay at home, thereby avoiding any potential "scenes" or disquieting conversations altogether. Unfortunately, taking extreme measures to avoid potential hassles has the secondary effect of eliminating opportunities to experience social support. CSOs typically do not realize the extent to which they have been withdrawing, and so before long they experience little relief from an overabundance of negative events and emotions. As a CRAFT therapist, you point out this consequence of their IPs' excessive substance use, and you encourage CSOs to pursue goals in the Social Life category (from the Happiness Scale and the Goals of Counseling form) in an effort to rebuild their support system.

Somewhere in the early stages of working with a CSO to develop new social activities (with or without the IP), the relevant issues of embarrassment and fear of rejection should be raised. Recall Katie, who was reluctant to invite a neighbor to take walks with her out of concern that the neighbor would turn her down due to the public commotions caused by her inebriated husband. The therapist was aware of these common CSO feelings, and so probed them. Since many CSOs will not readily volunteer such emotions, it is important to inquire about them and discuss them in advance. Otherwise you run the risk of delaying progress; CSOs will likely skip the assignment altogether and only reveal the real reason when later asked why. It is also helpful to practice role plays of upcoming interactions that could result in rejection, so that CSOs have the opportunity to process the feelings in advance.

IMPORTANCE OF DEVELOPING SOME SOCIAL ACTIVITIES INDEPENDENT OF THE IP

Most CSOs agree with the notion that their social life needs help. Most CSOs also assume that improving their social lives necessarily involves their IPs. Thus, it is important to discuss the benefits of carving out a piece of their social/recreational lives that is independent of their IP. Not only does this independence allow clients to have greater control over their quest for satisfaction and fun in this area, but it decreases the chance that the IP will interfere with the process in some manner. Despite these seemingly reasonable points, CSOs frequently experience guilt over the prospect of devoting session time to making their social lives happier in a way that excludes the IP. You may need to reassure them that a critical component in achieving a healthier relationship with their IP entails the CSOs taking better care of themselves. Having social outlets for stress reduction and overall support is an excellent way to accomplish this objective. At the same time, remind them that a considerable amount of therapy time and effort is regularly devoted to enhancing the shared social life of the CSO and IP, such as through planning increased pleasant time together when the IP is clean and sober.

Another issue to consider when talking with CSOs about developing independent aspects to their social lives is how their IPs will respond to the prospect. Certainly the primary concern is one of determining the potential for violence if the IP views this new CSO behavior as threatening to their relationship. If the risk is great, you would want to proceed very slowly, checking with the client about the least precarious behavior in this area that has been used before safely. If there does not appear to be an activity in which the CSO can safely participate alone, then you might want to conduct a problem-solving procedure. The main objective behind the notion of improving the CSO's social/recreational life would need to be kept in mind; namely, broadening the

CSO's support system. Clients who risk physical harm for socializing without their IP might need to include their IP at some level. In such a case, the activities would be planned for occasions when the IP is least likely to be under the influence of any abusive substances. Regardless of the risk for violence, you should discuss when and how (or if) to inform the IP about the planned independent social behavior and rehearse the interaction in a role play.

GENERATING A LIST OF ENJOYABLE, INDEPENDENT SOCIAL ACTIVITIES

For CSOs who agree to work on their social/recreational lives independent of their IP, the next step involves generating a list of activities they think would be enjoyable. Interestingly, the task appears to stump many CSOs. You might assist by suggesting they consider activities that in the past were done in the company of the IP, but which perhaps can now be attempted without him or her. Sometimes it is also useful to provide a few examples of other CSOs' selected activities (e.g., spending time with extended family members, volunteering at the library, walking the dog with a neighbor). Finally, you might have CSOs examine an instrument such as the Pleasant Events Schedule (MacPhillamy & Lewinsohn, 1982) to stimulate ideas.

If the CSO is able to offer a few suggestions, review them carefully. Ideally, these independent social/recreational activities should contain certain properties (summarized in Table 8.2), several of which overlap with the guidelines given for selecting reinforcers for the IP, and for narrowing down IP behaviors to reinforce (Chapter 6). To begin with, the objective is *not* simply to fill up the CSO's day with activities, but to add ones that are truly enjoyable. Furthermore, if the activity is too costly to

TABLE 8.2. GUIDELINES FOR SELECTING INDEPENDENT SOCIAL ACTIVITIES

The selected social activity should be one that:

1. Is *pleasurable* for the CSO.
2. Is *inexpensive*.
3. Is *easy to add* to the CSO's schedule.
4. Is *ongoing* or has been done in the *past* by the CSO.
5. *Involves other people*, particularly some who are acquaintances of the CSO.

undertake on a fairly regular basis, it does not have much potential for making a significant impact on the CSO's happiness. Also, the activity should be easy to add to the CSO's schedule. Even if only a few minor obstacles are encountered as the CSO attempts to engage in the activity, it is not likely to be completed. If possible, the activity should be one that is either ongoing, to some extent, or in which the CSO has participated previously. This familiarity makes the activity less intimidating and increases the chance that the CSO will actually attempt it. Ideally, the activity should involve other people, and at least some of these people should already be acquaintances of the CSO. Since the overall goal is to enhance the CSO's social life, access to other people is imperative. Furthermore, the chances of the CSO following through with the activity are increased if it is a matter of reviving an old friendship as opposed to starting a new one.

Occasionally, CSOs insist that they would rather try something totally new; that they cannot get excited about the prospect of picking up where they left off with any of their previous social outlets. This is not a problem, because sooner or later, all CSOs are encouraged to sample some novel recreational experiences. Whichever the preference, once a number of activities has been identified, ask the CSO to select one to add to her or his schedule in the upcoming week. Depending on the client, you may want to run through the problem-solving steps (see sample below) to ensure that the client will be able to handle any obstacles that might interfere with sampling the activity. Finally, you should check with the CSO at the next session to determine whether the assigned task was completed, and whether it served that all-important purpose of being *enjoyable*.

USING PROBLEM SOLVING TO IDENTIFY AND SELECT SOCIAL ACTIVITIES

For CSOs who are at a standstill in their efforts to identify reasonable, pleasurable, old *or* new social activities to add to their schedules, the problem-solving procedure (Chapter 7) is brought to bear. In other cases clients are able to generate a list of activities, but they are uncertain as to which one would be an appropriate choice due to unpredictable and possibly insurmountable obstacles. Again, the problem-solving procedure would be employed.

A sample problem-solving exercise for identifying and selecting a social activity is presented below. Assume that the CSO is a 55-year-old professional male who has been married to the IP for almost 25 years. The IP is a professional woman who has used pain pills and tranquilizers excessively in recent years and now is abusing alcohol as well. When the CSO tried to create a list of enjoyable activities that were (or could be) independent of his wife, he had trouble naming any that did not necessarily involve her *and* that he was still interested in doing. The therapist decided to utilize the problem-solving procedure. The CSO also was worried that he might resort to excuses to justify his failure to follow through with the activity. Problem solving was an appropriate exercise for this reason as well, since it helps CSOs anticipate obstacles to task completion and tackle them in advance.

The exercise starts with the operational definition of the problem at hand. The CSO's responses are provided, and brackets are placed around those comments that are not normally displayed on the worksheet but are considered informative here.

SAMPLE PROBLEM-SOLVING WORKSHEET

1. *Define the problem narrowly.*

   Must identify independent enjoyable activities for myself and try one.

2. *Brainstorm possible solutions.*

   - Attend local conferences.
   - Go to Al-Anon meetings.
   - Find someone to exercise (bike) with.
   - Start playing golf.
   - Have afternoon coffee with a colleague.
   - Play cards with some friends weekly.
   - Join a men's group.
   - Hang out at bars.
   - Coach a kids' soccer team.
   - Take a woodworking course.
   - Go fishing with a friend.

3. *Eliminate undesired suggestions.*

   Note: You will see from the reasons given (in brackets) for rejecting a potential solution that the CSO is actually following several of the guidelines for selecting an activity without necessarily being aware of it.

   - ~~Attend local conferences.~~ [Too infrequent to rely on.]
   - ~~Go to Al-Anon meetings.~~ [Not really an enjoyable activity.]
   - Find someone to exercise (bike) with. [Can't think of anyone it would be easy to schedule with.]
   - ~~Start playing golf.~~ [Doesn't seem like a pleasant activity; would rather try something else first.]

- Have afternoon coffee with a colleague. [Maybe, but already do this once in awhile.]
- Play cards with some friends weekly. [Maybe, a group has been asking me to join.]
- ~~Join a men's group.~~ [Too Yuppie for my taste.]
- ~~Hang out at bars.~~ [No way—not pleasant.]
- ~~Coach a kids' soccer team.~~ [Too much of a time commitment.]
- ~~Take a woodworking course.~~ [Someday, but not now.]
- Go fishing with a friend. [Maybe; inconvenient though.]

4. *Select one potential solution.*

   - Play cards with some friends weekly.

   [I have a few friends who've been trying to get me to play cards with them on Tuesday nights for a long time now. I've always come up with an excuse. I don't really like to go out during the week, but I like these guys a lot, and I do enjoy playing cards. I'll call Stu today and let him know I'm in for next week.]

5. *Identify possible obstacles.*

   - Too tired from work that day.
   - Need to finish up some work that evening.

6. *Address each obstacle.*

   - [Too tired from work that day. *Solution?*: I can take a nap when I get home from work if I'm really that tired. Sometimes a brisk walk helps wake me up, too.]
   - [Need to finish up some work that evening. *Solution?*: As long as I plan in advance to attend, I should be able to get my work done earlier. Stu always checks with us on Mondays, so it will be a good reminder to get everything off my plate for the next evening.]

7. *Decide on the assignment and do it.*

   - Call Stu today and tell him I'm interested in playing cards next Tuesday. I'll put it on my calendar so I can plan for it. Tuesday night—I'm there!

8. *Evaluate the outcome.*

   - [It was fun. The only problem with the activity is that I lost a lot of hands because I'm so out of practice. I guess the solution is to go every week! Good thing we don't bet a lot of money.]

This client's choice of a new independent recreational activity contained many favorable aspects to it. He knew he got pleasure out of card playing, and it appeared to be an inexpensive form of recreation for him. It was easy to add to his schedule, in the sense that the card-playing occasion was already up and running. And although he had never played cards with this particular group of individuals, he *was* a card player. Furthermore, the activity involved other people, and the people were already friends of his (guidelines 1–5, Table 8.2).

SYSTEMATIC ENCOURAGEMENT PROCEDURES

Sometimes CSOs are 100% willing, in theory, to try new activities or work on their support system, but when it comes down to actually changing their behavior in order to do so, they find it almost impossible to take that first step. The common emotional obstacles were already mentioned: CSO guilt, fear, anxiety, and depression. Sometimes there also are practical impediments, such as a lack of information as to what is available or whom to contact. For an individual who is somewhat ambivalent about making a change, *any* type of obstacle may be sufficient to prevent her or him from taking the first step.

The Community Reinforcement Approach has a procedure called Systematic Encouragement that appears useful in such situations (see Meyers & Smith, 1995). Systematic Encouragement consists of three basic recommendations that should be considered whenever a client is planning to sample something new but is at risk for *not* initiating the change:

1. *Never assume that the client will make the first contact independently.* Once a suitable activity has been decided upon, role play the initial phone call to the organization or individual. If an organization is the target of the call, the role play will allow you to see whether the CSO can determine whom to contact and her or his communication skill in terms of asking the appropriate questions. If a relative or friend is being called, behavioral rehearsal affords the opportunity for practice in a very different type of communication—one that may trigger an emotional reaction on the CSO's part. Once the CSO appears to be prepared emotionally and is sufficiently skillful, the phone call should be placed *during the session.* Most clients are surprised by this request, but with encouragement, they proceed. For others, being asked to actually make the call helps them realize that, for various reasons, they are not yet ready to do so.

2. *Whenever possible, arrange to have a contact person meet the CSO at the activity.* Oftentimes contact people are listed on community resource lists of organizations. Alternatively, a contact person can be requested when

the initial phone call is made to obtain information. This extra step of arranging for a specific person to meet the CSO at the function increases the chance that the CSO will attend for two reasons. First, most CSOs feel more comfortable about attending a new activity if they know someone will be available to show them around and make the initial introductions. Second, making a verbal commitment to meet a contact person serves as an inducement to follow through and honor the commitment.

3. *Review the experience at the next session.* First, you will need to find out if the CSO attended the activity. If not, the reason should be discussed, and problem-solving procedures can be used to prevent its recurrence. In some cases it becomes apparent that the particular activity is not suitable after all, and a new one should be selected. If the CSO *did* attend the function, find out whether it was enjoyable. An easy way to ascertain this is by asking if the CSO would like to attend again. If the CSO attended the activity but did not experience it as pleasurable, it would be unreasonable to urge the CSO to repeat the assignment. In the event that the CSO attended the planned activity *and* found it enjoyable, potential obstacles to participating in the future should be addressed, such as transportation or babysitters.

SUMMARY

This chapter presents a behavioral approach to working with CSOs who may be experiencing a variety of unique problems of their own. The procedures are part of the Community Reinforcement Approach program and largely revolve around its method for assessing clients' satisfaction with their lives (Happiness Scale) and developing treatment plans for setting appropriate goals (Goals of Counseling). Throughout, the emphasis is on simplifying and motivating. The task may involve structuring goals or strategies so that they will be likely to be successful, or it may involve supplying Systematic Encouragement procedures to help the CSO get "unstuck." The chapter also demonstrates other suitable occasions for introducing Community Reinforcement Approach procedures (e.g., problem solving, communication skills training). The overall importance of helping CSOs develop and act on a willingness to take care of themselves is the major theme.

FIGURE 8.1.

HAPPINESS SCALE

This scale is intended to estimate your *current* happiness with your life in each of the 10 areas listed below. Ask yourself the following question as you rate each area:

How happy am I with this area of my life?

Circle one of the numbers (1–10) beside each area. Numbers toward the left indicate various degrees of unhappiness, and numbers toward the right reflect various levels of happiness. In other words, state exactly how you feel today, using the numerical scale (1–10).

Remember: Try to exclude all feelings of yesterday and concentrate only on your feelings *today* in each of the areas. Also, try not to allow one category to influence your answers in the other categories.

	Completely Unhappy						**Completely Happy**			
Drinking/Drug Use	1	2	3	4	5	6	7	8	9	10
Job or Education Progress	1	2	3	4	5	6	7	8	9	10
Money Management	1	2	3	4	5	6	7	8	9	10
Social Life	1	2	3	4	5	6	7	8	9	10
Personal Habits	1	2	3	4	5	6	7	8	9	10
Marriage/Family Relationships	1	2	3	4	5	6	7	8	9	10
Legal Issues	1	2	3	4	5	6	7	8	9	10
Emotional Life	1	2	3	4	5	6	7	8	9	10
Communication	1	2	3	4	5	6	7	8	9	10
General Happiness	1	2	3	4	5	6	7	8	9	10

Name: _____   Date: _____

FIGURE 8.2.

GOALS OF COUNSELING

Name: _____ Date: _____

Problem Areas/Goals	Strategies	Time Frame
1. In the area of drinking/drug use, I would like:		
2. In the area of job/educational progress, I would like:		
3. In the area of money management, I would like:		
4. In the area of social life, I would like:		

5. In the area of personal habits, I would like:

_____

_____

_____

6. In the area of marriage/family relationships, I would like:

_____

_____

_____

7. In the area of legal issues, I would like:

_____

_____

_____

8. In the area of emotional life, I would like:

_____

_____

_____

9. In the area of communication, I would like:

_____

_____

_____

FIGURE 8.3.

GOALS OF COUNSELING: COMPLETED EXAMPLE

Name: __Katie__   Date: __July 1__

Problem Areas/Goals	Strategies	Time Frame
4. In the area of social life, I would like: To have coffee with a girlfriend (Amy, Penny) late Tuesday afternoon.	1. Call Amy tonight re coffee Tuesday (or call Penny at work tomorrow).	1 week (July 8th)
5. In the area of personal habits, I would like: To walk 30 mins. 4 days/wk.	1. Ask Julie to join me on walks. Set up day and time. 2. Walk 30 mins. with Julie 2 x/wk. 3. Take son (on bike) on 30-min. walks 2 x/wk.	2 weeks (July 15th)
6. In the area of marriage/family relationships, I would like: To help my son with his homework 30 mins/weeknight.	1. Tell son we're going to work together on his homework each night after dinner but before dessert. 2. Allow him to earn a star for working the full 30 mins., and help him make a chart for the stars. 3. Take son to Target to select a $2 prize once he's earned 5 stars.	1 month (Aug. 1st)

FIGURE 8.4.

GOALS OF COUNSELING: COMPLETED EXAMPLE

Name: Liz   Date: Aug. 1st

Problem Areas/Goals	Strategies	Time Frame
1. In the area of drinking/drug use, I would like:		
To drink sparkling water with dinner at home instead of wine.	1. Get cases of sparkling water at Costco this weekend.	1 month
	2. Have approx. 2 glasses of wine at home per wk (but not with dinner).	(Sept. 1st)
2. In the area of job/educational progress, I would like:		
To finish 1 course toward my nursing degree.	1. Pick up course catalog at bookstore and read.	4½ months
	2. Make appt. with academic advisor to check requirements.	(Dec. 15th)
	3. Enroll in 1 course that fits work schedule.	
	4. Meet with instructor 1st week to get study guidance, and later in semester if necessary.	
3. In the area of money management, I would like:		
To find a source of an additional $100/mo.	1. Ask Emily to contribute $50 the 1st month, then $75, and then $100. If she misses any of these payments, she will be asked to move out within the week. If necessary:	3 months
		(Nov. 1st)
	2. Post 100 flyers about clothing alterations.	
	3. Post 100 flyers about pet-sitting services.	

(cont.)

FIGURE 8.4. *(cont.)*

Problem Areas/Goals	Strategies	Time Frame
7. In the area of legal issues, I would like: To give Emily the name and number of the contact person for her legal problem.	1. Call county courthouse and ask for the correct contact person for handling Emily's type of legal problem. 2. Tell Emily that this is the extent of my help; encourage her to call.	1 week (Aug. 8th)
8. In the area of emotional life, I would like: To have 1 hour of relaxation (e.g., hiking, swimming, napping) each weekend.	1. Remind self that I don't need to feel guilty about time off to relax. 2. Get information about local hiking trails and pool hours/costs. 3. Invite Elise and Trish to join me in the activity and schedule a specific time/date.	1 month (Sept. 1st)
9. In the area of communication, I would like: To give a small compliment or be neutral toward Emily the majority of our conversations.	1. [Communication skills training for situations when angry at Emily.] 2. Generate a list of things to compliment Emily about.	1 month (Sept. 1st)

CHAPTER 9

INVITING THE IDENTIFIED
PATIENT TO ENTER TREATMENT

From the moment they begin CRAFT training, most CSOs anxiously anticipate the day they will be ready to invite their IP to enter treatment. Considering that CSOs, on average, successfully engage their IPs in less than five CSO sessions (Meyers et al., 1999; W. Miller et al., 1999), most individuals do not have long to wait. In preparation for this day, the foundation is laid by teaching the series of skills-based procedures presented in the previous chapters (e.g., positive communication training, problem-solving procedures, domestic violence precautions). This groundwork ensures that each CSO is competent and confident to tackle the task at hand, and that personal safety issues have been addressed.

Ideally, a number of factors should be in place before CSOs invite their IP to sample treatment. Eager or impatient CSOs need to be cautioned to proceed slowly, because premature invitations have a higher rate of refusal. The specifics regarding when and how CSOs should extend the therapy invitation to their IPs are outlined in Table 9.1 and covered fully in the chapter.

CHOOSING A TIME OF HIGHER IP MOTIVATION

Despite the fact that IPs are, by definition, treatment refusers, you should not assume that their level of motivation to sample therapy is equally low (or nonexistent) at all times. According to the research literature within the last two decades, individuals' motivation to change their behavior is *not* akin to an on/off switch. Rather, motivation for treatment is better understood as a dynamic process that, at times, moves in the direction of deciding to

TABLE 9.1. ACCOMPLISHMENTS REQUIRED PRIOR TO A CSO SUGGESTING TREATMENT

1. The CSO has learned to identify times of *higher IP motivation* for treatment, and to stress key motivational points (engagement *"hooks"*) within the request.

2. The CSO has mastered the relevant *positive communication skills* for delivering the therapy invitation, knows when and where to present it, and how to respond to problematic repercussions.

3. At least one *viable treatment option* has been arranged, in advance, for the IP.

4. As a precaution, the CSO has been prepared for a potential treatment *refusal* or a premature *dropout*.

5. The necessity for *continued CSO support* after the IP is engaged in treatment has been explained.

---

change, whereas at other times moves away from it (Miller, 1985, 2003; Prochaska & DiClemente, 1982, 1986). Borrowing from the language of the transtheoretical model of change presented by Prochaska and DiClemente (1982, 1986), treatment-resistant IPs fall within one of the first three stages of change: precontemplation, contemplation, or preparation. If the CRAFT procedures have been somewhat effective, we might expect that IPs have moved beyond the precontemplation stage and are fluctuating between contemplation and preparation—stages that at least include ambivalence about changing. The implication is that IPs are more open to a therapy invitation during some periods of time than others.

CSOs would not be able to determine precisely when their IPs are in the contemplation or preparation stages of change and therefore (presumably) more approachable. Nonetheless, there are a few noteworthy IP behaviors that represent a more open attitude characteristic of these stages and thus merit exploration as prime times for suggesting treatment.

WINDOWS OF OPPORTUNITY

1. *The IP acting remorseful about causing a drinking- or drug-related crisis.* Some individuals feel guiltier about, and more disgusted with, their substance use if it is responsible for an emergency of some type. Does this remorse translate into an increased openness to the suggestion of treatment? Sometimes. Studies have found that individuals were, on average, more agreeable to substance abuse treatment after experiencing an alco-

hol-related physical injury (Bombardier, Ehde, & Kilmer, 1997; Longabaugh et al., 1995). Research also has shown that people were more likely to enter and complete marital or family therapy after a crisis, especially if the relationship were threatened in some way (O'Farrell & Fals-Stewart, 2003). Therefore, we might surmise that it would be reasonable to approach IPs in the aftermath of an alcohol or drug incident marked by salient negative consequences. However, this line of thinking is not to suggest that CSOs should wait until their IPs "hit rock bottom" before intervening, but only that they should be prepared to respond with a treatment invitation if such an event does occur. Examples of typical substance-associated dilemmas include: an alcohol- or drug-related arrest (e.g., DWI; drunken disorderly, assault, possession of illegal drugs); losing a promotion or a job as a consequence of substance-related absences; spending the family's entire monthly expense allotment on drugs; battering a loved one while under the influence.

2. *The IP appearing upset over a totally unexpected remark about his or her substance use.* Periodically, IPs are quite taken aback when they hear a comment about their substance use from someone they believed had no knowledge of it. In fact, some IPs even make resolutions, on the spot, to "cut back." Considering that this shift in attitude might occur, CSOs could be ready with a specific suggestion for counseling. Examples of these situations that surprise and disturb IPs include the following: An IP's boss says coworkers have reported smelling alcohol on the IP's breath; an IP's child says that his schoolmates are afraid to come over to the house because they might run into his stoned dad; the IP's parents ask suspiciously about why the IP needs to borrow money again this month; an IP's neighbor naively asks if the IP has been having a lot of quiet parties, because she's noticed empty liquor bottles outside the door each morning.

3. *The IP inquiring about the CSO's (CRAFT) treatment.* Obviously this only applies to cases in which the IP knows that the CSO is in treatment. Examples of "promising" questions by the IP that open the door to mention treatment include: "What goes on during those sessions of yours?"; "Why, exactly, are you in treatment?"; "What do you and your therapist talk about?"; "Do you talk about me during sessions?"; and "So, is your therapy helping?"

4. *The IP questioning why the CSO's behavior has changed.* Although IPs who question their CSO's out-of-character behavior often have not been informed directly about their CSO's involvement in CRAFT, a fair number suspect some type of professional influence. Typically the inquiring IPs are referring to their CSO's ongoing positive reinforcement of sober behavior or their withdrawal of reinforcement from using behavior.

Examples of IP queries that could pave the way for a therapy invitation include: "Why are you acting so strange/funny/weird?"; "What are you up to?"; "How come you're being so nice all of a sudden?"; "You're no fun anymore. Why won't you join in on the partying?"; and "You've been acting really different lately. You must want something."

Each of these examples represents a valuable opportunity for the CSO to respond to the IP's question or concern with a suggestion of treatment. As far as identifying other suitable occasions for extending an invitation, CSOs should fall back on the suggestions for selecting a time to make a request of the IP, in general (Chapter 5). In other words, ideally both the CSO and IP should be in reasonably good moods, and the IP should be clean/sober and not experiencing a hangover. Regardless of *when* the invitation is made, considerable communication training (including role plays) is required to prepare most clients for this momentous step. However, it is not uncommon for CSOs to find themselves faced with a "window of opportunity" similar to those noted previously, *before* their communication training is complete. Consequently, early in CRAFT treatment it is worthwhile to assist the CSO in preparing a reasonable, preliminary response, and to introduce the more formal positive communication training as soon as possible.

Illustrations of solid CSO responses during the "windows of opportunity" just presented are listed below, and the relevant components of a positive communication are referenced (from Figure 5.1). In each case a preview is also given of an even more comprehensive response that would be practiced as therapy progresses and the special inducements, to be outlined shortly, are acquired. However, since one of these motivational "hooks" is so commonly used, it was built into several of these basic examples. It entails the CSO suggesting that the IP meet the CSO's therapist. The rationales for this and other relevant treatment engagement hooks are presented later in the chapter.

1. *The IP acting remorseful about causing a drinking- or drug-related crisis.*

IP: Come on. I didn't mean to run up our credit card. I just get a little crazy sometimes when I'm high. You know how much I care about you, right? Let me make it up to you.

CSO: I can think of one really good way for you to show me you care, but it's asking quite a bit. Would you come with me to one of my sessions so you can meet my therapist and see what we've been working on?

Positive communication components: The request is brief, positive, specific, and contains an understanding statement. With more training the CSO would know to mention that the IP would have his or her own therapist and would have major input into the treatment goals and plan.

2. *The IP appearing upset over a totally unexpected remark about his or her substance use.*

IP: Did you hear what little Jamaal said to me the other day—that his friends were afraid to come around his "druggie" dad? Is my smoking that noticeable? Did *you* say something to him about it?

CSO: No, I haven't said a word. Babe, that's gotta be upsetting. Listen, I imagine this is hard for you to hear, but I care so much about you and Jamaal that I have to say it anyway. What do you think about getting some professional help for the sake of the family?

Positive communication components: The request is positive, specific, and contains a feelings statement and two understanding statements. Advanced training could teach the wife also to suggest that the IP simply sample treatment initially.

3. *The IP inquiring about the CSO's (CRAFT) treatment.*

IP: So, are you ever going to tell me what you and that therapist of yours have been up to? I bet some of it has to do with me.

CSO: Sure. I probably should have told you already. But I'd rather have you come down and meet my therapist. He'll tell you all about the program I've been in, plus another one that you might even be interested in. It would really mean a lot to me if you gave this a try.

Positive communication components: This request is positive, specific, and contains both a feelings and a partial responsibility statement. With further practice the CSO would know to mention, for instance, that the IP could have his own therapist.

4. *The IP questioning why the CSO's behavior has changed.*

IP: You seem really different. How come you've been extra nice lately?

CSO: I've started to feel better because I've been going to therapy. I've been trying out some new ways to help us, because I want our relationship to be better. I think it could really be good again. It would mean an awful lot to me if you'd try something like it. What do you say?

Positive communication components: The request is positive, specific, and contains a feelings statement. Additional skills training would show the CSO the utility of further clarifying how therapy could be used for non-substance-related issues (i.e., their relationship).

HOOKING IPs INTO THE IDEA OF SAMPLING TREATMENT

In several of the CRAFT studies, IPs who were successfully engaged in treatment were asked to describe the factors that eventually led them to agree to try therapy (Meyers et al., 1999, 2002). Internal reasons were the most frequently cited (e.g., "I want to feel good about myself"), yet it is unclear what prompted IPs to respond to those thoughts by seeking treatment precisely when they did (E. Miller, Ogle, Anderson, Meyers, & Miller, 1999). However, some of the comments did refer directly to changes in CSO behavior (i.e., as a result of the CSOs' CRAFT training). One young male IP stated, "My mom was being so nice all of a sudden, that I felt like I owed it to her to see what the program was about." Additionally, IPs frequently mentioned appealing features of the therapy proposed for them or indisputable rewards associated with a successful therapy outcome. Several of these treatment engagement hooks are explored below.

MOTIVATIONAL HOOKS

1. *Being offered the chance to informally meet the CSO's therapist.* Although a treatment-engaged IP would not ordinarily be assigned the CSO's therapist, an invitation to meet the CSO's counselor by joining the two of them informally (e.g., for a cup of coffee) is appealing to some curious IPs. The fact that IPs can get a glimpse of a treatment program with "no strings attached" and from a person who has been playing a significant role in their CSO's life is tempting. This relatively nonthreatening visit provides a valuable "foot-in-the-door," as it offers an excellent opportunity for the CSO's therapist to play a more direct role in the engagement process.

2. *Hearing that the standard practice would be for them to see a therapist other than their CSO's therapist.* Depending on your theoretical orientation, you might automatically assume that you would *not* be doing individual work with the loved one of an established client. Interestingly, IPs in the studies routinely (erroneously) assumed that they *would be* expected to see their CSO's therapist. Anecdotally, many IPs became much more receptive to the idea of therapy when they were informed that they would have their own (a different) therapist. One might surmise they were concerned about their CSO's therapist being biased against them.

3. *Being given the option to simply "sample" treatment.* As a reminder, the sampling concept capitalizes on the belief that an intimidating task will appear less overwhelming if individuals are invited to try it in small, manageable pieces (Meyers & Smith, 1995). In line with this notion, IPs in the CRAFT studies responded favorably to the suggestion that they agree

only to a session or two of treatment up front and decide about a longer-term commitment later. They also appreciated hearing that their therapy would be time limited, regardless; it was not going to last for years.

4. *Being told that they would have major input into the treatment goals and plan.* It is not unusual for clients, in general, to prefer some degree of control over their treatment plans. Perhaps this desire is even more understandable for clients who, until that moment, were outright treatment-refusers. CRAFT therapists regularly give IPs the same message at an introductory meeting that CSOs were given when they started: "You won't have to do anything in this program that you don't want to do." Naturally, this promise can only be made if it can be backed by the available treatment for IPs.

Some counselors might question the logic of promising substantial control over treatment goals, since it could result in a seriously substance-dependent IP choosing moderate use over abstinence. There are several reasons to proceed with these promises, nonetheless. A sizeable group of individuals with substance abuse problems elects moderation initially but then subsequently chooses abstinence (Miller, Leckman, Delaney, & Tinkcom, 1992). Although the reasons for the change are not always known, at least a subset of them switches to an abstinence goal because a trial period of social drinking has failed (Alcoholics Anonymous, 1976; Hester, 2003). Interestingly, research findings show no long-term differences in outcome for those randomly assigned a goal of moderation versus those assigned a goal of abstinence (Graber & Miller, 1988; Sanchez-Craig, Annis, Bornet, & MacDonald, 1984). In other words, people decide on their own treatment goal, regardless of a program's mandate (Hester, 2003), so you only stand to gain by being receptive to the IPs' proposed goals. Fortunately, many therapists are willing to work with clients despite not agreeing with their stated treatment goal of moderation. Some behavioral therapists negotiate contracts whereby these clients agree to switch to a goal of abstinence if a trial of moderation is unsuccessful (Hester, 2003; Meyers & Smith, 1995). Other therapists request that clients "sample sobriety" from the onset for a brief period so that they can make an informed decision about whether it might be acceptable to them after all (Azrin et al., 1982; Meyers & Smith, 1995).

5. *Having the option to work on* non-*substance-related areas as part of treatment.* IPs responded approvingly to the prospect of receiving assistance with job searches, depression or anxiety, marital issues, legal problems, children's difficulties at school, or psychotropic medication referrals. Conceivably, IPs who were not ready to "admit" that they had a significant substance abuse problem also felt they were saving face by agreeing to seek therapy for other reasons. Given that these problem areas were always at least indirectly associated with IPs' substance abuse,

most IPs brought up the alcohol or drug problem themselves rather quickly anyway.

6. *Seeing the connection between getting clean/sober via therapy and obtaining something else of value as a consequence.* As emphasized throughout this book, individuals are more likely to change their behavior, including finally entering treatment, if it offers them something they value. To distinguish this hook from the types of reinforcers just outlined, the reinforcer in this instance is *not* an appealing feature of the therapy itself but an objective reward that results from actually decreasing the drinking or drug use. As part of this presentation, a sense of immediacy is often stressed by linking the available remaining period for sobriety with an upcoming valued occasion. For instance, a CSO might tell her husband (IP) that their extended family would reconsider and agree to come for the holiday meal that was scheduled for next month if they knew he had been sober several weeks already.

USE OF POSITIVE COMMUNICATION SKILLS WHEN INVITING THE IP TO SAMPLE TREATMENT

As noted in previous chapters, the manner and timing of the communication are critical when making a request of the IP. A request for an IP to enter treatment is certainly no exception. In an effort to contrast new, improved strategies with more negative attempts to engage the IP, it is helpful to start this discussion with a review of the unsuccessful types of past communications employed by CSOs when trying to get their IP to agree to therapy. Frequently, these "requests" would more accurately be described as threats and accusations, and their tone as nagging and ridiculing:

- "That's it! I can't take it anymore. Get help or get out!"
- "*I'm* going to treatment because of *your* drug problem. The least you could do is go, too."
- "How many times do I have to ask you to do something about your drinking? Do you get some perverse pleasure out of hearing me beg?"
- "Your smoking is driving me over the edge; I'm in therapy now. You'd better join me or it's over!"
- "Thanks to *you*, our family is falling apart. Are you ever going to step up and do anything about it?"

In reviewing a sample of CSOs' earlier attempts to engage their IP in treatment, ask them to determine whether they used any of the positive communication skills recently learned (Figure 5.1). Since in all probability, few (if any) of the seven elements of a positive communication were employed, have CSOs start by incorporating several of the components into their typical request for the IP to enter therapy. Reinforce their efforts and shape the behavior in the process. Assume, for example, that a CSO begins with her standard (negative) request for her husband to get help. Through her therapist's praise and feedback, it progresses through the following iteration:

- *First attempt*: "That's it! I can't take it anymore. Get help or get out!"

Positive communication components: The request is brief and feelings are mentioned (albeit in a negative, indirect way).

- *Second attempt*: "Your drinking every night is really stressing me out. I know your job is extra tough these days, but isn't there another way to handle it?"

Positive communication components: The request is still brief, her feelings are mentioned in a less negative manner, a specific behavior (nightly drinking) is referred to, and an understanding statement is offered.

- *Third attempt*: "Your drinking every night really upsets me. And I miss talking to you. I know that work is extra tough these days. How about I help you figure out another way to handle the stress? I have some ideas."

Positive communication components: The request is brief, a specific behavior is still referred to, it contains a feelings statement, a positive comment is added, an understanding statement remains, and an offer to help is added.

Most IPs would not be particularly defensive in response to this final communication. In fact, chances are that a number of them would participate in a conversation about alternative ways to manage their stress. This is an excellent opening for suggesting treatment. In the event that this hypothetical IP already knew his wife was in therapy, the CSO would be trained next to say something that incorporated this fact. Notice that in these more advanced samples of treatment engagement conversations that follow, (motivational) hooks are added as well:

- *Sample (if the IP already knows about the CSO being in treatment)*: "I can see why you've been so stressed out these days. But you've got me worried! We've talked about how *I've* been getting help for the stuff that stresses me. Hey, what do you think about coming down and meeting my therapist? I know he could offer you some options as far as getting help for *your* stress."

Positive communication components: The request is positive and contains a feelings statement, an understanding statement, and an offer to help. Hook 1 is presented: meeting the CSO's therapist. Hook 5 is also used: the option to seek therapy for a problem area other than substance abuse.

Although the discussion in this scenario was prompted by the CSO's concerns about the IP's drinking, the invitation left the topic of the therapy wide open. Depending on the CSO and the IP, it may be reasonable to specifically mention the substance abuse as well as the other possible topics for treatment:

- *Alternative (if the IP already knows about the CSO being in treatment)*: "I discuss all sorts of things with my therapist, and I end up feeling better. I know you have a lot on your mind. If you went into therapy, *you* could talk about any number of things, too; it wouldn't be only about drugs. You could talk about whatever's bothering you. Why don't you just give it a try?"

Positive communication components: The request is positive, specific, and contains both feelings and understanding statements. Hook 5 is used again, and the suggestion to sample treatment (hook 3) is added.

When CSOs have not already informed their IP about their own treatment, sharing this fact may be the first step toward encouraging the IP to begin therapy. This may be revealed separately or presented in combination with a request for the IP to attend. Sample conversations follow:

- *Sample (if the IP is first learning about the CSO being in therapy)*: "Honey, I want you to know that I started therapy about a month ago. I wasn't dealing with things very well, and I was really missing what our relationship used to be like when you were sober. It's helped me feel quite a bit better. What do you think about seeing someone for the things that are bothering you? My therapist could help you get that set up with somebody."

Positive communication components: The request is positive, specific, and includes a feelings statement and an offer to help. Hook 5 is employed again, and hook 2 is introduced: IPs can have their own therapists. Another version of such a request, which incorporates several different positive communication steps, might be:

- *Alternative (if the IP is first learning about the CSO being in therapy)*: "You've probably been wondering why I've been acting different lately. Maybe I should have told you from the start, but I've been going to therapy for a few weeks now. I'm learning ways to reconnect with the "old you." Listen, I know you've been dealing with an awful lot of stuff, especially at work. Why don't you come with me to my next appointment? My therapist knows some really good counselors who let their clients have a big say in what they work on. We could all have a cup of coffee and see what she has to say."

Positive communication components: The request is positive and includes an understanding statement, a partial responsibility statement, and an offer to help. Hook 2 is used again, along with hook 1: meeting the CSO's therapist. And hook 4 is added: IPs can have significant input into their treatment goals and plans.

Some of the previous illustrations included reinforcing characteristics of the treatment itself, such as noting that the IP could obtain help for a variety of life stressors by beginning therapy. As outlined earlier in hook 6, CSOs also could highlight the benefits associated with the sobriety that ideally would result from entering treatment. Furthermore, they could provide a motivating rationale for starting therapy *now*. Examples for hook 6 are demonstrated in the excerpts below:

- *Sample*: "I know you're not really interested in therapy, and I guess I understand. But I wonder if you'd consider it . . . even if it's just for medical reasons. I keep thinking about what the doctor said the last time he saw you. He made it sound like things needed to change in a hurry. I'm afraid I'm going to lose you!"

Positive communication components: The request is brief, positive, specific, and includes a feelings and an understanding statement. Hook 6 is used, with physical health as the reinforcer. The next example uses access to a loved one as the reinforcer.

- *Sample*: "I know your 'ex' said you weren't welcome to attend your son's tournament next month if you were still getting high. Maybe this would be a good time to get into treatment. I know it wouldn't be easy, but with some clean and sober time under your belt, your 'ex' wouldn't have any reason to keep you away. I've got the names of some highly recommended therapists. What do you think?"

Positive communication components: The request is specific, offers an understanding statement, and includes an offer to help. Hook 6 is used again, along with hook 2: IPs can have their own therapist.

After reviewing the components of a positive communication and giving examples of how they can be incorporated into an invitation for the IP to enter treatment, you should enact several role plays. As always, remind CSOs that rehearsing the conversation should allow them to feel more relaxed and confident when delivering the message in their emotionally charged home atmosphere. Discuss how, although most IPs are unlikely to become overly defensive or angry in response to this type of positive communication, CSOs nevertheless should consider the possibility of a threatening IP reaction and plan accordingly.

ILLUSTRATIVE CASE OF A CSO (WIFE) INVITING HER IP (HUSBAND) TO SAMPLE TREATMENT

Assume that a CSO (wife) has been attending CRAFT sessions for 5 weeks. Her husband (IP) is a high-functioning chronic marijuana user. Imagine that, at this point, both the CSO and her therapist have decided that the time is right for inviting the IP to enter treatment, and the CSO is fully prepared (as specified in Table 9.1). The dialogue begins with the therapist guiding the CSO in her selection of the time and the wording for this conversation with the husband:

THERAPIST: Erica, since we're both agreeing that this is generally a good time to invite Craig to treatment, let's go ahead and nail down a specific time or two this week when it would be ideal to ask him. Do you remember how we've talked before about the best times to approach him? Which times have worked the best so far? When has he been able to listen and not get real defensive? And it goes without saying now that he shouldn't be high.

CSO: I think I'd like to try Sunday night after dinner. I've had some luck with that already. He never gets high Sunday night because he doesn't want to have trouble getting up for work on Monday. As far as a backup time . . . let's say Monday morning at breakfast.

Note: To reiterate: An ideal time to make a request is when the IP is sober and has no hangover, and both the CSO and IP are in reasonably good moods. Note that the CSO has learned to select a backup occasion.

THERAPIST: Excellent. You're a step ahead of me on this, which convinces me that you're ready to have this conversation with Craig. Of course, we'll practice first. Hopefully you'll be able to use a few of the pieces of a positive communication and also incorporate some of the motivational hooks we've discussed, like tying in his reinforcers.

CSO: I've thought about that. See how this sounds. (*In role play*) Craig, is this a good time to talk to you about something important?

THERAPIST: (*As husband*) Uh-oh. Why do I have the feeling I'm going to get into trouble?

CSO: (*In role play*) This doesn't have anything to do with you getting in trouble. It has to do with me caring so much about you that I want you to be happy and healthy.

Note: The CSO uses various components of a positive communication throughout the dialogue (Figure 5.1). Here she emphasizes the positive (i.e., wanting the IP to be happy and healthy) instead of the negative (i.e., the IP's marijuana use) and offers her feelings.

THERAPIST: (*As husband*) What are you talking about?

CSO: (*In role play*) I should start at the beginning. I've gotten the impression that you're curious about why I've started to act differently toward you when you're high. But you never said anything. Have you noticed something's up?

THERAPIST: (*As husband*) I'm not dense. I noticed. I really didn't want to know. I figured it was bad news for me.

CSO: (*In role play*) I don't look at it as bad news, but I can see how you'd be worried about it. Maybe I should have come right out and told you from the start. I've been seeing a therapist.

Note: The CSO uses an understanding statement and accepts partial responsibility. She also alludes to one of the standard occasions for mentioning treatment; namely, when the IP notices the CSO's behavior changing (item 4 in "Windows of Opportunity," p. 231).

THERAPIST: (*As husband*) Really? Who's paying for it? I figured you'd gone to one of those fancy assertiveness classes or something. OK. So what does it have to do with me now?

CSO: (*In role play*) I feel like I've gotten a lot out of therapy. I'm less depressed . . .

THERAPIST: (*As husband*) You were depressed? You always said *I* was the depressed one.

CSO: (*In role play*) I *do* think you're depressed. But I was too, and the therapy helped. So I'm thinking it could probably help you, too. It hurts to see you so down all the time.

Note: The CSO introduces hook 5: presenting therapy as an opportunity to explore non-substance-related areas of interest to the IP (i.e., depression). She also offers statements of her feelings again.

THERAPIST: (*As husband*) I know exactly what a therapist would say though; stop smoking. And I don't want to do that.

CSO: (*In role play*) Maybe so. I'm not sure. I only know that my therapist gives me a lot of choices. She gives guidance, too, but the final decision about which steps I'm going to take is up to me. And I bet it would be the same thing for you too . . . especially if you let my therapist help you get hooked up with a similar kind of therapist for yourself.

Note: The CSO uses two more motivational hooks. First, she reassures her husband that he will have ultimate control over any major decisions regarding his substance use. Second, she alludes to the fact that he can have his own therapist (hooks 4 and 2). The latter is done within the framework of an offer to help.

THERAPIST: (*As husband*) I don't know. I'm not sure I want to bother. I've got so much going on that I can hardly see straight.

CSO: (*In role play*) I can't argue with that. I've never seen a busier person. But what would you think about just giving it a try? If you didn't like the therapist or the therapy, you could stop going. In the meantime, would you be willing to meet *my* therapist, just to see what I've been up to?

Note: The CSO makes another understanding statement, and then adds hooks 2 (the sampling idea) and 1 (meeting her therapist).

THERAPIST: (*As husband*) Well, maybe. I'll go meet your therapist. No promises beyond that.

CSO: (*In role play*) Fair enough!

The therapist would ask the client to critique her own performance, then offer her feedback and reinforce the effort. Given the unusually high quality of this conversation, the role play probably would be repeated only if the CSO wanted additional practice in order to feel more comfortable, or if she believed it would be helpful to have the therapist portray her husband acting more "difficult."

ILLUSTRATIVE CASE OF A CSO (MOTHER) INVITING HER IP (SON) TO SAMPLE TREATMENT

The next case portrays a single mother (CSO) who is trying to get her 29-year-old son (IP) to accept treatment. Assume that after losing yet another job, the polydrug-abusing son has returned home to live with his mother and 16-year-old sister. The mother has attended seven CRAFT sessions and now appears ready to ask her son to sample treatment. Notice that in contrast to the previous illustration, this CSO struggles with the wording of the request. Also, since the CSO believes her son will still be rather resistant to the idea, the therapist portrays the son accordingly. Given these factors, the therapist spends more time providing feedback and assisting with the planned communication:

CSO: I think maybe I should ask Leroy to start therapy. This might be a good time. He asked me the other day why I was being so nice to him, like he was suspicious about what I was up to. It was after I'd told him how much I liked talking with him over dinner. Remember? I was supposed to compliment him if he joined me for dinner without being high. Anyway, I started to tell him about my therapy, but he got a phone call to go pick up his friend. He split. Maybe it was better that way, because I wasn't being very clear. I was nervous! But I think I could get us back on the topic.

THERAPIST: Good for you, Vanessa. First of all, you followed through again with a plan to reward his nonusing behavior. You're really good at that! And then you recognized one of those ideal times we've spoken about, to invite Leroy to enter treatment. Excellent! Don't worry that you stumbled a bit with the wording. We'll work on that today, and the practice should help with your nervousness, too. OK. So, do you remember some of the hooks we talked about keeping in mind when asking Leroy to attend?

Note: The therapist reinforces the client for complying with an assignment and for recognizing a window of opportunity for mentioning treatment.

CSO: Since Leroy is out of work again, I was thinking about how you said most therapists can help with things besides just drug abuse. But I'm not sure my son thinks he needs help getting a job. Anyway, the program you helped me line up is one that lets people decide whether they want to shoot for abstinence or moderation. Leroy would never agree to a program if they required abstinence, so I definitely want to mention that to him.

THERAPIST: You're right on track, Vanessa. You mentioned two key motivational points: First, the fact that he can have a major voice in deciding his goals—in this case, choosing moderate use over abstinence—and second, he can work on other areas that are important to him in therapy, such as a getting a job. As far as the job topic, I bet you can come up with a way of mentioning this without him getting too defensive. Why don't we go ahead and give the conversation a try. Should we review some of the positive communication points we've practiced? They're really handy when it comes to making an "unpopular" request.

Note: Besides being prepared to use two motivational hooks (pp. 234–236), the CSO already had a program lined up for her son in the event that he agreed to treatment (outlined in "Rapid Intake Process" later in this chapter).

CSO: Here, I've got my card with the seven steps listed. (*Pulls out index card.*) Not like I remember to use it, though! I think I'd like to just go ahead and give it a try. And I think I'll bring it up when he's sober at dinner again. I'm pretty sure I'll have a chance in a day or so.

THERAPIST: Sounds good. I'll start it off. (*As son*) Ma, pass me more of those 'taters.

CSO: (*In role play*) Sure, Leroy. Hey, remember the other day I started to tell you about me being in therapy?

THERAPIST: (*As son*) It's none of my business what you do. I don't need to know that stuff.

CSO: (*In role play*) That's OK. Actually, I wanted to tell you about it, because it's about *you.*

THERAPIST: (*As son*) Well, that sounds like a waste of time and money. So you've been telling your therapist horror stories about your delinquent son? Hope it makes you feel better. (*Said sarcastically.*)

CSO: (*In role play*) No, that's not the point. (*To therapist*) That's just about what he'll say. He won't want to listen to me. What was I thinking? I didn't even have a chance to use any of these things. (*Waves index card.*)

THERAPIST: Don't let him throw you off course. He's being sarcastic, but so far he's still listening. Hang in there. Remind yourself about the points you wanted to make. Oh . . . and you might not want to start off by saying that the therapy is about him. It *is*, but people often feel uncomfortable and get defensive when that's the first thing they hear. Besides, therapy is definitely about *you*, too, in a lot of ways. So how about starting from the top again? Go ahead and glance at your index card when you need to. (*As son*) I must be starving tonight. How about a few more of those spuds?

Note: The therapist believes it is premature to highlight too many communication errors at this point, as the CSO barely got started before she gave up. Instead, he primarily offers her encouragement and a fresh start. Depending on the quality of her next role play, he may insist on selecting and preparing several positive communication components prior to repeating the role play.

CSO: (*In role play*) Glad you've got your appetite back. Hey, Leroy, remember when I started to tell you that I was in therapy the other day? I'd like to talk to you about it.

THERAPIST: (*As son*) Why should I hear about your therapy? That's your own business.

CSO: (*In role play*) You're right, it *is* my own business. It's been good for me. I've had a lot of stuff to work on, but a lot of the time I've been working on figuring out a way to get you to see that you need help. I know you've said your life is pretty messed up now, right? What do you think? I've got a good program picked out for you.

THERAPIST: (*As son*) Whoa! I bet you do! I knew you were up to something. Why can't you stop trying to run my life for me? I'm almost 30, ya know.

CSO: (*In role play*) Yeah, and you're living at home again. (*To therapist*) Shoot! I slid back into our old ways of "talking" again. Yup, that's what happens.

THERAPIST: It's easy to fall back into old, familiar ways of doing things. Vanessa, don't get discouraged. Keep in mind that I'm purposely giving you a hard time because I know that's what you expect from Leroy. Let's take a quick break from the role play and look at your conversation so far. Tell me what you liked about your conversation.

CSO: I didn't start off by saying therapy was about him this time. I don't think the rest was very good though.

THERAPIST: You definitely were off to a good start. But you did say a couple of things that I, in my role as Leroy, reacted to. Maybe we can work on your conversation, so your son can continue to listen without getting defensive. For instance, you said something like "I'm trying to get you to see you need some help." Do you see why Leroy might react negatively to that?

CSO: I said that? That's no good. Leroy doesn't like it when *anybody* tries to get him to do *anything*. And he'd hate the part about *needing* help. Ya know, this stuff always makes so much sense when you point it out to me. But how am I ever going to get it right when I really need to?

THERAPIST: You will. You've come a long way with your conversations. It's *hard*, but that's why we're practicing. The more we practice, the more automatic it should be when you're actually in the situation with Leroy. So how might you bring up the topic of treatment in a way that's easier for him to hear? Let's see if we can add some specific steps of a positive communication.

Note: The therapist relies on his own natural reactions to the client's communication to guide his feedback. Then, given the relatively low level of skill displayed by the CSO, he spends time helping her carefully map out a positive conversation before moving forward to repeat the role play. He reinforces her efforts and reminds her of one of the main purposes of role plays.

CSO: I could say I'd like him to try therapy; that I think he might get something out of it. Hey, look at this! Wouldn't I be using numbers 1–3 with that? (*Points to index card.*) It's brief, positive, and specific . . . at least, in terms of what *I* want him to do.

THERAPIST: You're absolutely right. That has a much better feel to it, too. It sounds more like an invitation that way. And "trying" therapy is a suggestion to "sample" it, which is one of our motivational hooks. Good. So what will you follow it up with if he asks you *why* he should go?

CSO: I'm not sure how I'd bring this up, but I heard his younger sister say something to her friends the other day about his pot smoking. It really bothered me, because she was bragging about it. Leroy thinks she doesn't even know he smokes. I'm worried that she's going to start doing drugs. Maybe she already has.

THERAPIST: Do your son and daughter have a good relationship? Does he care a lot about her?

CSO: They've always been close. He looks out for her, and she looks up to him.

THERAPIST: Maybe that's the real hook we need, then. He might not see treatment as being important for himself, but perhaps he might view his own treatment as a good move *for his sister*. Of course, you wouldn't want to place blame on him. You'd have to be careful how you worded it. Go ahead and take a peek at your index card again. These steps will be very important in this delicate situation.

CSO: OK. (*Glances at index card.*) Let's see. I could say something positive about his relationship with his sister; how he's always looked out for her.

THERAPIST: Good start. That's item number 2 on the positive communication list. What else?

Note: The CSO is hoping to appeal to her son to enter treatment so that he can become a better role model for his sister. The notion of being a good role model is a reinforcer (hook 6) because his sister's welfare is important to him. At the same time, the wording of the request is being polished.

CSO: Hmmm. Everything else I can think of sounds negative. I'd like to get him to accept partial responsibility for her bragging about his pot smoking, because if he wasn't smoking, she wouldn't be bragging about it.

THERAPIST: So you're trying to use communication item 6: Accept partial responsibility. I see. But, Vanessa, when it says to "accept partial responsibility," it means for *you* to accept it, not for your son. It's a way to make somebody else less defensive. Do you see what I mean?

CSO: Oh, right. I remember you explaining this to me before. So *I'd* have to accept partial responsibility. OK. I could say that maybe I've relied on him too much to look out for her, but that I've come to count on it.

THERAPIST: Hey, that's good, really good. Go ahead. Now how will you bring up the treatment request?

CSO: Can't I just say something like, I want his sister to admire him but *not* for doing drugs? And that treatment might be worth trying for his sister's sake right now. How's that sound?

THERAPIST: Quite good. I'll have you put it all together in a minute. Let me just comment on one other statement you made in your role play a few minutes ago, because it could easily come up again. You said you'd picked out a program for him. How does that strike you?

CSO: Hmmm. It sounds sort of pushy. He always wants to make his own decisions. I could say I have some suggestions, if he'd like to hear 'em.

THERAPIST: You're on a roll! That's an offer to help—#7 from your communication list. Now, you also planned to mention the fact that moderate drinking was a reasonable goal for some of the programs you'd checked out, but you didn't quite get to it. That's one of those important hooks.

CSO: Oh, that's right. Like I said, I got nervous. I can fix that, though.

THERAPIST: I know you can. A little more practice here and you'll be set. Shall we start from the top? Don't forget: Try not to let it turn into an argument. Think positive!

Note: Most of the problems involved the CSO's negative style of speaking—a style of which she was not fully aware. The therapist did not mention every problematic segment of the conversation, because he did not want to risk overwhelming and discouraging her.

THERAPIST: (*As son*) Ma, where's Sis? How come she's not eating supper with us again?

CSO: (*In role play*) Oh, she's just being a teenager. Tonight she's busy doing an after-school project at Lucy's house.

THERAPIST: (*As son*) Well, she better not be screwing up her grades.

CSO: (*In role play*) So far, she's doing OK. I'm a little worried, though. I heard her bragging to her friend about your drinking and smoking the other day. I'm afraid that if she starts in with that herself, her grades will suffer.

THERAPIST: (*As son*) I'm sure you'll blame that one on me if it happens.

CSO: (*In role play*) Leroy, I didn't bring this up so that I could blame you. I just know how much you care about your sister. And you just said that you want her to do well in school.

THERAPIST: (*As son*) I *do* care about her. I can always look at the bright side: If she starts smoking, maybe it will get you off *my* back for a while. (*Tries to joke.*)

CSO: (*In role play*) Maybe I do get on your back about things too much. I just want things to go well for you, for you to be happy.

THERAPIST: (*As son*) A little money would make me happy. Uh-oh. Now you're gonna give me the lecture about getting a job.

CSO: (*In role play*) No lectures. I don't know if you want to hear this, but like I started to say the other day, I've been going to therapy for a few weeks now, and one of the things I learned is that therapists can help people get jobs.

THERAPIST: (*As son*) So can Job Corp, and it's probably cheaper. Is this your sneaky way to try to get me to see a therapist?

CSO: (*In role play*) I'm not trying to be sneaky. You already know that I want you to see a therapist. I just thought this might be a good time to get help. The job is part of it, but I'm worried about your sister bragging about your smoking. She really looks up to you. I'd like her to admire other things about you besides your smoking and drinking.

THERAPIST: (*As son*) And so I have to give up all my "vices" just so she can find something else to admire in me? Maybe there isn't anything else.

CSO: (*In role play*) Sure there is. You're a smart, caring, big brother. Oh, and I also found out that some therapists are willing to work with people who want to smoke or drink socially; they don't require you to quit totally. I even know of a program like that. Want to hear about it?

THERAPIST: (*As son*) Not really. Well, maybe later.

In reality, it probably would have taken a client such as this one more than a few role plays to arrive at this point, given her communication skills at the onset. Regardless, the CSO eventually was able to avoid making negative "digs" at her son. She utilized three motivational hooks (4–6) and six components of a positive communication. Since both of these numbers are likely to drop appreciably at the time of the actual conversation with the IP, it is preferable to strive for an elevated rate during a session.

OTHER FORMATS FOR INVITING
AN IP TO ENTER TREATMENT

Although the norm is for *one* CSO to work with a CRAFT therapist, peri-odically that individual is joined by others. Some CSOs decide they want the emotional support of additional family members as they work toward IP engagement, and others believe they need the "extras" offered by a sec-ond CSO. These "extras" may include fresh ideas for motivating or invit-ing the IP, or the special influence that this particular family member may have on the IP. The suggestion to bring other loved ones into the CSO's sessions can be made by either you or your client.

Occasionally CSOs make convincing cases for devising a method to invite their IPs to sample treatment other than by speaking to them face to face. Some CSOs strongly prefer having their therapist "available" dur-ing the conversation. This preference can be approximated by having the CSO deliver the therapy invitation to the IP during a phone call made within a therapy session. The advantage of this option is that the conversa-tion can be rehearsed immediately prior to placing the call, and you are present to coach, provide moral support, and process the outcome. Still, this is not viewed as a preferable mode for extending the invitation to IPs, since CSOs ultimately need to be willing to tackle difficult conversations in person and independently.

Given that learning good verbal communication skills is an essential element of CRAFT, a request to circumvent its application altogether would be supported only after careful consideration. One example of a reasonable exception might be an unassertive CSO who, despite ulti-mately profiting from many role plays over numerous sessions, remains concerned about her ability to get her point across clearly to her obstrep-erous, impatient husband. Assume she *does* feel comfortable, however, inviting him to enter therapy via a short note. In this situation, you would likely ask the CSO to draft a note as an assignment, and you would review and finalize it together during a session. Role plays would be conducted in anticipation of handling the IP's reaction to reading the note.

Another unorthodox CRAFT method for inviting an IP to begin treatment is one in which the *therapist* calls the IP. Again, the circum-stances for this option would be unusual but not inconceivable. For instance, a timid CSO might state, with conviction, that the IP would lis-ten to you because of your position of authority. If you made the decision to call the IP, you would do so during a CSO session. The call might start off sounding something like the following:

"Hello, I'm _____. I know your wife told you she was in therapy. I'm her therapist. I'm calling because I've had the chance to get to know your wife, and I'd like the opportunity to get to know you a little, too."

"Hi. This is _____, your mom's therapist. She's here with me now. Listen, I wonder if I could talk to you a minute? One of the things we've been working on is finding ways to make the relationship between you and your mom enjoyable again. Would you be willing to come down just once to talk about that?"

Notice that the invitation remains as nonthreatening as possible; the topic of alcohol or drug use is avoided altogether. The notion of getting a separate therapist for the IP would be raised when the IP met the CSO's counselor, unless, of course, the issue was broached by the IP on the phone. The outcome of the telephone conversation would be processed immediately with the CSO. Importantly, you would call an IP only with the CSO's permission and backing, because issues of confidentiality and safety would be of utmost concern.

RAPID INTAKE PROCESS

It is extremely important to move quickly once an IP agrees to begin treatment. The old adage "Strike while the iron is hot" is apropos, given that individuals' motivation to address their substance abuse problem often waxes and wanes (Miller, 1985; Prochaska & DiClemente, 1982, 1986). According to CRAFT, "rapid intake" means that an IP attends a first session with his or her *own* therapist within 48 hours of the IP's stated willingness to sample therapy. Since this expressed willingness may occur in the middle of a weekend, when clinics and professional offices are closed, CSOs may need access to an emergency number for the scheduling of IP appointments. Obviously considerable groundwork must be laid in order for an individual both to get an appointment arranged with a new therapist and for the session to take place within the designated 48-hour time frame. The rapid intake process is easier if you have access to qualified colleagues within your own counseling service, group practice, etc. However, insurance limitations or other constraints may preclude relying on coworkers, thereby necessitating another plan at times.

In preselecting a possible therapist for the IP, you should consider practical complications, such as whether the IP would likely be placed on a waiting list. Sometimes colleagues circumvent this problem by having standing agreements to see IPs for each other immediately. Additionally, you would want a therapist who is also willing to act as the Intake worker, so that the IP and the therapist actually meet and start the therapy process at the time of the IP's first session. Rapport building can thus begin immediately—a critical component when working with treatment-resistant clients. Within an agency setting, it also ensures that an ambivalent IP will not spend the entire session simply completing paperwork, because the therapist can monitor this process and delay segments of it until the next session, if necessary. Furthermore, since the therapist is hearing the client's "story" firsthand, it reduces client frustration by minimizing the number of times a client has to repeat him- or herself.

An important clinical consideration is the theoretical orientation of the IP's therapist. Given that CSOs have received primarily behavioral training through CRAFT, it is helpful to stay within this (or a cognitive-behavioral) framework for their IPs. Doing so allows both CSOs and IPs to conceptualize treatment and understand change strategies in similar ways, which should increase the chance that they will support each other's programs emotionally and behaviorally. Additionally, to some extent, you have assumed that the IP would see a cognitive-behavioral or behavioral therapist, inasmuch as you taught the CSO to describe treatment characteristics in line with such programs as an incentive for the IP to enter therapy. Specifically, you encouraged the CSO to discuss the fact that the IP would have control over the goals of the program, would have significant input into the course of treatment, and would be able to focus on problems other than substance abuse. Although these features certainly might be descriptive of other theoretical orientations, they definitely are not congruous with all approaches. There is no doubt that these treatment components and objectives are part of CRAFT's companion program, the Community Reinforcement Approach (Azrin et al., 1982; Hunt & Azrin, 1973; Meyers & Smith, 1995). Moreover, the Community Reinforcement Approach and other behavioral/cognitive-behavioral interventions for alcohol problems have received high rankings in meta-analytic reviews over the years (Finney & Monahan, 1996; Holder, Longabaugh, Miller, & Rubonis, 1991; Miller et al., 1995, 2003), which further argues for selecting a behaviorally or cognitive-behaviorally oriented therapist for the IP.

In narrowing down prospective IP therapists, another consideration is whether the counselors are qualified and willing to do couples work. CSOs in the CRAFT studies (Meyers et al., 1999, 2002; W. Miller et al., 1999) were routinely encouraged to participate in a few couples sessions with the IP's therapist. Not only does CSOs involvement demonstrate support for IP therapy, but the literature also suggests that behaviorally oriented couples therapy can be a highly successful treatment modality for substance abuse problems (Epstein & McCrady, 1998; Fals-Stewart et al., 2001; O'Farrell & Fals-Stewart, 1999; 2003). And whereas it may not be standard practice for one therapist to see both an individual *and* that individual as part of a couple, practical issues must be considered. Specifically, an IP and CSO would otherwise need three therapists: one each for the CSO and IP, and a couples therapist. Given that most couples would find this arrangement "overkill," it appears reasonable to settle for the next best option, particularly since this type of couples work typically lasts only a few sessions anyway. Table 9.2 summarizes the factors to consider when choosing a therapist for the IP.

Inasmuch as CSOs in the studies were much more willing to join couples therapy conducted by the IP's therapist than vice versa, this arrangement should be suggested first. Interestingly, it was fairly common for IPs *not* to want their CSOs to join them for a couples session until they were well into their own individual therapy. Based on this finding, the opportunity for couples therapy is not routinely dangled as an inducement when attempting to engage IPs into treatment.

HANDLING REFUSAL BY AN IP TO ENTER TREATMENT

It is imperative to prepare CSOs for the realistic possibility that their IP may refuse treatment, despite the fact that the CSOs have been trained to deliver the request in an appealing and timely manner. The preparation entails role plays of treatment refusals and discussions of the implications. These rehearsals allow CSOs to experience the perceived rejection in a somewhat naturalistic way. Characteristically, the feeling is one of failure. The feeling of failure may be magnified if the CSO is thinking about the fact that the majority of CSOs employing CRAFT techniques have successfully engaged their IPs in treatment. Therefore, it is very important to remind them that CRAFT-based procedures do not necessarily work *the first time* with every IP. It is fairly common for trained CSOs to find it necessary to make multiple, carefully orchestrated requests before their IP agrees to sample therapy. So encourage CSOs to be patient and remain optimistic and assure them that other treatment-engagement opportunities invariably will present

TABLE 9.2. CHOOSING A THERAPIST FOR THE IP

In selecting a potential therapist for the IP, ideally this individual should be:

1. Willing to see the IP *within 48 hours* of the time the IP agrees to treatment.
2. Willing to serve as the *Intake worker* to handle preliminary paperwork.
3. Primarily *behavioral/cognitive-behavioral* in orientation.
4. Skilled at conducting *couples therapy*.

themselves. If necessary, utilize cognitive restructuring techniques to challenge any overpowering negative thoughts that surface after the perceived rejection (e.g., Beck, 1976). In addition, the simple act of repeated exposure to the upsetting feelings triggered by the "rejection" role plays should decrease the impact of these feelings on the CSO.

During the course of ongoing CRAFT sessions, it is informative for CSOs to supply the details of any new interactions in which they have just *un*successfully approached their IPs about starting therapy. You are interested in knowing whether the CSOs delivered the conversation in the manner and at the time planned, and in learning precisely how the IPs reacted. Gathering this information allows you to determine if aspects of the communication should be changed prior to the next attempt. A common ineffectual scenario is one in which the CSO begins the conversation, as practiced, but then is stunned by unexpected or hurtful remarks by the IP. Frequently the CSO responds with an angry retort, which derails the positive communication and renders the therapy invitation unsalvageable. In such a situation your job is to (1) briefly explore the CSO's angry, bruised feelings, (2) then discuss whether the CSO could approach the topic in the future in a manner that might be less likely to elicit such a disquieting response from the IP. At the same time, practice role plays in which the IP responds similarly, so that the CSO has the opportunity to prepare a reply that keeps the conversation moving forward. During the process, motivate the CSO with reminders about the specific rewards that await her or him once the IP enters treatment.

Although CSOs do not routinely execute the request *exactly* as planned, you cannot assume that this variance is the reason why their IP refused treatment—so listen for cues that might provide insight. For instance, consider a CSO who reports that her husband became very agitated when she mentioned, as part of her therapy invitation, that *she* had been in therapy for several weeks already. He complained bitterly about being the last person in the family to know what was going on, and he accused her of plotting behind his back. If the wife thought her husband truly *was* concerned about the "plotting behind his back," you would encourage her to share the specifics of her CRAFT work, as it related to him, and would remind her to mention that he could have his own "unbiased" therapist. Assume "being the last person in the family to know what was going on" meant that the husband resented not being afforded what he perceived as the appropriate amount of respect or control in his family. You would ask the CSO to find a comfortable response that would increase the chance of his treatment engagement. Depending on the husband's values, the CSO might inform him that taking charge of his substance abuse problem was the best way, in her view, for him to resume his position as head of the household. In reviewing these possible options for future interactions, you would keep in mind that it is unclear whether it would have made a difference if the husband had known, in advance, that his wife was in treatment. He simply might have been intentionally steering the conversation off course so that it did not focus on him and his substance abuse problem. Regardless, the wife's next conversation with the IP could begin with an acceptance of partial responsibility for any problems created by not telling him about her therapy from the start.

Periodically, a CSO questions whether it is worthwhile to continue inviting the IP to treatment, given the repeated refusals. There are many factors to consider. Although across several studies the average number of CSO sessions prior to successful engagement was less than five (Meyers et al., 1999; W. Miller et al., 1999), *average* means that some individuals took longer. Not only were some IPs engaged late in the course of the CSO's sessions, but sometimes the IPs were only engaged *after* the CSO's therapy had ended (Meyers et al., 1999; W. Miller et al., 1999). Thus, the passage of time and the number of CSO sessions alone are insufficient for drawing any final conclusions.

CSOs may independently decide to temporarily stop asking their IPs to sample therapy, when they perceive the need for a break in order to recover from the disappointment and frustration of repeated refusals. This is certainly an understandable decision. The hiatus allows you to carefully review the tactics being employed, and to develop a revised plan. The time is also used to help CSOs make their own personal reinforcement a priority for a while. The Happiness Scale is revisited and their Goals of Counseling plan is updated. It should be stressed that the "break" from extending therapy invitations should *not* encompass a break from the other CRAFT procedures, such as the use of positive reinforcement for clean and sober behavior. If these procedures are, in fact, helping to reduce the alcohol or drug use, there would be no standard reason to discontinue them.

When deciding whether it is advisable for CSOs to stop inviting their IP permanently, a prime consideration is how comfortable CSOs are with the alternatives, given that their IP may never seek therapy. Your discussion of possible outcomes should include a review of the status of the IP's current use, the CSO–IP relationship, and the CSO's own personal functioning. If you have not been regularly monitoring progress in these areas, you could gather this information by readministering the relevant instruments introduced at the Intake (see Chapter 2, "Reviewing Standard Assessment Material," pp. 11–14). When possible, contrast CSOs' current scores with their Intake scores, so that signs of progress (or lack thereof) are evident. Whether CSOs elect to stay involved with their IP or end the relationship altogether, they may need your guidance and support to plan the next step.

PREPARING FOR THE POSSIBILITY
OF A PREMATURE DROPOUT

Sometimes clients are so relieved when their IPs finally agree to sample treatment that they lose sight of the fact that premature termination is a realistic outcome. Although you will have raised the issue previously, it is important to remind CSOs about this possibility once treatment engagement seems imminent. Your objective is to help them understand that, for some individuals, treatment entry is a gradual process characterized by multiple starts and stops along the way. This is one of the reasons why the CSO should be involved in the IP's treatment at some level; namely, to know immediately if the IP ceases attending. You should agree on a plan of action for the CSO in the event that this occurs.

In dealing with CSOs who are still in treatment when their IP drops out, spend a little time examining the factors that appeared to lead to this IP decision. If a practical problem seems largely responsible (e.g., inconvenient session times), there are usually practical solutions. More often than not, the reason is more complicated and includes factors such as an IP's fear of losing a (maladaptive) coping strategy, concern about resultant changes in the marriage, or the surfacing of an underlying IP depression. Treatment termination is unfortunate, as more therapy (couples, individual) is often the obvious solution. Nevertheless, CSOs are not helpless; they can always reinstate the CRAFT procedures that laid the foundation for treatment engagement in the first place. Furthermore, problem solving can generate fresh ideas and a plan for engaging the IP once again. Some CSOs choose to employ their new communication skills to directly ask their IPs what it would take to get them back into treatment.

Since IP treatment dropout may occur after CSOs have completed their own therapy, you should review the relevant CRAFT procedures in advance. If you have an "open door" policy, be sure to tell CSOs that returning for a few "emergency" planning sessions is an option as well.

Although CSOs tend to be quite motivated for treatment, occasionally they become less interested in attending once their IP has entered treatment. Premature CSO termination should be discouraged, since additional CSO training in the CRAFT procedures that support clean and sober behavior is often helpful for IPs during their struggle. Also, the

CRAFT goal that focuses on the CSO's own happiness may get over-looked if the CSO stops attending sessions.

CSO'S SUPPORT OF IP'S THERAPY

Many CSOs are participants in at least one IP session eventually, and thus ideally you should discuss in advance what to expect. This is yet another reason to be familiar with the orientation of the IP's prospective therapist and his or her attitude toward temporarily involving the CSO in the IP's treatment. A Community Reinforcement Approach therapist, for example, typically includes a couples therapy component in which the partner of the substance-abusing individual is asked to participate in several sessions (see Meyers & Smith, 1995, Chapter 9). The couple first completes a Relationship Happiness Scale (Figure 2.1, p. 39). After choosing a problem area to target, the Perfect Relationship form is used to set small relationship-based goals for each individual (see Meyers & Smith, 1995, Appendix 9.D). Other components of the Community Reinforcement Approach's relationship therapy include training in communication skills and in learning to reintroduce some of the subtle ways in which the partners used to be kind to each other (see Daily Reminder To Be Nice; Meyers & Smith, 1995, Appendix 9.G). In the event that the IP is going to use disulfiram (Antabuse) or naltrexone (ReVia) as a tool, the CSO would attend a session in order to be trained as the medication monitor (Meyers & Smith, 1995). If the IP's therapist is not using the Community Reinforcement Approach, but is behavioral or cognitive-behavioral in orientation, you would still prepare the CSO to expect some type of goal negotiation and skills training.

If the engagement plan calls for couples therapy as the main treatment format for the IP, you can provide CSOs with specific details about this therapy in advance as well, particularly if it entails empirically supported behavioral couples therapy (O'Farrell & Fals-Stewart, 2003; Miller et al., 2003). CRAFT-trained CSOs would already be familiar with several procedures similar to those incorporated into most behavioral couples programs: for example, communication training, problem solving, and learning to share positive activities (O'Farrell & Fals-Stewart, 2003). They would also have experience with components of "alcohol focused spouse involvement" (McCrady et al., 1986). This is a spouses program that utilizes a number of strategies comparable to several found in CRAFT, such as carefully rewarding abstinence and allowing the natural negative consequences of a person's drinking to emerge.

Regardless of whether the ultimate plan is for the CSO to attend any couples sessions, discuss the need for the CSO to support the IP's therapy emotionally and behaviorally, and determine the manner in which this support can best be offered. Some IPs appreciate well-timed encouragement or praise for their commitment to sobriety. Support may also begin with a CSO's broad offer to help in some way. In response, a CSO might be asked to do any number of (hopefully) reasonable things, such as preparing a favorite dinner on the IP's therapy appointment day, so that this can be anticipated as an evening reward. Another IP might ask his CSO to help plan enjoyable weekend activities to compete with drinking—a task that the CSO should already be doing, to some extent, given her CRAFT training.

SUMMARY

This chapter outlines the foundation that needs to be securely in place before CSOs are viewed as ready to invite their IPs to begin treatment. Examples of positive requests to sample treatment are demonstrated, with suggestions about enhancing the IPs' inclination to accept. Importantly, the need to prepare CSOs for possible refusals is discussed, as is the significance of staying supportive.

CHAPTER 10

EMPIRICAL SUPPORT
FOR CRAFT

The previous chapters provided detailed instructions in the use of CRAFT, as well as representative case illustrations. This final chapter presents CRAFT's scientific support. The findings demonstrate the degree to which CRAFT has outperformed the traditional treatments for CSOs in terms of engaging treatment-refusing individuals into substance abuse therapy. In the process of describing the other available interventions for CSOs, it covers a few more recently developed ones that share some similarities with CRAFT. The chapter also offers details on the types of clients who participated in the studies, those who were excluded, and the instruments used to collect much of the data. Finally, preliminary facts about the IPs, as reported by the CSOs, are presented.

TRADITIONAL INTERVENTIONS FOR CSOs

For many years the main treatment option extended by substance abuse facilities to CSOs who have requested help for a resistant loved one has been a 12-step program such as Al-Anon (Al-Anon Family Groups, 1984) or Nar-Anon (Narcotics Anonymous, 1993). As noted in Chapter 1, 12-step programs teach CSOs to detach from the drinker or drug user and to accept the fact that they are unable to control their IP's unhealthy behavior. Instead, CSOs are encouraged to focus on themselves. One study that exclusively examined Al-Anon (Dittrich & Trapold, 1984) discovered that when 23 wives of untreated alcoholic husbands were randomly assigned to either immediate or delayed Al-Anon group therapy, the wives in the former condition showed greater improvement in both mood and self-concept in 8 weeks than the wives in the latter. However, in this and other Al-

Anon studies, the IPs neither entered treatment nor decreased their substance use (Barber & Gilbertson, 1996; Sisson & Azrin, 1986). The studies in which Al-Anon was used as one of the comparison treatments are covered later in the chapter.

A second treatment option that has been available to CSOs, but to a more limited degree, is the Johnson Institute Intervention (Johnson, 1986). Known simply as the "Intervention," this program entails having a therapist meet with a CSO for the purpose of planning a "surprise" confrontational meeting with the substance abuser. For several weeks the CSO and other supportive individuals prepare statements describing how they have been negatively affected by the IP's use. During the confrontation with the IP, the messages are delivered and the IP is told that transportation to a treatment center has been arranged and is waiting. In essence, the philosophy behind the Johnson Institute Intervention is diametrically opposed to that of 12-step programs, since the former believes that CSOs *can* and *should* influence an individual's decision to seek professional help. The results from one study of the Intervention showed high rates of treatment engagement (86%) for those who actually carried it out, but given that only 29% of the CSOs even completed the training component of the Intervention, the overall success of the program was merely 24% (Liepman, Nirenberg, & Begin, 1989). The primary reason for the high attrition appeared to be CSOs' discomfort with the highly confrontational role expected of them, which they perceived as potentially injurious to their relationship with the drinker (Barber & Gilbertson, 1997). Of additional concern is some tentative evidence suggesting that clients who received the Intervention are more likely to relapse than clients who have experienced less confrontational techniques (Loneck, Garrett, & Banks, 1996a). The one study that used the Intervention as a comparison condition is reviewed later in this chapter (see "CRAFT: Alcohol Treatment Studies").

UNILATERAL FAMILY THERAPY APPROACHES

The newer, less traditional approaches for CSOs have often been collectively labeled as "unilateral family therapy" (Thomas & Santa, 1982). In general, they involve teaching the CSOs strategies to promote change in the IPs' substance use and improve the chance that they will enter treatment. The majority of the studies of these approaches has focused on individuals with alcohol problems. Thomas and colleagues (Thomas & Santa, 1982; Thomas, Santa, Bronson, & Oyserman, 1987) were among the first to demonstrate the success of a unilateral family intervention with spouses of IPs. Their treatment focused on modifying the CSOs' customary behavior toward the IP as an initial step, so that the marital relationship could be calmed and enhanced prior to the introduction of any treatment directives. CSOs later received instruction for carrying out a programmed confrontation rather similar to that in the Intervention (Johnson, 1986), but only if they agreed to follow through with serious consequences (e.g., separation) in the event that their husbands still refused treatment (Thomas & Santa, 1982). Without this agreement, a programmed request was taught instead.

The original clinical trial had a somewhat unusual design, as it involved 15 CSOs who were randomly assigned to receive either immediate or delayed unilateral family therapy, and then another 10 CSOs who were followed as a nonrandom, no-treatment control group. The available outcome data for 13 (of the 15) treated cases and for six (of the 10) no-treatment controls demonstrated that almost two-thirds of the drinkers whose CSOs were in the treated condition *either* entered treatment or decreased their drinking by at least 53%. In contrast, none of the control cases showed either of these improvements (Thomas et al., 1987). A larger subsequent study also obtained support for unilateral family therapy (Thomas & Ager, 1993). A total of 55 spouses of alcohol-abusing partners were randomly assigned either to an immediate ($n = 27$) or a delayed ($n = 28$) treatment of unilateral family therapy for 6 months. Spouses whose IPs did not want them to participate in the treatment were again followed as a nonrandom, no-treatment control group ($n = 14$). The findings showed significant differences in engagement rate in the expected direction immediately after spouse treatment. However, this difference was reduced to a trend at the 18-month assessment, when the final engagement rate was 57% for the spouses who had received treatment and 31% for the no-treatment condition. Improved functioning in the nondrinking spouses in the treatment condition included positive changes in psychopathology, life distress, marital adjustment, and marital satisfaction. Nonrandom assignment to the control group was the major limitation of both studies.

Researchers in Australia have received promising results with a unilateral family therapy program called Pressures to Change (PTC; Barber & Crisp, 1994; Barber & Gilbertson, 1997). The lower "levels" in this approach involve teaching CSOs various ways to provide environmental pressures for their drinkers to alter their behavior. One example is having CSOs plan activities that are incompatible with drinking. If these efforts do not satisfactorily reduce the drinkers' alcohol use or prompt them to enter treatment, the CSOs' training is moved up a level. Originally, the final level was a confrontation similar to the Johnson Institute Intervention, but currently it entails teaching CSOs to prepare other members of their social network to administer the different levels of pressure. Their first controlled study compared the outcomes of 32 CSOs randomly assigned to individual PTC, group PTC, or a waiting list control group (Barber & Crisp, 1995). Seven of the 16 drinkers with CSOs in one of the PTC conditions (44%) began treatment, and another three decreased their drinking (19%). There were no similar signs of progress for the drinkers in the control condition. Surprisingly, there was no substantial improvement in CSO functioning in general—a fact that the researchers believed was the result of CSOs' discomfort with the pressure to confront in the final level of the program.

The next PTC study involved 48 CSOs who were randomly assigned to one of the same three groups already described (Barber & Crisp, 1995) or to a fourth condition: Al-Anon. The results were very similar to those of the earlier trial: About two-thirds of the drinkers with partners in the PTC conditions again *either* sought treatment or reduced their alcohol use, whereas none of those associated with Al-Anon or the waiting list did (Barber & Gilbertson, 1996). This study also detected improvements in CSO functioning, but only for those women in the individualized version of PTC or in Al-Anon. The most recent study obtained favorable results for a self-help form of PTC as well (Barber & Gilbertson, 1997). These small sample studies require replication. Future research also may want to investigate the reasons why the CSOs' functioning did not improve in the group version of PTC.

The number of programs that has worked with family members in an attempt to influence the behavior of a treatment-resistant individual who abuses *illicit drugs* is even more limited. The relatively new ARISE (A Relational Intervention Sequence for Engagement) program offers specific treatment engagement advice for family members of drug-addicted individuals, but the IPs are not necessarily treatment refusers. ARISE evolved from the Johnson Institute Intervention, and yet there are important distinctions. For example, much of the early coaching of CSOs is done over the telephone. Additionally, the drug-abusing individual is informed about the meetings between the therapist and the CSOs from the start, and is regularly invited to join them. Also, there are multiple, small confrontations that build up to the more traditional Intervention only if the IP continues to offer resistance (Garrett et al., 1998). ARISE has offered many promising case findings but no controlled studies, to date (Garrett et al., 1999; Landau et al., 2000; Loneck et al., 1996b).

CRAFT STUDIES: GENERAL METHODOLOGY

Given that the basic methodology was similar for most of the CRAFT studies (Meyers et al., 1999, 2002; W. Miller et al., 1999), it is described next prior to presenting the findings.

RECRUITMENT AND SCREENING

In the majority of the CRAFT projects, CSOs were recruited primarily through newspaper ads, but local substance abuse programs periodically referred callers when they were CSOs of treatment-refusers. Common inclusion criteria for CSOs stipulated that they had to be close relatives or intimate partners (heterosexual or homosexual) of the IP and have regular contact with the IP (e.g., at least 40% of the time). It was necessary to require that a CSO and IP have a close relationship for two reasons: (1) It increased the likelihood that a CSO's estimate of IP use was accurate (Project MATCH Research Group, 1997); (2) it presumably ensured greater knowledge of, and access to, reinforcement contingencies for the IP. An additional inclusion criterion stated that CSOs had to describe the IP in a manner consistent with the diagnosis for a psychoactive substance use disorder in the fourth edition of the *Diagnostic and Statistical Manual of Mental Disorders* (DSM-IV; American Psychiatric Association, 1994). Also, CSOs had to be at least 18 years of age, and with the exception of the adolescent study (Waldron et al., 2003), the IPs did as well.

CSOs were excluded from participating if they met the DSM-IV criteria for a substance use disorder, were diagnosed as psychotic or otherwise too impaired to participate in treatment, or were unable to read at a sixth-grade level. CSOs also were excluded if they stated that their IP actually was *willing* to accept treatment, had received treatment (other than detoxification) for substance abuse problems in the prior 3 months, or was court mandated to receive treatment. As noted in Chapter 4, CSOs were excluded if they reported that their IP had engaged in domestic violence or had committed criminal assault in the prior 2 years, or had a history of severe violence, such as involving a weapon or resulting in hospitalization.

THERAPISTS

In the more recent studies, behaviorally oriented therapists delivered CRAFT, 12-step counselors conducted the Al-Anon Facilitation therapy, and the Johnson Institute Intervention was offered by experts in that treatment (Meyers et al., 1999, 2002; W. Miller et al., 1999). Although this nesting of therapists was a deviation from the procedure used in the earliest CRAFT study (Sisson & Azrin, 1986), it was considered an improvement because nested therapists are theoretically committed to, and therefore presumably more passionate about, their own therapeutic approach (Leake & King, 1977). In terms of formal training, therapists of all orientations held bachelor's or master's degrees in psychology or counseling. Their experience varied greatly within treatment conditions, with therapists having accumulated anywhere from 0 to 16 years of experience in the alcohol or drug field. Importantly, therapists in the CRAFT conditions tended to be the least experienced overall, with the typical therapist having 0–3 years of experience with substance-abusing clients. All therapists received ongoing weekly supervision from an expert in the particular technique. Individual therapy sessions were routinely videotaped in order to allow supervisors to randomly monitor protocol adherence.

TREATMENT FOR IPS

Whenever an IP agreed to seek treatment, the standard procedure was to have either the CSO or the IP call the project office during business hours to schedule an appointment, or the 24-hour access pager after hours or on weekends. It was made clear to CSOs that they should not delay scheduling the appointment once a commitment was obtained from the IP. In turn, every effort was made to schedule the IP's assessment session as soon as possible, typically within 24–48 hours. All IPs who were interested in participating in the study were included if they contacted the program within 6 months of the CSO's first session. Referrals were made to other local programs if an IP was no longer interested in participating upon hearing the details of the treatment study, or if an IP called after the 6-month window had closed.

CRAFT: ALCOHOL TREATMENT STUDIES

The early version of CRAFT was called CRT: Community Reinforcement Training. CRT was first used in a small, randomized study with the female CSOs of 12 male problem drinkers in rural Illinois (Sisson & Azrin, 1986). Each of the CSOs had contacted a local alcoholism treatment program about a family member's severe alcohol problem. The CSOs were wives of the IPs ($n = 9$), sisters ($n = 2$), or daughters ($n = 1$). The seven women assigned to CRT received the standard CRAFT procedures. The five women assigned to the control condition received disease-concept-based traditional treatment consisting of weekly individual counseling sessions and referrals to Al-Anon meetings. The referrals were always followed up with Systematic Encouragement, an established Community Reinforcement Approach behavioral procedure (see Meyers & Smith, 1995, pp. 141–143) that had already proven to be effective at increasing the likelihood of attendance at meetings (Sisson & Mallams, 1981).

In terms of the main outcome, six of the seven drinkers whose CSOs were assigned to CRT (86%) entered treatment, compared to none of the five drinkers whose CSOs received disease-concept-based traditional treatment. According to the CSOs' estimates, taken from their daily recording charts, these six treatment-engaged drinkers significantly decreased their alcohol consumption prior to even beginning therapy, when just their

CSO was in CRT treatment. In contrast, the drinking pattern of the IPs in the control condition remained largely unchanged. The study was limited by the small sample size, the absence of any CSO functioning data, and the fact that CRT participants attended a higher average number of sessions (7.2) compared to the comparison group (3.5). Still, in a short period of time these CRT-trained family members were able to obtain the skills necessary to engage their severely alcohol-dependent loved ones in treatment and to favorably influence their drinking from the start.

The National Institute on Alcohol Abuse and Alcoholism (NIAAA) funded a large study, conducted in Albuquerque, New Mexico, with 130 CSOs of alcohol-dependent individuals (W. Miller et al., 1999). CSOs were randomly assigned either to CRAFT (n = 45), Al-Anon Facilitation (n = 45), or the Johnson Institute Intervention (n = 40). The Johnson Institute Intervention was set up in the manner described earlier. Al-Anon Facilitation involved an individual form of 12-step treatment that was aimed at securing CSOs' attendance at Al-Anon meetings; it was modeled after the Project MATCH 12-step Facilitation therapy (Nowinski, Baker, & Carroll, 1992). CSOs assigned to this condition were taught that they were powerless to control their IP's substance use, and so they needed to detach from him or her and focus on strengthening their own mental health. The basic program components included (1) acquainting CSOs with the12-step concepts and readings, (2) teaching loving detachment, (3) reducing CSOs' enabling behavior, (4) helping CSOs work through the beginning steps of Al-Anon, and (5) increasing the likelihood that CSOs would attend 12-step meetings by using Systematic Encouragement procedures (Sisson & Mallams, 1981). In addition to deviating from traditional Al-Anon programs by offering one-on-one professional help as opposed to a self-help group format, Al-Anon Facilitation also considered IP engagement as part of its charge.

Relationship status of the recruited CSOs included IP spouses (59%), parents (30%), girlfriends/boyfriends (8%), children (1.5%), and grandparents (1.5%). The vast majority were females (91%). The ethnic breakdown was white, non-Hispanic (53%), Hispanic (39%), Native American (6%), African American (1%), and "other" (1%). On average, CSOs were 47 years of age and had 14 years of education. They tended to be employed either full time (51%) or part time (17%). In terms of attendance for the 12 hours of individual treatment, there were no significant differences between the percentage of completed sessions for those in CRAFT (89%) versus those in Al-Anon Facilitation (95%). However, CSOs in the Johnson Institute Intervention attended only 53% of the sessions; these participants commonly stating that they terminated therapy because they had decided against going through with the family confrontation.

The primary interest of the study was to determine the engagement outcome across treatment conditions. *Engagement* was defined as an IP completing the 4-hour Intake assessment and at least one therapy session. CRAFT-instructed CSOs were significantly more successful at engaging their IPs in treatment during the 6-month window (64%), compared to those trained in the Johnson Institute Intervention (30%) or Al-Anon Facilitation (13%). Interestingly, parents were significantly more likely to successfully engage their IP in treatment (51%) than were spouses (32%). For the engaged drinkers, the average number of sessions completed by their CSOs prior to IP engagement was similar across CRAFT (4.7 sessions), the Johnson Institute Intervention (4.7 sessions), and Al-Anon Facilitation (5.7 sessions). The median length of stay for IPs who entered treatment was 10.5 out of 12 sessions.

Overall, CSOs showed marked improvement in their own functioning as well as that of their relationship, but there were no group differences. These significant changes over time occurred for depression, as measured by the Beck Depression Inventory (BDI; Beck et al., 1988); for anger, as measured by the State–Trait Anger Expression Inventory (STAXI; Spielberger, 1988); for family cohesion and family conflict, on the Family Environment Scale (FES; Moos & Moos, 1986), and for relationship happiness, on the Relationship Happiness Scale (Azrin et al., 1973). Furthermore, these improvements were *not* limited to those CSOs who had engaged their IPs in treatment.

In addition to providing a large sample, the study offered several other methodological advantages over previous studies. These included efforts to ensure that the IPs were diagnosable as alcohol dependent or abusive and were initially treatment-refusers. Furthermore, the therapists were committed ideologically to their particular therapeutic approach, and each treatment was manual-guided. Lastly, follow-ups were conducted by interviewers who were uninformed regarding group status, and follow-up rates were high (e.g., 94% at 12 months).

CRAFT: DRUG TREATMENT STUDIES

The CRAFT (and CRT) programs have been applied to drug-abusing populations in several recent studies. For example, the National Institute on Drug Abuse (NIDA) sponsored a project conducted in Philadelphia and Camden, New Jersey, by Kirby and colleagues (1999). Thirty-two CSOs of drug users were randomly assigned to either individual CRT training sessions or to 12-step meetings. The CSOs generally consisted of women (94%) who were the spouses of the drug users (56%), their parents (38%), or their siblings (6%). CSOs were 40 years of age, on average, and their ethnicity was white (75%), African American (22%), or "other" (3%). They had a mean of 14.5 years of education, and employment status tended to be full time (50%) or part time (25%). The drug of choice for their IPs was most often cocaine (56%), followed by heroin (22%).

Significant differences in IP treatment engagement rates were detected at the conclusion of the 10-week program, when the CSOs who had received individual CRT training sessions (64% engaged) were contrasted with CSOs who had attended 12-step meetings (17% engaged). It is unclear whether this finding was influenced by the fact that 86% of the CSOs in the CRT condition completed the minimum number of required therapy hours (approximately 15), whereas only 39% in the 12-step condition did so. The CSOs' psychosocial functioning in both conditions improved from baseline to the posttreatment assessment. Positive changes were noted on many variables, including each of the scales from the Profile of Mood States (McNair, Lorr, & Droppleman, 1971, 1992) and two (Family Unit, Social Leisure) from the Social Adjustment Scale (Weissman & Bothwell, 1976; Weissman, Paykel, & Prusoff, 1990). In general, CSOs also showed significant reductions in problems related to their IP's drug use on the Family Impact Survey (Kirby et al., 1999) in two areas: financial and health issues. The improvement on the FES (Moos & Moos, 1986; Moos, 1987) was more restricted, as only three subscales (Expressiveness, Intellectual–Cultural, Organization) out of 10 showed significant baseline-to-posttest changes.

Limitations of the study included a relatively small sample size, few minority participants (25%), and a reliance on CSOs' self-report regarding IP treatment engagement. Also, treatment formats differed across conditions, with CSOs in CRT receiving individual sessions and CSOs in the 12-step program participating in group meetings. Nevertheless, this promising and well-conducted study was the first published controlled CRAFT trial with illicit drug users.

The next study was a NIDA-funded uncontrolled CRAFT trial with 62 CSOs of treatment-refusing drug users that was carried out at the Center on Alcoholism, Substance Abuse, and Addictions (CASAA) in Albuquerque, New Mexico (Meyers et al., 1999). The sample was primarily female (97%) and averaged 45 years of age. Ethnic self-identification was diverse: 48% Hispanic, 47% white, non-Hispanic, 3% Native American, and 2% African American. With regard to the relationship between the CSOs and their IP, 56% of the CSOs were parents of an IP, 34% were spouses, 6% were siblings, and 4% were children. According to the IPs' own reports when they entered treatment, drugs of choice included marijuana (43%), cocaine (32%), stimulants (14%), opiates (9%), and tranquilizers (2%).

CSOs were administered a battery of assessment instruments that covered CSO functioning, IP functioning, and the CSO–IP relationship.

The four categories of instruments administered to CSOs about them-selves included:

1. *CSO's emotional state*: BDI (Beck et al., 1988); State–Trait Anxiety Inventory (STAI; Spielberger et al., 1983); State–Trait Anger Expression Inventory (STAXI; Spielberger, 1988); and State Self-Esteem Scale (Heatherton & Polivy, 1991).
2. *CSO's substance use*: Form-90-DI (Miller & DelBoca, 1994; Miller, 1996); and the Inventory of Drug Use Consequences (InDUC; Tonigan & Miller, 2002).
3. *CSO's social adaptation*: Social Functioning and Resources Scale (from the Health and Daily Living Form, Moos et al., 1987); and Purpose in Life Scale (Crumbaugh, 1968).
4. *CSO's physical health*: Physical Symptoms (Moos et al., 1987).

It was necessary to collect the CSOs' impressions of their IP's func-tioning, since these would serve as the only information available on IP status for those IPs who never entered treatment (Meyers et al., 1999; W. Miller et al., 1999). Research has shown that collaterals typically give information about a drinker's alcohol consumption that is highly corre-lated with the drinker's own self-report (Sobell & Sobell, 1992). The col-lection of data from CSOs, using time line interviewing about a loved one's drug use, appears to be effective as well (Anglin, 1988; Day & Robles, 1989). With these points in mind, CSOs were asked to complete the following measures about their IP in two categories:

1. *IP's substance use*: Form-90-DC (Drug Collateral; Miller, 1996); and the InDUC-SO (Significant Other; Tonigan & Miller, 2002).
2. *IP's motivation for treatment*: Readiness Ruler (Rollnick, Heather, Gold, & Hall, 1992); and Barriers to Treatment (Anderson, Ogle, Miller, Meyers, & Miller, 1999).

With regard to the CSO–IP relationship, CSOs completed a number of instruments that appeared most appropriate for assessing the quality of the dyad, given that different types of relationships with the IPs were expected. These instruments included:

1. *Characterization of the CSO–IP relationship*: FES (Moos & Moos, 1986); Dyadic Adjustment Scale (Spanier, 1976; for those in inti-mate relationships); and Relationship Happiness Scale (Azrin et al., 1973; Sisson & Azrin, 1986).
2. *CSO–IP conflict resolution strategies*: Conflict Tactics Scales (Straus, 1979).

The CSOs completed a mean of 10.4 sessions out of their possible 12. The average length of CSO treatment before their IP was engaged was 4.8 sessions. These CRAFT-trained CSOs were successful at engaging their IP into treatment in 74% of the cases. Once engaged, IPs attended an average of 7.6 out of 12 available sessions. As in the alcohol study (W. Miller et al., 1999), parents overall were significantly more successful (83%) than were non-parents (63%) at engaging their IP. CSOs' functioning improved as well, with symptoms of depression, anxiety, anger, and physical ailments dropping, on average, to within the normal range over the course of the 6-month follow-up. Improvements in the CSOs' evaluation of their relationship status were not as pronounced, although some signs of progress were detected in general relationship happiness and diminished family conflict.

The primary purpose of a recent, experimentally controlled NIDA-funded CRAFT study conducted in Albuquerque, New Mexico, was to determine whether the CSOs who were assigned to the CRAFT program would be more successful at engaging their treatment-resistant drug-abusing IP than would the CSOs who were randomly placed in an Al-Anon/Nar-Anon Facilitation therapy (Al-Nar FT) program (Meyers et al., 2002). The Al-Nar FT condition was essentially the same program as that described for the CRAFT alcohol trial (W. Miller et al., 1999), with the added recognition of Nar-Anon as another appropriate self-help group for these CSOs. A secondary interest was to ascertain whether the CRAFT outcome could be improved if a group aftercare component were added that roughly paralleled the Al-Anon or Nar-Anon meetings for Al-Nar FT participants. To test this question, CRAFT + Aftercare was introduced as a second CRAFT condition, which offered ongoing group support for up to 6 months once the individual CRAFT sessions had ended. These open-ended groups utilized the same treatment principles as the CRAFT individual sessions and were conducted by the same therapists.

Several of the limitations of earlier studies also were addressed with this clinical trial. For example, both CRAFT and Al-Nar FT were conducted in individual session formats, as opposed to having one of them available only in a group setting. Additionally, objective verification of IP treatment engagement was required, and the follow-up period (18 months) was longer than the norm for this type of study (Kirby et al., 1999). As in previous CRAFT studies, it was expected that CSOs assigned to either CRAFT condition would be significantly more successful at engaging their IPs in treatment than would CSOs assigned to Al-Nar FT. Secondly, CRAFT + Aftercare CSOs were predicted to have higher engagement rates than CSOs in both the CRAFT alone and the Al-Nar FT interventions. Thirdly, based on the results of the earlier alcohol study (W. Miller et al., 1999), CSOs across all conditions were expected to show significant improvements in functioning over time.

The 90 CSOs in the study were distributed in the following manner: CRAFT (n = 29), CRAFT + Aftercare (n = 30), and Al-Nar FT (n = 31). This primarily female sample (88%) averaged 47 years of age and 14 years of education. They were an ethnically diverse group, with approximately an equal number of Hispanic (49%) and white, non-Hispanic participants. Regarding employment status, 51% worked full time and 21% part time, 17% were retired, and 11% were either homemakers or unemployed. There were no significant group differences on any of these variables. In terms of the relationship of these CSOs to the IPs, 53% of the CSOs were the IPs' parents, 30% were intimate partners, 10% were their siblings, and 7% were "other" (e.g., their children, friends). According to the CSOs, the primary categories of illicit drugs being used by the IPs included marijuana (67%), cocaine (63%), stimulants (30%), and opiates (19%).

CSOs attended, on average, 10.6 out of a possible 12 sessions. There were no differences across treatments. An examination of the main interest of the study—that is, engagement rates—detected an overall significant difference in CSO group assignment: CRAFT (58.6% engaged), CRAFT + Aftercare (76.7%), and Al-Nar FT (29.0%). Both CRAFT interventions had significantly higher engagement rates than the Al-Nar FT group when contrasted individually with it. An analysis indicated that there were no significant differences in engagement rates between the two CRAFT conditions, so they were combined for all subsequent analyses. The results showed that the CSOs in the combined CRAFT conditions were significantly more successful (67% engaged) than the CSOs in the Al-Nar FT condition (29% engaged) at influencing their IPs to enter treatment. Unlike two earlier studies (Meyers et al., 1999; W. Miller et al., 1999), parents were not significantly more successful than spouses at engaging their IPs in treatment. Engaged IPs attended an average of 7.6 out of 12 therapy sessions. Follow-up rates were high, with the lowest rate (96%) occurring at 12 months. Pre–post improvement was detected for several measures of CSO functioning, again regardless of treatment condition, albeit significance was lost when corrections for multiple tests were used.

This large-scale controlled study demonstrated that treatment-refusing individuals with a wide variety of illicit drug problems were more likely to be engaged in treatment when CSOs were trained in CRAFT procedures than Al-Nar FT procedures. Although the results were clearly in the predicted direction, the hypothesis that CSOs in the CRAFT + Aftercare condition would show significantly higher engagement rates than the CRAFT alone condition was not supported. In order to understand this finding, we should first note that only 47% of the eligible CSOs ever attended any of the aftercare groups once their individual sessions had ended. In part, this low attendance was probably due to the fact that 79% of the CSOs in this condition had already successfully engaged their IP in treatment. In terms of the seven CSOs in the CRAFT + Aftercare condition who had *not* gotten their IP to begin treatment, only three of these CSOs attended any aftercare groups. Since none of these three CSOs ever engaged their IP, it showed that the addition of the aftercare group did nothing to improve CRAFT engagement rates.

Preliminary results are available from an uncontrolled NIDA-funded trial of CRAFT with adolescent drug abusers as the treatment-refusing IPs (Waldron et al., 2003). The 43 CSOs were the parents of these teenagers, the vast majority being their mothers (80%). A total of 49% of the IPs were from two-parent families. The CSOs averaged almost 46 years of age and had a mean family income of $44,000. The ethnic breakdown was 48% Hispanic, 47% white, non-Hispanic, and 5% Native American. The treatment engagement rate was comparable to that of other CRAFT studies, with 71% of the CSOs able to get their treatment-refusing teenager to enter treatment. On average, these successfully engaged IPs were 16.5 years of age, and 77% were boys. They attended an average of 8.1 out of 12 possible sessions.

The psychosocial functioning of the CSOs of the engaged IPs improved significantly on a number of dimensions from baseline to 3- and 6-month follow-ups, whereas the functioning of the CSOs of nonengaged IPs did not. Specifically, significant decreases in parents' depression, anxiety, and physical symptoms were demonstrated, along with significant increases in their self-esteem. This first CRAFT study with adolescent IPs offers promising findings for this younger population of resistant substance abusers. It requires replication in the context of a controlled trial.

SUMMARY OF RESEARCH EVIDENCE AND FUTURE DIRECTIONS

Traditional treatment options for CSOs are problematic. The two studies of the Johnson Institute Intervention showed that although CSOs who completed treatment had high engagement rates, only a small percentage of CSOs apparently felt comfortable going through with the surprise confrontation (Liepman et al., 1989; W. Miller et al., 1999), thereby leaving the engagement rates at 30% or less. For the six studies that included Al-Anon (or Al-Anon Facilitation therapy), the majority of CSOs demonstrated significant improvements in functioning over time, which frequently equaled that of the other treatments. However, the IP engagement rates were low, ranging from 0 to 29%. Among the unilateral family therapy studies, Thomas and colleagues showed encouraging results with engagements rates near 57%, but several methodological problems limited enthusiasm somewhat (Thomas & Ager, 1993; Thomas et al., 1987). Additionally, their program was lengthier than most and geared exclusively for spouses. The Pressures to Change program likewise reported interesting early findings for IP engagement (44% engaged) and improved CSO functioning (Barber & Gilbertson, 1996), but research with larger samples still needs to be conducted. Furthermore, since the final level of the program no longer involves confrontation, the outcome of studies with this revised program is of particular interest. The ARISE program offers promise as well, in part because it addresses some of the main criticisms of the Intervention, on which it is based. For instance, it has eliminated the surprise element and the confrontation is now more gradual (Garrett et al., 1999; Landau et al., 2000). An adequate evaluation of the ARISE program would require controlled studies and clarification regarding the percentage of IPs who are actually treatment-refusers.

The CRAFT program is backed by four well-controlled studies and two pilot projects, to date. The IP engagement rates for CRAFT (64–86%) were superior to those of traditional treatments when directly contrasted in studies, and they consistently exceeded the rates of other unilateral family therapy programs, as reported in the literature. Moreover, these successful CSOs represented a highly diverse group in terms of age, ethnicity, and the type of relationship they had with the IP (e.g., parent, spouse). Furthermore, CSO functioning typically improved, regardless of whether the IP agreed to enter treatment. Importantly, CRAFT was the only unilateral family therapy program proven to be effective with IPs who have either alcohol or illicit drug problems. It was also efficient: CSOs averaged only 4.7–7.2 sessions prior to engaging their IPs in treatment. Finally, though they were regularly supervised, most of the CRAFT therapists were relatively inexperienced clinicians.

Despite the highly favorable scientific support for CRAFT, many research questions remain. For instance, the fact that parents were more successful than spouses at engaging their IPs in two of the studies (Meyers et al., 1999; W. Miller et al., 1999) merits investigation. Future studies might also focus on *including* some of the *excluded* but interested CSOs, such as those with substance abuse problems themselves, or even those struggling with domestic violence issues with their IP. Although recruiting the latter sample could raise controversy, it could be argued that the decision to systematically exclude these individuals is equally controversial, given the unacceptable alternatives for these CSOs (Caetano et al., 2003; Sullivan et al., 1992). Potentially, CRAFT could be applied to a host of problems outside the substance abuse realm, such as with treatment-refusing individuals who have anorexia nervosa, those suffering from paranoid ideation, or even patients with chronic medical problems (e.g., diabetes, morbid obesity) who resist seeking the medical attention they desperately need.

REFERENCES

Abbott, J., Johnson, R., Koziol-McLain, J., & Lowenstein, S. R. (1995). Domestic violence against women: Incidence and prevalence in an emergency room population. *Journal of the American Medical Association, 273,* 1763–1767.

Acierno, R., Resnick, H. S., & Kilpatrick, D. G. (1997). Health impact of interpersonal violence: Prevalence rates, case identification, and risk factors for sexual assault, physical assault, and domestic violence in men and women. *Behavioral Medicine, 23,* 53–64.

Akillas, E., & Efran, J. S. (1995). Symptom prescription and reframing: Should they be combined? *Cognitive Therapy and Research, 19,* 263–279.

Al-Anon Family Groups. (1984). *Al-Anon faces alcoholism.* New York: Author.

Alcoholics Anonymous. (1976). *Alcoholics Anonymous.* New York: Alcoholics Anonymous World Services.

American Psychiatric Association. (1994). *Diagnostic and statistical manual of mental disorders* (4th ed.). Washington, DC: Author.

Anderson, R., Ogle, R., Miller, E., Meyers, R., & Miller, W. (1999, November). *Why won't they come in? A questionnaire to assess barriers to seeking treatment among substance abusers.* Poster presented at the meeting of the Association for Advancement of Behavior Therapy, Toronto, Canada.

Anglin, M. D. (1988). The efficacy of civil commitment in treating narcotic addiction. In C. Leukefeld & F. Tims (Eds.), *Compulsory treatment of drug abuse: Research and clinical practice* (pp. 8–34). Rockville, MD: National Institute on Drug Abuse.

Ascher, L. M., & Turner, R. M. (1979). Paradoxical intention and insomnia: An experimental investigation. *Behaviour Research and Therapy, 17,* 408–411.

Azrin, N. H. (1976). Improvements in the community reinforcement approach to alcoholism. *Behaviour Research and Therapy, 14,* 339–348.

Azrin, N. H., Naster, B. J., & Jones, R. (1973). Reciprocity counseling: A rapid learning-based procedure for marital counseling. *Behaviour Research and Therapy, 11,* 365–382.

Azrin, N. H., Sisson, R. W., Meyers, R. J., & Godley, M. (1982). Alcoholism treatment by disulfiram and community reinforcement therapy. *Journal of Behavior Therapy and Experimental Psychiatry, 13,* 105–112.

Barber, J. G., & Crisp, B. R. (1994). The effects of alcohol abuse on children and the partner's capacity to initiate change. *Drug and Alcohol Review, 13*, 409–416.

Barber, J. G., & Crisp, B. R. (1995). The 'pressures to change' approach to working with the partners of heavy drinkers. *Addiction, 90*, 269–276.

Barber, J. G., & Gilbertson, R. (1996). An experimental study of brief unilateral intervention for the partners of heavy drinkers. *Research on Social Work Practice, 6*, 325–336.

Barber, J. G., & Gilbertson, R. (1997). Unilateral interventions for women living with heavy drinkers. *Social Work, 42*, 69–78.

Beck, A. T. (1976). *Cognitive therapy and the emotional disorders*. New York: International Universities Press.

Beck, A. T., Rush, A. J., Shaw, B. F., & Emery, G. (1979). *Cognitive therapy of depression*. New York: Guilford Press.

Beck, A. T., Steer, R. A., & Garbin, M. G. (1988). Psychometric properties of the Beck Depression Inventory: Twenty-five years of evaluation. *Clinical Psychology Review, 8*, 77–100.

Berlinger, J. S. (2001). Domestic violence: How you can make a difference. *Nursing, 31*, 58–63.

Bombardier, C. H., Ehde, D., & Kilmer, J. (1997). Readiness to change alcohol drinking habits after traumatic brain injury. *Archives of Physical Medicine and Rehabilitation, 78*, 592–596.

Bowers, T. G., & Al-Rehda, M. R. (1990). A comparison of outcome with group/marital and standard/individual therapies with alcoholics. *Journal of Studies on Alcohol, 51*, 301–309.

Brown, J. M., & Miller, W. R. (1993). Impact of motivational interviewing on participation and outcome in residential alcoholism treatment. *Psychology of Addictive Behaviors, 7*, 211–218.

Brown, T. G., Kokin, M., Seraganian, P., & Shields, N. (1995). Models of helping and coping. *American Psychologist, 37*, 368–384.

Busby, D. M., Crane, D. R., Larson, J. H., & Christensen, C. (1995). A revision of the Dyadic Adjustment Scale for use with distressed and nondistressed couples: Construct hierarchy and multidimensional scales. *Journal of Marital and Family Therapy, 21*, 289–308.

Caetano, R., Field, C. A., & Scott, N. (2003). Association between childhood physical abuse, exposure to parental violence, and alcohol problems in adulthood. *Journal of Interpersonal Violence, 18*, 240–257.

Caetano, R., Schafer, J., & Cunradi, C. B. (2001). Alcohol-related intimate partner violence among white, black, and Hispanic couples in the United States. *Alcohol Research and Health, 25*, 58–65.

Carroll, K. M., Nich, C., Sifry, R. L., Nuro, K. F., Frankforter, T. L., Ball, S. A., Fenton, L., & Rounsaville, B. J. (2000). A general system for evaluating therapist adherence and competence in psychotherapy research in the addictions. *Drug and Alcohol Dependence, 57*, 225–238.

Centers for Disease Control and Prevention. (1994). Physical violence during the 12 months preceding childbirth—Alaska, Maine, Oklahoma, and West Virginia, 1990–1991. *Morbidity and Mortality Weekly Report, 43*, 132–137.

Chermack, S. T., Stoltenberg, S. F., & Fuller, B. E. (2000). Gender differences in the development of substance-related problems: The impact of family history of alcoholism, family history of violence and childhood conduct problems. *Journal of Studies on Alcohol, 61,* 845–852.

Children of Alcoholics Foundation. (1996). *Helping children affected by parental addiction and family violence: Collaboration, coordination, and cooperation.* New York: Author.

Christensen, A., & Jacobson, N. S. (2000). *Reconcilable differences.* New York: Guilford Press.

Collins, R. L., Leonard, K., & Searles, J. (Eds.) (1990). *Alcohol and the family.* New York: Guilford Press.

Connors, G. J., Carroll, K. M., DiClemente, C. C., Longabaugh, R., & Donovan, D. M. (1997). The therapeutic alliance and its relationship to alcoholism treatment participation and outcome. *Journal of Consulting and Clinical Psychology, 65,* 588–598.

Council on Scientific Affairs. (1992). Violence against women: Relevance for medical practitioners. *Journal of the American Medical Association, 267,* 3184–3189.

Crumbaugh, J. C. (1968). Cross-validation of the Purpose of Life Test based on Frankl's concepts. *Journal of Individual Psychology, 24,* 74–81.

Cunningham, J. A., Sobell, L. C., Sobell, M. B., & Kapur, G. (1995). Resolution from alcohol treatment problems with and without treatment: Reasons for change. *Journal of Substance Abuse, 7,* 365–372.

Day, N. D., & Robles, N. (1989). Methodological issues in the measurement of substance use. *Annals of New York Academy of Sciences, 562,* 8–13.

Dittrich, J. E., & Trapold, M. A. (1984). A treatment program for the wives of alcoholics: An evaluation. *Bulletin of the Society of Psychologists in Addictive Behaviors, 3,* 91–102.

D'Zurilla, T. J., Chang, E. C., Nottingham, E. J., & Faccini, L. (1998). Social problem-solving deficits and hopelessness, depression, and suicide risk in college students and psychiatric inpatients. *Journal of Clinical Psychology, 54,* 1–17.

D'Zurilla, T. J., & Goldfried, M. R. (1971). Problem solving and behavior modification. *Journal of Abnormal Psychology, 78,* 107–126.

Emery, R. E., Fincham, F. D., & Cummings, E. M. (1992). Parenting in context: Systemic thinking about parental conflict and its influence on children. *Journal of Consulting and Clinical Psychology, 60,* 909–912.

Epstein, E. E., & McCrady, B. S. (1998). Behavioral couples treatment of alcohol and drug use disorders: Current status and innovations. *Clinical Psychology Review, 18,* 689–711.

Falkowski, C. L. (2003). *Dangerous drugs* (2nd ed.). Center City, MN: Hazelden.

Fals-Stewart, W., Birchler, G. R., & O'Farrell, T. J. (1996). Behavioral couples therapy for male substance-abusing patients: Effects on relationship adjustment and drug-using behavior. *Journal of Consulting and Clinical Psychology, 64,* 959–972.

Fals-Stewart, W., O'Farrell, T. J., & Birchler, G. R. (2001). Behavioral couples therapy for male methadone maintenance patients: Effects on drug-using behavior and relationship adjustment. *Behavior Therapy, 32,* 391–411.

Fals-Stewart, W., O'Farrell, T. J., Feehan, M., Birchler, G. R., Tiller, S., & McFarlin, S. K. (2000). Behavioral couples therapy versus individual-based treatment for male substance-abusing patients: An evaluation of significant individual change and comparison of improvement rates. *Journal of Substance Abuse Treatment, 18,* 249–254.

Finney, J. W., & Monahan, S. C. (1996). The cost-effectiveness of treatment for alcoholism: A second approximation. *Journal of Studies on Alcohol, 57,* 229–243.

Foote, F. H., Szapocznik, J., Kurtines, W. M., Perez-Vidal, A., & Hervis, O. K. (1985). One-person family therapy: A modality of brief strategic family therapy. In R. Ashery (Ed.), *Progress in the development of cost-effective treatment for drug abusers* (pp. 51–65). Rockville, MD: National Institute on Drug Abuse.

Garrett, J., Landau, J., Shea, R., Stanton, M. D., Baciewicz, G., & Brinkman-Sull, D. (1998). The ARISE intervention: Using family and network links to engage addicted persons in treatment. *Journal of Substance Abuse Treatment, 15,* 333–343.

Garrett, J., Stanton, M. D., Landau, J., Baciewicz, G., Brinkman-Sull, D., & Shea, R. (1999). The "concerned other" call: Using family links and networks to overcome resistance to addiction treatment. *Substance Use and Misuse, 34,* 363–382.

Goldfried, M. R. (1982). Resistance and clinical behavior therapy. In P. L. Wachtel (Ed.), *Resistance: Psychodynamic and behavioral approaches* (pp. 95–114). New York: Plenum Press.

Gondolf, E. W., & Foster, R. A. (1991). Wife assault among VA alcohol rehabilitation patients. *Hospital and Community Psychiatry, 42,* 74–79.

Graber, R. A., & Miller, W. R. (1988). Abstinence and controlled drinking goals in behavioral self-control training of problem drinkers: A randomized clinical trial. *Psychology of Addictive Behaviors, 2,* 20–33.

Graham-Bermann, S. A., & Brescoll, V. (2000). Gender, power, and violence: Assessing the family stereotypes of the children of batterers. *Journal of Family Psychology, 14,* 600–612.

Greenfeld, L. A. (1998). *Alcohol and crime: An analysis of national data on the prevalence of alcohol involvement in crime.* Report prepared for Assistant Attorney General's National Symposium on Alcohol Abuse and Crime. Washington, DC: U.S. Department of Justice.

Grisso, J. A., Schwarz, D. F., Hirschinger, N., Sammel, M., Brensinger, C., Santanna, J., Lowe, R., Anderson, E., Shaw, L. M., Bethel, C. A., & Teeple, L. (1999). Violent injuries among women in an urban area. *New England Journal of Medicine, 341,* 1899–1905.

Heatherton, T. F., & Polivy, J. (1991). Development and validation of a scale for measuring state self-esteem. *Journal of Personality and Social Psychology, 60,* 895–910.

Hester, R. K. (2003). Behavioral self-control training. In R. K. Hester & W. R. Miller (Eds.), *Handbook of alcoholism treatment approaches* (3rd ed., pp. 152–164.). Boston: Allyn & Bacon.

Hingson, R., Mangione, T., Meyers, A., & Scotch, N. (1982). Seeking help for drinking problems: A study in the Boston metropolitan area. *Journal of Studies on Alcohol, 43,* 271–288.

Hohman, M. M., & Butt, R. L. (2001). How soon is too soon? Addiction recovery and family reunification. *Child Welfare, 80,* 53–67.

Holder, H., & Blasé, J. D. (1986). Alcoholism treatment and total health care utilization and costs. *Journal of the American Medical Association, 256,* 1456–1460.

Holder, H., Longabaugh, R., Miller, W. R., & Rubonis, A. V. (1991). The cost-effectiveness of treatment for alcoholism: A first approximation. *Journal of Studies on Alcohol, 52,* 517–540.

Hunt, G. M., & Azrin, N. H. (1973). A community-reinforcement approach to alcoholism. *Behaviour Research and Therapy, 11,* 91–104.

Institute of Medicine. (1990). *Broadening the base of treatment for alcohol problems.* Washington, DC: National Academy Press.

Jacob, T., Krahn, G. L., & Leonard, K. (1991). Parent–child interactions in families with alcoholic fathers. *Journal of Consulting and Clinical Psychology, 59,* 176–181.

Jacob, T., & Seilhamer, R. A. (1985). Adaptation of the Areas of Change Questionnaire for parent–child relationship assessment. *American Journal of Family Therapy, 13,* 28–38.

Johnson, V. E. (1986). *Intervention: How to help those who don't want help.* Minneapolis: Johnson Institute.

Joint Commission on Accreditation of Healthcare Organizations. (1992). *Accreditation manual for hospitals, 1* (standards). Oakbrook Terrace, CA: Author.

Kahn, M. (1997). *Between therapist and client.* New York: Freeman.

Kirby, K. C., Marlowe, D. B., Festinger, D. S., Garvey, K. A., & LaMonaca, V. (1999). Community reinforcement training for family and significant others of drug abusers: A unilateral intervention to increase treatment entry of drug users. *Drug and Alcohol Dependence, 56,* 85–96.

Kyriacou, D. N., Anglin, D., Taliaferro, E., Stone, S., Tubb, T., Muelleman, R., Barton, E., & Kraus, J. F. (1999). Risk factors for injury to women from domestic violence. *New England Journal of Medicine, 341,* 1892–1898.

Landau, J., Garrett, J., Shea, R. R., Stanton, M. D., Baciewicz, G., & Brinkman-Sull, D. (2000). Strength in numbers: Using family links to overcome resistance to addiction treatment. *American Journal of Drug and Alcohol Abuse, 26,* 379–398.

Larson, D. B., Hohmann, A. A., Kessler, L. G., Meador, K. G., Boyd, J. H., & McSherry, E. (1988). The couch and the cloth: The need for linkage. *Hospital and Community Psychiatry, 39,* 1064–1069.

Leake, G. J., & King, A. S. (1977). Effect of counselor expectations on alcoholic recovery. *Alcohol Health and Research World, 11,* 16–22.

Leonard, K. (2000, June). *Domestic violence and alcohol: What is known and what do we need to know to encourage environmental interventions.* Paper presented at the National Crime Prevention Council, Washington, DC.

Levin, S. M., & Greene, J. A. (Eds.). (2000). *Linking substance abuse treatment and domestic violence services: A guide for administrators.* Treatment Improvement Protocol (TIP) Series, U.S. Department of Health and Human Services, Substance Abuse and Mental Health Services Administration, Washington, DC.

Liepman, M. R., Nirenberg, T. D., & Begin, A. M. (1989). Evaluation of a program designed to help family and significant others to motivate resistant alcoholics into recovery. *American Journal of Drug and Alcohol Abuse, 15,* 209–221.

Lipsey, M. W., Wilson, D. B., Cohen, M. A., & Derzon, J. H. (1997). Is there a causal relationship between alcohol use and violence? A synthesis of the evidence. In M. Galanter (Ed.), *Recent developments in alcoholism. Vol. 13. Alcohol and violence: Epidemiology, neurobiology, psychology, and family issues* (pp. 245–282). New York: Plenum Press.

Loneck, B., Garrett, J. A., & Banks, S. M. (1996a). The Johnson Intervention and relapse during outpatient treatment. *American Journal of Drug and Alcohol Abuse, 22,* 363–375.

Loneck, B., Garrett, J. A., & Banks, S. M. (1996b). A comparison of the Johnson Intervention with four other methods of referral to outpatient treatment. *American Journal of Drug and Alcohol Abuse, 22,* 233–246.

Longabaugh, R., Minugh, A., Nirenberg, T., Clifford, P., Becker, B., & Woolard, R. (1995). Injury as a motivator to reduce drinking. *Academy of Emergency Medicine, 2,* 817–825.

MacPhillamy, D. J., & Lewinsohn, P. M. (1982). The Pleasant Events Schedule: Studies on reliability, validity, and scale intercorrelation. *Journal of Consulting and Clinical Psychology, 50,* 363–380.

Maisto, S. A., McKay, J. R., & O'Farrell, T. J. (1995). Relapse precipitants and behavioral marital therapy. *Addictive Behaviors, 20,* 383–393.

Maisto, S. A., O'Farrell, T. J., Connors, G. J., McKay, J., & Pelcovits, M. A. (1988). Alcoholics' attributions of factors affecting their relapse to drinking and reasons for terminating relapse events. *Addictive Behaviors, 13,* 79–82.

Malott, R. W., & Trojan Suarez, E. A. (2004). *Principles of behavior* (5th ed.). Upper Saddle River, NJ: Pearson Prentice Hall.

McCrady, B. S. (1989). Outcomes of family-involved alcoholism treatment. In M. Galanter (Ed.), *Recent developments in alcoholism* (Vol. 7, pp. 165–182). New York: Plenum Press.

McCrady, B. S., Noel, N.E., Abrams, D. B., Stout, R. L., Nelson, H. F., & Hay, W. N. (1986). Comparative effectiveness of three types of spouse involvement in outpatient behavioral alcoholism treatment. *Journal of Studies on Alcohol, 47,* 459–467.

McCrady, B. S., Stout, R., Noel, N., Abrams, D., & Nelson, H. F. (1991). Effectiveness of three types of spouse-involved behavioral alcoholism treatment. *British Journal of Addiction, 86,* 1415–1424.

McNair, D. M., Lorr, M., & Droppleman, L. F. (1971). *Profile of mood states manual.* San Diego, CA: Educational and Industrial Testing Service.

McNair, D. M., Lorr, M., & Droppleman, L. F. (1992). *Manual for the profile of mood states* (rev. ed.). San Diego, CA: Educational and Industrial Testing Service.

Meyers, R. J., Dominguez, T. P., & Smith, J. E. (1996). Community reinforcement training with concerned others. In V. B. Van Hasselt & M. Hersen (Eds.), *Sourcebook of psychological treatment manuals for adult disorders* (pp. 257–294). New York: Plenum Press.

Meyers, R. J., Miller, W. R., Hill, D. E., & Tonigan, J. S. (1999). Community reinforcement and family training (CRAFT): Engaging unmotivated drug users in treatment. *Journal of Substance Abuse, 10,* 1–18.

Meyers, R. J., Miller, W. R., & Smith, J. E. (2001). Community reinforcement and family training (CRAFT). In R. J. Meyers & W. R. Miller (Eds.), *A community reinforcement approach to addiction treatment* (pp. 147–160). Cambridge, UK: Cambridge University Press.

Meyers, R. J., Miller, W. R., Smith, J. E., & Tonigan, J. S. (2002). A randomized trial of two methods for engaging treatment-refusing drug users through concerned significant others. *Journal of Consulting and Clinical Psychology, 70,* 1182–1185.

Meyers, R. J., & Smith, J. E. (1995). *Clinical guide to alcohol treatment: The community reinforcement approach.* New York: Guilford Press.

Meyers, R. J., & Smith, J. E. (1997). Getting off the fence: Procedures to engage treatment resistant drinkers. *Journal of Substance Abuse Treatment, 14,* 467–472.

Meyers, R. J., Smith, J. E., & Miller, E. J. (1998). Working through the concerned significant other. In W. R. Miller & N. Heather (Eds.), *Treating addictive behaviors* (2nd ed., pp. 149–161). New York: Plenum Press.

Meyers, R. J., & Wolfe, B. L. (2004). *Get your loved one sober: Alternatives to nagging, pleading, and threatening.* Center City, MN: Hazelden.

Miller, B. A., & Downs, W. R. (2000). Domestic violence and rape. In M. B. Goldman & M. C. Hatch (Eds.), *Women and health* (pp. 529–540). San Diego, CA: Academic Press.

Miller, B. A., Wilsnack, S. C., & Cunradi, C. B. (2000). Family violence and victimization: Treatment issues for women with alcohol problems. *Alcoholism: Clinical and Experimental Research, 24,* 1287–1297.

Miller, E., Ogle, R., Anderson, R., Meyers, R., & Miller, W. (1999, November). *Barriers to treatment and reasons for seeking treatment.* Poster presented at the meeting of the Association for Advancement of Behavior Therapy, Toronto, Canada.

Miller, W. R. (1985). Motivation for treatment: A review with special emphasis on alcoholism. *Psychological Bulletin,* 98, 84–107.

Miller, W. R. (1986). Haunted by the Zeitgeist: reflections on contrasting treatment goals and concepts of alcoholism in Europe and the United States. *Annals of the New York Academy of Sciences, 472,* 110–129.

Miller, W. R. (1996). *Manual for Form 90: A structured assessment interview for drinking and related behaviors* (Project MATCH Monograph Series, Vol. 5). Rockville, MD: National Institute on Alcohol Abuse and Alcoholism.

Miller, W. R. (2003). Enhancing motivation for change. In R. K. Hester & W. R. Miller (Eds), *Handbook of alcoholism treatment approaches: Effective alternatives* (3rd ed., pp. 131–151). Boston: Allyn & Bacon.

Miller, W. R., Benefield, R. G., & Tonigan, J. S. (1993). Enhancing motivation for change in problem drinking: A controlled comparison of two therapist styles. *Journal of Consulting and Clinical Psychology, 61,* 455–461.

Miller, W. R., Brown, J. M., Simpson, T. L., Handmaker, N. S., Bien, T. H., Luckie, L. F., Montgomery, H. A., Hester, R. K., & Tonigan, J. S. (1995). What works?

A methodological analysis of the alcohol treatment outcome literature. In R. K. Hester & W. R. Miller (Eds.), *Handbook of alcoholism treatment approaches: Effective alternatives* (2nd ed., pp. 12–44). Boston: Allyn & Bacon.

Miller, W. R., & Brown, S. A. (1997). Why psychologists should treat alcohol and drug problems. *American Psychologist, 52,* 1269–1279.

Miller, W. R., & DelBoca, F. K. (1994). Measurement of drinking behavior using Form 90 Family of Instruments. *Journal of Studies on Alcohol* (Suppl. 12), 112–117.

Miller, W. R., & Hester, R. K. (1995). Treatment for alcohol problems: Toward an informed eclecticism. In R. K. Hester & W. R. Miller (Eds.), *Handbook of alcoholism treatment approaches: Effective alternatives* (2nd ed., pp. 1–11). Boston: Allyn & Bacon.

Miller, W. R., Leckman, A. L., Delaney, H. D., & Tinkcom, M. (1992). Long-term follow-up of behavioral self-control training. *Journal of Studies on Alcohol, 53,* 249–261.

Miller, W. R., & Meyers, R. J. (2001). Summary and reflections. In R. J. Meyers & W. R. Miller (Eds.), *A community reinforcement approach to addiction treatment* (pp. 161–170). Cambridge, UK: Cambridge University Press.

Miller, W. R., Meyers, R. J., & Tonigan, J. S. (1999). Engaging the unmotivated in treatment for alcohol problems: A comparison of three strategies for intervention through family members. *Journal of Consulting and Clinical Psychology, 67,* 688–697.

Miller, W. R., & Rollnick, S. (1991). *Motivational interviewing: Preparing people to change addictive behavior.* New York: Guilford Press.

Miller, W. R., Taylor, C. A., & West, J. C. (1980). Focused versus broad spectrum behavior therapy for problem drinkers. *Journal of Consulting and Clinical Psychology, 48,* 590–601.

Miller, W. R., Wilbourne, P. L., & Hettema, J. E. (2003). What works? A summary of alcohol treatment outcome research. In R. K. Hester & W. R. Miller (Eds), *Handbook of alcoholism treatment approaches: Effective alternatives* (3rd ed., pp. 13–63). Boston: Allyn & Bacon.

Monti, P. M., Abrams, D. B., Binkoff, J. A., Zwick, W. R., Liepman, M. R., Nirenberg, T. D., & Rohsenow, D. J. (1990). Communication skills training, communication skills training with family and cognitive behavioral mood management training for alcoholics. *Journal of Studies on Alcohol, 51,* 263–270.

Monti, P. M., Kadden, R. M., Rohsenow, D. J., Cooney, N. L., & Abrams, D. B. (2002). *Treating alcohol dependence: A coping skills training guide* (2nd ed.). New York: Guilford Press.

Monti, P. M., & Rohsenow, D. J. (2003). Coping skills training and cue exposure treatment. In R. K. Hester & W. R. Miller (Eds.), *Handbook of alcoholism treatment approaches: Effective alternatives* (3rd ed., pp. 213–236). Boston: Allyn & Bacon.

Moos, R. H. (1987). *The social climate scales: A user's guide.* Palo Alto, CA: Consulting Psychologists Press.

Moos, R. H., Cronkite, R. C., Billings, A. G., & Finney, J. W. (1987). *Health and Daily Living Form manual.* Palo Alto, CA: Social Ecology Laboratory, VA Medical Center.

Moos, R. H., & Moos, B. S. (1986). *Family Environment Scale manual* (2nd ed.). Palo Alto, CA: Consulting Psychologists Press.

Murphy, C. M., & O'Farrell, T. J. (1997). Couple communication patterns of maritally aggressive and nonagressive male alcoholics. *Journal of Studies on Alcohol, 58,* 83–90.

Narcotics Anonymous. (1993). *Narcotics Anonymous: It works–how and why.* Van Nuys, CA: N.A. World Services.

Nowinski, J., Baker, S., & Carroll, K. (1992). *12–step facilitation therapist manual: A clinical research guide for therapists treating individuals with alcohol abuse and dependence.* (Project MATCH Monograph Series, Vol. 1). Rockville, MD: National Institute on Alcohol Abuse and Alcoholism.

O'Farrell, T. J. (1995). Marital and family therapy. In R. K. Hester & W. R. Miller (Eds.), *Handbook of alcoholism treatment approaches: Effective alternatives* (2nd ed., pp. 195–220). Boston: Allyn & Bacon.

O'Farrell, T. J., & Birchler, G. R. (1987). Marital relationships of alcoholic, conflicted, and nonconflicted couples. *Journal of Marital and Family Therapy, 13,* 259–274.

O'Farrell, T. J., Cutter, H. S., & Floyd, F. J. (1985). Evaluating behavioral marital therapy for male alcoholics: Effects on marital adjustment and communication from before to after therapy. *Behavior Therapy, 16,* 147–167.

O'Farrell, T. J., & Fals-Stewart, W. (1999). Treatment models and methods: Family models. In B. S. McCrady & E. E. Epstein (Eds.), *Addictions: A comprehensive guidebook* (pp. 287–305). New York: Oxford University Press.

O'Farrell, T. J., & Fals-Stewart, W. (2000). Behavioral couples therapy for alcoholism and drug abuse. *Journal of Substance Abuse Treatment, 18,* 51–54.

O'Farrell, T. J., & Fals-Stewart, W. (2003). Marital and family therapy. In R. K. Hester & W. R. Miller (Eds.), *Handbook of alcoholism treatment approaches: Effective alternatives* (3rd ed., pp. 188–212). Boston: Allyn & Bacon.

O'Farrell, T. J., & Murphy, C. M. (1995). Marital violence before and after alcoholism treatment. *Journal of Consulting and Clinical Psychology, 63,* 256–262.

O'Farrell, T. J., & Murphy, C. M. (2002). Behavioral couples therapy for alcoholism and drug abuse: Encountering the problem. In C. Wekerle & A. M. Wall (Eds.), *The violence and addiction connection: Theoretical and clinical issues in substance abuse and relationship violence* (pp. 293–302). Philadelphia: Brunner/Mazel.

Orford, J., & Harwin, J. (1982). *Alcohol and the family.* London: Croom Helm.

Otto, R. K., & Borum, R. (1998, July). *Assessing and managing violence risk: A workshop for clinicians.* Workshop presented at the meeting of the American Psychological Association, San Francisco, CA.

Paolino, T. J., & McCrady, B. S. (1977). *The alcoholic marriage: Alternative perspectives.* New York: Grune & Stratton.

Pierce, W. D., & Epling, W. F. (1995). *Behavior analysis and learning.* Englewood Cliffs, NJ: Prentice-Hall.

Project MATCH Research Group. (1992). *Cognitive-behavioral coping skills therapy manual.* Rockville, MD: National Institute on Alcohol Abuse and Alcoholism.

Project MATCH Research Group. (1997). Matching alcoholism treatments to client heterogeneity: Project MATCH posttreatment drinking outcomes. *Journal of Studies on Alcohol, 58,* 7–29.

Prochaska, J. O., & DiClemente, C. C. (1982). Transtheoretical therapy: Toward a more integrative model of change. *Psychotherapy: Theory, Research, and Practice, 19,* 276–288.

Prochaska, J., & DiClemente, C. (1986). Toward a comprehensive model of change. In W. R. Miller & N. Heather (Eds.), *Treating addictive behaviors: Process of change* (pp. 3–27). New York: Plenum Press.

Roberts, K. S., & Brent, E. E. (1992). Physician utilization and illness patterns in families of alcoholics. *Journal of Studies on Alcohol, 43,* 119–128.

Rogers, C. P. (1957). The necessary and sufficient conditions of therapeutic personality change. *Journal of Consulting Psychology, 21,* 95–103.

Rogers, E. M. (1995). *Diffusions of innovations* (4th ed.). New York: Free Press.

Rollnick, S., Bell, A., & Heather, N. (1992). Negotiating behavior change in medical settings: The development of brief motivational interviewing. *Journal of Mental Health, 1,* 25–37.

Rollnick, S., Heather, N., Gold, R., & Hall, W. (1992). Development of a short "readiness to change" questionnaire for use in brief, opportunistic interventions among excessive drinkers. *British Journal of Addiction, 87,* 734–754.

Romijn, C. M., Platt, J. J., Schippers, G. M., & Schaap, C. P. (1992). Family therapy for Dutch drug users: The relationship between family functioning and success. *International Journal of Addictions, 27,* 1–14.

Room, R. (1987, June). *The U.S. general population's experience with responses to alcohol problems.* Paper presented at the Alcohol Epidemiology Section of the International Congress on Alcohol and Addictions, Aix-en-Provence, France.

Rosenberg, M. (1965). *Society and adolescent self-image.* Princeton, NJ: Princeton University Press.

Ryan, J. G., Verardo, L. T., Kidd, J. M., Horbatuk, E. L., Bonanno, R., Fahrenwald, R., Kirsch, S., & Stretch, G. V. (1997). Health outcomes of women exposed to household alcohol abuse: A family practice training site research network (FPTSRN) study. *Journal of Family Practice, 45,* 410–417.

Sanchez-Craig, M., Annis, H. M., Bornet, A. R., & MacDonald, K. R. (1984). Random assignment to abstinence and controlled drinking: Evaluation of a cognitive-behavioral program for problem drinkers. *Journal of Consulting and Clinical Psychology, 52,* 390–403.

Sarason, I. G., Sarason, B. R., Shearin, E. N., & Pierce, G. R. (1987). A brief measure of social support: Practical and theoretical implications. *Journal of Social and Personal Relationships, 4,* 497–510.

Schornstein, S. L. (1997). *Domestic violence and health care: What every professional needs to know.* Thousand Oaks, CA: Sage.

Schuckit, M. A. (1995). *Educating yourself about alcohol and drugs: A people's primer.* New York: Plenum Press.

Senft, R. A., Polen, M. R., Freeborn, D. K., & Hollis, J. F. (1995). *Drinking patterns and health: A randomized trial of screening and brief intervention in a primary care setting.* Final report to the National Institute on Alcohol Abuse and Alcoholism (Grant No. AA08976). Portland, OR: Center for Health Research, Kaiser Permanente.

Sisson, R. W., & Azrin, N. H. (1986). Family-member involvement to initiate and promote treatment of problem drinkers. *Behavior Therapy and Experimental Psychiatry, 17,* 15–21.

Sisson, R. W., & Mallams, J. H. (1981). The use of systematic encouragement and community access procedures to increase attendance at Alcoholics Anonymous and Al-Anon meetings. *American Journal of Drug and Alcohol Abuse, 8,* 371–376.

Smith, J. E., Laframboise, D., & Bittinger, J. (2002). Intervening through social support networks. In W. R. Miller & C. M. Weisner (Eds.), *Changing substance abuse through health and social systems* (pp. 211–224). New York: Kluwer Academic/Plenum Publishers.

Smith, J. E., Meyers, R. J., & Delaney, H. D. (1998). The community reinforcement approach with homeless alcohol-dependent individuals. *Journal of Consulting and Clinical Psychology, 66,* 541–548.

Smith, J. E., Meyers, R. J., & Milford, J. L. (2003). Community reinforcement approach and community reinforcement and family training. In R. K. Hester & W. R. Miller (Eds.), *Handbook of alcoholism treatment approaches: Effective alternatives* (3rd ed., pp. 237–258). Boston: Allyn & Bacon.

Snow, M. G., Prochaska, J. O., & Rossi, J. S. (1992). Stages of change for smoking cessation among former problem drinkers: A cross-sectional analysis. *Journal of Substance Abuse, 4,* 107–116.

Sobell, L. C., & Sobell, M. B. (1992). Timeline follow-back: A technique for assessing self-reported alcohol consumption. In R. Z. Litten & J. P. Allen (Eds.), *Measuring alcohol consumption: Psychosocial and biochemical methods* (pp. 41–72). Totowa, NJ: Humana Press.

Spanier, G. B. (1976). Measuring dyadic adjustment: New scales for assessing the quality of marriage and similar dyads. *Journal of Sex and Marital Therapy, 38,* 15–28.

Spear, S., & Mason, M. (1991). Impact of chemical dependency on family health status. *International Journal of Addictions, 26,* 179–187.

Spiegler, M. D., & Guevremont, D. C. (2003). *Contemporary behavior therapy* (4th ed.). Belmont, CA: Wadsworth/Thomson Learning.

Spielberger, C. D. (1988). *State–Trait Anger Expression Inventory: Professional manual.* Odessa, FL: Psychological Assessment Resources.

Spielberger, C. D., Gorsuch, R. L., Lushene, R., Vagg, P., & Jacobs, G. A. (1983). *Manual for State–Trait Anxiety Inventory (STAI Form Y).* Palo Alto, CA: Consulting Psychologists Press.

Stanton, M. D. (1982). Appendix A: Review of reports on drug abusers' family living arrangements and frequency of family contact. In M. D. Stanton, T. C. Todd, & Associates (Eds.), *The family therapy of drug abuse and addiction* (pp. 427–432). New York: Guilford Press.

Stanton, M. D., & Heath, A. (1997). Family and marital therapy. In J. H. Lowinson, P. Ruiz, B. Millman, & J. G. Langrod (Eds.), *Substance abuse: A comprehensive textbook* (3rd ed., pp. 448–454). Baltimore: Williams & Wilkins.

Stanton, M. D., & Shadish, W. R. (1997). Outcome, attrition, and family/couples treatment for drug abuse: A meta-analysis and a review of controlled, comparative studies. *Psychological Bulletin, 122,* 170–191.

Stith, S. M., Crossman, R. K., & Bischof, G. P. (1991). Alcoholism and marital violence: A comparative study of men in alcohol treatment programs and batterer treatment programs. *Alcoholism Treatment Quarterly, 8,* 3–20.

Straus, M. A. (1979). Measuring intrafamily conflict and violence: The Conflict Tactics Scales. *Journal of Marriage and the Family, 41,* 75–86.

Sullivan, C. M., Basta, J., Tan, C., & Davidson, W. S. II. (1992). After the crisis: A needs assessment of women leaving a domestic violence shelter. *Violence and Victims, 7,* 267–275.

Thomas, E. J., & Ager, R. D. (1993). Unilateral family therapy with the spouses of uncooperative alcohol abusers. In T. J. O'Farrell (Ed.), *Treating alcohol problems: Marital and family interventions* (pp. 3–33). New York: Guilford Press.

Thomas, E. J., & Santa, C. A. (1982). Unilateral family therapy for alcohol abuse: A working conception. *American Journal of Family Therapy, 10,* 49–58.

Thomas, E. J., Santa, C., Bronson, D, & Oyserman, D. (1987). Unilateral family therapy with spouses of alcoholics. *Journal of Social Service Research, 10,* 145–163.

Thomas, E. J., Yoshioka, M. R., & Ager, R. D. (1994a). Spouse Enabling Inventory (SEI). In J. Fischer & K. Corcoran (Eds.), *Measures for clinical practice: A sourcebook: Vol. 1. Couples, families, and children* (2nd ed., pp. 177–182). New York: Free Press.

Thomas, E. J., Yoshioka, M. R., & Ager, R. D. (1994b). Spouse Sobriety Influence Inventory (SSII). In J. Fischer & K. Corcoran (Eds.), *Measures for clinical practice: A sourcebook: Vol. 1. Couples, families, and children* (2nd ed., pp. 183–189). New York: Free Press.

Tonigan, J. S., & Miller, W. R. (2002). The Inventory of Drug Use Consequences (InDuC): Test–retest stability and sensitivity to detect change. *Psychology of Addictive Behaviors, 16,* 165–168.

Valle, S. K. (1981). Interpersonal functioning of alcoholism counselors and treatment outcome. *Journal of Studies on Alcohol, 42,* 783–790.

Velleman, R., Bennett, G., Miller, T., Orford, J., Rigby, K., & Tod, A. (1993). The families of problem drug users: A study of 50 close relatives. *Addiction, 88,* 1281–1289.

Veroff, J., Kulks, R. A., & Douvan, E. (1981). *Mental health in America: Patterns of help seeking from 1957–1976.* New York: Basic Books.

Waldron, H. B., Turner, C. W., Ozechowski, T., & Hops, H. (2003, June). *"Treatment-elusive" vs. traditional outpatient adolescent substance abusers: Baseline and treatment outcome differences.* Paper presented at the College on Problems of Drug Dependence, Miami, FL.

Weiner, I. B. (1975). *Principles of psychotherapy.* New York: Wiley.

Weissman, M., & Bothwell, S. (1976). Assessment of social adjustment by patient self-report. *Archives of General Psychiatry, 33,* 1111–1115.

Weissman, M. M., Paykel, E. S., & Prusoff, B. A. (1990). *Social Adjustment Scale handbook.* New York: Research Foundation for Mental Hygiene, New York Psychiatric Institute.

White, H. R., & Chen, P. (2002). Problem drinking and intimate partner violence. *Journal of Studies on Alcohol, 63*, 205–214.

Wilson, G. T., & O'Leary, K. D. (1980). *Principles of behavior therapy.* Englewood Cliffs, NJ: Prentice Hall.

Winters, J., Fals-Stewart, W., O'Farrell, T. J., Birchler, G. R., & Kelley, M. L. (2002). Behavioral couples therapy for female substance-abusing patients: Effects on substance use and relationship adjustment. *Journal of Consulting and Clinical Psychology, 70*, 344–355.

Zweben, A. (1986). Problem drinking and marital adjustment. *Journal of Studies on Alcohol, 47*, 167–172.

INDEX